FOOLS AND IDIOTS?

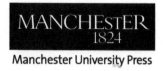

MANCHESTER
1824

Manchester University Press

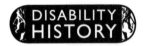

Series editors
Dr Julie Anderson, Professor Walton Schalick, III

This new series published by Manchester University Press responds to the growing interest in disability as a discipline worthy of historical research. The series has a broad international historical remit, encompassing issues that include class, race, gender, age, war, medical treatment, professionalisation, environments, work, institutions and cultural and social aspects of disablement including representations of disabled people in literature, film, art and the media.

FOOLS AND IDIOTS?

INTELLECTUAL DISABILITY IN THE MIDDLE AGES

Irina Metzler

Manchester University Press

Published by Manchester University Press
Altrincham Street, Manchester M1 7JA, UK

www.manchesteruniversitypress.co.uk

British Library Cataloguing-in-Publication Data
A catalogue record for this book is available from the British Library

Library of Congress Cataloging-in-Publication Data applied for

ISBN   978 0 7190 9636 5 hardback

ISBN   978 0 7190 9637 2 paperback

First published 2016

The publisher has no responsibility for the persistence or accuracy of URLs for any external or third-party internet websites referred to in this book, and does not guarantee that any content on such websites is, or will remain, accurate or appropriate.

Typeset in 10/12pt Arno Pro by
Servis Filmsetting Ltd, Stockport, Cheshire
Printed in Great Britain by
TJ International Ltd., Padstow

Contents

Figures

Series editors' foreword

You know a subject has achieved maturity when a book series is dedicated to it. In the case of disability, while it has co-existed with human beings for centuries the study of disability's history is still quite young.

In setting up this series, we chose to encourage multi-methodologic history rather than a purely traditional historical approach, as researchers in disability history come from a wide variety of disciplinary backgrounds. Equally 'disability' history is a diverse topic which benefits from a variety of approaches in order to appreciate its multi-dimensional characteristics.

A test for the team of authors and editors who bring you this series is typical of most series, but disability also brings other consequential challenges. At this time disability is highly contested as a social category in both developing and developed contexts. Inclusion, philosophy, money, education, visibility, sexuality, identity and exclusion are but a handful of the social categories in play. With this degree of politicisation, language is necessarily a cardinal focus.

In an effort to support the plurality of historical voices, the editors have elected to give fair rein to language. Language is historically contingent, and can appear offensive to our contemporary sensitivities. The authors and editors believe that the use of terminology that accurately reflects the historical period of any book in the series will assist readers in their understanding of the history of disability in time and place.

Finally, disability offers the cultural, social and intellectual historian a new 'take' on the world we know. We see disability history as one of a few nascent fields with the potential to reposition our understanding of the flow of cultures, society, institutions, ideas and lived experience. Conceptualisations of 'society' since the early modern period have heavily stressed principles of autonomy, rationality and the subjectivity of the individual agent. Consequently we are frequently oblivious to the historical contingency of the present with respect to those elements. Disability disturbs those foundational features of 'the modern'. Studying disability history helps us resituate our policies, our beliefs and our experiences.

Julie Anderson
Walton O. Schalick, III

Acknowledgements

This book is the result of a research fellowship generously supported by the Wellcome Trust [grant number 098848 Cognitive Impairment in the Middle Ages: Uncovering medical and cultural aspects of intellectual disabilities according to medieval normative texts] through the funding stream in Medical Humanities, while I was based at Swansea University.

Thanks are due to Chris Goodey for correspondence and cordial disagreements on the subject of intellectual disability past and present, to Wendy Turner for discussions on the finer points of medieval jurisprudence, to Julie Anderson for embracing this topic for the Disability History series, to the members of the Research Group on Health, History and Culture at Swansea, and especially to Anne Borsay (who, sadly, passed away before this project could be completed) and to David Turner for a shared interest in disability history, to Iona McCleery and the attendees of my seminar at the University of Leeds for invigorating interrogation, to Kurt Lampe at Bristol University for helping with some particularly tricky medieval Latin, to Anne Bailey for drawing my attention to the miracle of Giles the 'idiot' and to Adam Mosley at Swansea for debating medieval natural philosophy with me.

My gratitude naturally extends to my family and friends, who yet again patiently put up with the quirks and foibles of an academic in the ups and downs of immersive engagement with the notoriously slippery topic that is pre-modern disability.

Abbreviations

CCSL	Corpus Christianorum Series Latina (Turnhout: Brepols, 1953–)
CIH	*Corpus Iuris Hibernici*, ed. D. A. Binchy (Dublin, 1978)
CIM	*Calendar of Inquisitions Miscellaneous (Chancery), Henry III–Henry V*, 7 vols (London: HMSO, 1916–68)
CIPM	*Calendar of Inquisitions Post Mortem and Other Analogous Documents Preserved in the Public Record Office*, 20 vols (London: HMSO, 1904–70)
CPR	*Calendar of the Patent Rolls Preserved in the Public Record Office, 1216–1509*, Public Record Office, 52 vols (London: HMSO, 1891–1901)
CSEL	*Corpus Scriptorum Ecclesiasticorum Latinorum* (Vienna, 1866–)
DSM-5	*Diagnostic and Statistical Manual of Mental Disorders*, American Psychiatric Association (Washington, DC: American Psychiatric Association, 5th edition 2013)
ID	intellectual disability
OED	*Oxford English Dictionary*, at www.oed.com/
PL	*Patrologiae cursus completus, series latina*, ed. J. P. Migne, 221 vols (Paris, 1841–64)
ST	Thomas Aquinas, *Summa theologiae*, numerous editions, English available at www.newadvent.org/summa; Latin at www.corpusthomisticum.org; cited following convention Part, Question, Article, objection/response/adversus
TNA	The National Archives: Public Record Office, Kew, London

I

PRE-/CONCEPTIONS: PROBLEMS OF DEFINITION AND HISTORIOGRAPHY

Intellectual disability means a significantly reduced ability to understand new or complex information and to learn and apply new skills (impaired intelligence). This results in a reduced ability to cope independently (impaired social functioning), and begins before adulthood, with a lasting effect on development. Disability depends not only on a child's health conditions or impairments but also and crucially on the extent to which environmental factors support the child's full participation and inclusion in society.[1]

This is the World Health Organisation's definition of intellectual disability, which incorporates social and environmental factors, and is one attempt at an inclusive definition of a notoriously ambiguous conceptual category – variously called mental retardation, cognitive disability or, most recently, intellectual disability (ID). The terminology immediately prompts a series of questions. What is ID as applied to the Middle Ages? Would a person whom our modern society diagnoses as autistic have been noticed as someone different from the 'norm' back in the Middle Ages? Could one, then, even say that autism existed as an illness in those times? And in more general terms, if we do not have a category or label for an entity such as a disease, does that disease exist? Do these different words (medieval versus modern usage) in actuality express roughly the same underlying 'true' or 'real' concept? Or do all these different terms mean many, just as different concepts? Are medieval medical texts as concerned with establishing strict biological or psychological categories as modern ones? What cultural factors fed into the generation of statements surrounding mental disability in medieval medical texts; e.g. can we say the development of a forensic process in the medieval judicial system (by questioning people as to their mental capacities) had an impact on the way medical professionals described mental disability? The present volume tries to put some of these modern assumptions to the test against medieval evidence.

For this purpose, the conditions defined in modern medical terms as IDs will be the focus of interrogation for their medieval counterparts.

While physical disability in the Middle Ages (c. 500 to c. 1500) has become a rapidly emerging topic for scholarly engagement since the mid-2000s, mental or intellectual disability has not yet been adequately researched. 'Even the most radical historians have only ever treated "intellectual disability" either as a footnote to the history of *mental* pathology dominated by mental *illness*, or of disability dominated by the *physical* disability.'[2] In part this lacuna has been due to a lack of interest among both medical and social/cultural historians, but also due to the difficulties of uncovering narratives of ID in medieval sources. Since the medieval fool, for argument's sake the approximate equivalent of the person with ID, often had lifelong mental limitations and hence no fluctuating changes from sanity to insanity, no recoverance of mental faculties, the fool and the madman might frequently be linked,[3] but the overarching interest of historians has been in the more glamorous acquired madness rather than folly or idiocy. Research is also hampered by lack of documentation, especially institutional records, pertaining to ID – unlike the mad, the mentally disabled were rarely locked up. For early modern Britain it has been claimed that the absence of institutions for what was then often called 'idiocy' was less about lack of diagnostics or distinction from insanity; 'It was also a result of prevailing policies towards the disabled, which designated idiots (and other groups deemed to be chronically disabled or ill) as unfit for therapy and incarceration because untreatable and harmless.'[4]

In his study of madness in late medieval English literature, Harper concluded that 'the tendency of critics to conflate the concepts of madness and folly has led to alarmingly widespread disagreement about the meaning of madness'; all too many historians regarded madness as synonymous with folly, whereas, in fact, a closer look at medieval legal, theological and literary sources demonstrates quite clearly that medieval authorities 'distinguished madness from folly in all of its forms', with madness more commonly implying mania or melancholia.[5] The whole question as to whether mental afflictions are categorised as illnesses or not is of course a crucial one. Mental illness, although now a medical category in the modern Western world, was not always such, and was, and to an arguable extent still is, a social construct, based on social ideas about acceptable and unacceptable social deviance. Even with a modern medical knowledge base, it is not entirely clear whether mental illnesses fall into the category of diseases (which can be remedied by giving medicine) or of problems of individual socialisation and perception, which might be remedied by counselling and therapy.[6] Even should we successfully untangle folly from madness in medieval sources, we are still left with the fool overshadowing the person with ID. We still know comparatively little about mental disability in the pre-modern past because 'scholarship has remained so preoccupied with the literary figure of the "fool" and the cultural meanings of "folly", tending to eschew hard analysis of the social problems of the mentally disabled'.[7] Unfortunately, for the medieval period, the evidence that would permit such 'hard analysis' is elusive, to say the least. The historian's problems 'are multiform when it comes to actually identifying the mentally disabled amongst the ranks of all those described as having some sort of mental defect or affliction'.[8]

Medical and psychiatric definitions

The main focus will be on concepts and categories of ID as used in the medieval period. As part of this, the book will highlight the problem of imposing modern definitions of cognitive/intellectual/mental disability onto the past. Hence a few words about modern definitions are in order. It has been claimed that the modern concept of ID, as 'perceived by cognitive, developmental and educational psychologists and in much everyday thinking', is defined according to five criteria:

> (1) It is a deficit in the 'intelligence' specific to humans, defined more or less as an (in)ability to think abstractly. (2) This deficit occurs in the mind, as a natural realm distinct from the body; in this sense it differs from physical or sensory disability. (3) The deficit is incurable and thus defines the person, from birth or an early childhood onset until death; in this sense it differs from mental illness. (4) The people thus identified are a tiny, abnormal minority at the lowest extreme from the norm of intelligence. (This holds true whether or not the norm is measurable, by IQ for example.) (5) The causes of the deficit are natural in a deterministic sense, i.e. 'nature' implies 'necessity'. (This holds true whether or not nurture is perceived to have an influence.)[9]

This stands in contrast to the American Psychiatric Association's *Diagnostic and Statistical Manual of Mental Disorders* (DSM), which since the mid-twentieth century and over successive editions has become a standard reference for clinical practice in the mental health field. This 'bible' of modern psychiatry classifies cognitive disorders according to neurodevelopmental and neurocognitive disorders. Neurodevelopmental disorders cover broadly what tend to be called IDs, as well as communication, autism spectrum, attention-deficit/hyperactivity and motor disorders, plus the very modern educationalists' concept of specific learning disorders relating to reading, writing and mathematics. For the sake of argument, my study focuses on disabilities related to this broad category of neurodevelopmental disorders. The one thing in common, regardless for the moment of the question of how applicable these disorders might be for the medieval period, is that they are all developmental, in other words either congenital or connected to specific developmental stages of infancy, childhood or adolescence – they all manifest before adulthood and then remain with the person for life. In medical language, they are 'nonprogressive' (although in some genetic disorders such as Rett syndrome there are periods of worsening followed by stabilisation, and in San Phillipp syndrome progressive worsening of intellectual functions).[10] The two most common and well-known IDs today are autism spectrum disorder (formerly Asperger spectrum) and Down syndrome. In French, Down syndrome is referred to as *trisonomie*, after the triplication (usually spontaneous) of chromosome 21, which causes the syndrome. Down syndrome is the most common genetic cause of neurodevelopmental disorder, with around one in every 600 live births affected.[11] Today, around 50 per cent of infants with Down syndrome are born with 'significant congenital heart defects', which require life-saving surgery.[12] That was obviously not available in the past, so it is likely that if similar incidences of heart problems occurred in the past, then at least half of all infants with Down syndrome would have died during infancy. However, turn this statistic around, and it follows that about half of Down syndrome babies do not (and did not in the past) have heart problems, so one can assume that this half of the infants could survive into adulthood. With regard to autism spectrum, it has been observed that making psychiatric distinctions between the phenomenology of autism and the pathologies and behaviours of persons with (severe) ID is very difficult in those people with genetic syndromes of ID, since 'complex cognitive, communicative, behavioral, emotional, and physical difficulties … may mask or emulate' autism, but according to '*a pragmatic perspective, the etiology of the behavior presentation is, arguably, unimportant*'[13] [emphasis added]. Mental retardation can be associated with major chromosomal abnormalities or single-gene disorders such as fragile X and Williams syndromes. But again, the range and categorical diversity is rather stunning, and, interestingly for the medievalist familiar with 'loose' categories and nebulous ('unscientific') definitions, around two-thirds of the people diagnosed today as having some form of ID cannot be squeezed into any of these scientific or medical categories other than one of a general 'sub-standard' level of intelligence.[14] Somehow the inability of modern science and medicine to precisely label and categorise ID, despite the enormous advances since the 1990s, with even monthly developments, in the biological sciences in general and genetics in particular, appears worrying and troublesome to researchers and medical specialists.

   All these just-cited conditions fall under what the 5th edition of the *Diagnostic and Statistical Manual of Mental Disorders* [DSM-5] termed neurodevelopmental disorders. In contrast, I will not be discussing neurocognitive disorders, which not only tend to manifest in adulthood, but are due to disease (e.g. Alzheimer's, Parkinson's, Huntington's), intoxication (alcoholism) or traumatic brain injury – these are all conditions that may affect a person much later in life and have a fairly clear causality. There is of course scope for an overlap between neurodevelopmental and neurocognitive disorders: 'Intellectual disability may result from an acquired insult during the developmental period from, for example, a severe head injury, in which case a neurocognitive disorder also may be diagnosed.'[15] As aetiologies for ID, *DSM-5* lists genetic syndromes, congenital metabolic disorders, brain malformations, maternal disease and environmental influences such as alcohol, toxins and teratogens, all of which would have been likely risks during the medieval or any other periods. Similarly, problems during labour could lead to neonatal encephalopathy in all times and places. 'Postnatal causes include hypoxic ischemic injury, traumatic brain injury, infections, demyelinating disorders, seizure disorders (e.g., infantile spasms), severe and chronic social deprivation, and toxic metabolic syndromes and intoxications (e.g., lead, mercury).'[16] All of these are scenarios that are more than plausible for the medieval period, too. *DSM-5* presents a summary argument for the *physicality* of some IDs, and the reason why it is highly likely, in the absence of evidence to the contrary, that the same kinds of genetic disorders occurred in the Middle Ages, and probably in the same proportions to the rest of the population as in the early twenty-first century. If we assume that humans have been anatomically modern for at least 30,000 years, then surely during the past 1,500 to as recent as 500 years they were equally as 'modern' in the anatomical sense. Therefore similar disease and developmental patterns will have been in existence in the Middle Ages. The genetic and physiological causes of ID will have changed little, historically, thus ID cannot simply be dismissed as a purely 'modern disorder'.

Social constructionism and ID

At this point it is apposite to briefly introduce a philosophical critique, primarily expounded by Hacking, of the preponderance in Western academia to claim that nigh on everything, whether people, objects or ideas, is socially constructed. The question of social constructionism in medical history elicited two important articles by Jordanova and Harley, the latter arousing a lively debate, all in the journal *Social History of Medicine*.[17] Jordanova argued for the usefulness of social constructionism for medical history, considering the link between cultural history and medical history especially fruitful. Harley in turn emphasised semiotic frames of reference as lying at the heart of medical diagnosis, therapy and prognosis. Though of course they were important contributions in their own right to the field of the social history of medicine, these articles had little concern with disability. In contrast, Hacking devoted considerably more space to disability in general and psychiatric phenomena in particular.

In a nutshell, Hacking's critique is initially directed at sloppy semantic usage by the social constructionists, but he makes some important points concerning the apparent physicality and permanence of ID, as opposed to the transience of mental illness. With regard to 'disability' as a concept, Hacking criticises that many authors who write on disability as socially constructed do not distinguish sufficiently or rigorously enough between product and process. Presumably, in my attempt to simplify Hacking's analysis, 'disability' is a product, while discrimination is a process that creates 'disability'. Where it gets really interesting is in Hacking's chapter on madness, asking if it is a phenomenon that is biological or constructed. Pertinent to the theme of ID is that what Hacking calls 'transient' mental illnesses may be contrasted with conditions such as schizophrenia or mental retardation. Transient illnesses, in his definition, do not just mean 'that they last only for a time in the life of an individual' but that 'they show up only at some times and some places, for reasons which we can only suppose are connected with the culture of those times and places'.[18] The classic example he gives is late nineteenth-century hysteria from France, or anorexia in contemporary Argentina. Unlike such an illness, Hacking asserts, conditions such as mental retardation are in effect constant, immutable and 'real'.

But here Hacking is refuting his own observation of a few passages earlier, in that a fair number of psychiatric diagnostic labels are 'not a diagnosis but a disciplinary device'.[19] Why should all conditions subsumed under the label of ID (or learning difficulties, or mental retardation) suddenly be based in biological 'fact', when it is just as likely that many of these are just labels and classifications, and hence subject to social and cultural change? What evidence is there for Hacking's claim that 'there is a widespread conviction that these disorders [e.g. mental retardation, childhood autism, schizophrenia] are here to stay, and were with us long before they were named'?[20] The biological camp would see these as immutable realities, or, as Hacking puts it, 'indifferent kinds' of illness, while the constructionists regard them as changeable and hence 'interactive kinds' of illness. The classificatory concept of the 'feeble mind' is used by Hacking to demonstrate that mental retardation 'was an idea waiting for a social-construction thesis to happen to it'.[21] Despite his sarcasm, Hacking has to concede that the idea of mental retardation carries ideological baggage with it, used to control people perceived as 'difficult'. The historical horizon in all this discussion is of course limited to the modern period, with its special schools and institutions. Only at the end of his sketch of feeble-mindedness does Hacking draw attention to the belief that only now, in contemporary twenty-first-century science, are we truly understanding ID, while pretending it is an immutable phenomenon. In contrast to this is the biological approach.

> There is a deep-seated conviction that retarded children, schizophrenics, and autistic people suffer from one or more fundamental neurological or biochemical problems which will, in the future, be identified. It is not claimed that every person now diagnosed will have the same problem. ... No one maintains that mental retardation is a single disorder, but many believe that specific types of retardation have clear biological causes, to the extent that we can say these disorders simply are biological in nature.[22]

Aside from the ill-judged use of the word 'suffer', the attraction of Hacking's claim here is that it allows some justification for historical inquiry – if we can assume a biological basis for certain phenomena, think Down syndrome, then at least we can assume they existed as phenomena in the not-so-distant past; and in biological terms the Middle Ages are positively contemporary.

In all this, Hacking hits the nail on the head when he points out that 'an issue that troubles many cautious people [is] the idea that something can apparently be both socially constructed and yet "real"'.[23] One may respond that medieval theologians and natural philosophers would have had no problem with such an apparent contradiction, which therefore highlights how a mode of thinking or analysis is itself a product of culture. Hacking felt the need to present a highly complex and incomprehensible 'semantic way for a philosopher to make peace with the dilemma'.[24] Medieval intellectuals had an easier job, by splitting a single monolithic 'truth' into a number of 'truths', according to divine or human, natural or otherworldly modes of understanding. Teleology, the reading and interpretation of texts, primarily the Bible, at different levels, is the prime example here.

In medieval medical language, neurocognitive disorders would have been seen as caused by external factors impinging on and upsetting the internal humoral balance, while neurodevelopmental disorders presented a more puzzling aetiology, which is perhaps one reason why medieval medical texts say next to nothing on IDs as defined in modern clinical parlance. It is reasonably straightforward to make an association between receiving a bump on the head and observing the consequent cognitive changes that come under the modern category of traumatic brain injury, which therefore are reflected in antique and medieval medical texts; the fevers, rashes and other readily observable somatic signs of diseases such as meningitis could also readily be causally linked with a subsequent mental impairment; and intoxication, too, has well-observed and described cognitive effects in the pre-modern period. The neurocognitive degeneration affecting the elderly, which classical and medieval medicine lumped under the general heading of senility, was equally observed, even if now the differential diagnoses have become more sophisticated. But prior to the advent of modern psychiatry, neurodevelopmental disorders will have been far more difficult to attach to a medical causality, and hence much less prone to medical, as opposed to social or religious, diagnosis.

Socio-cultural reactions to ID

So much for the physiology. What about reactions, especially reactions by the parents of a mentally disabled child? Anthropological studies have rarely looked at disabilities in general, with an equally small number of cross-cultural studies concerned with pre-industrial societies. Based on the Human Relation Area File, ethnographers report that 'in 21 of 35 societies studied, infanticide was attributed to the presence of an infant who was "deformed or very ill"', and infanticide is occasionally justified by allusion to supernatural influences.[25] With regard to the historical myth of infanticide in times past that were infamously 'nasty, brutish and short', one may observe with Berkson that, firstly, 'individuals with mental and physical disabilities have been members of society since the emergence of Homo sapiens and probably well before that'; secondly, the 'development of agrarian societies brought with them an increase of certain diseases and the appearance of new disabilities', and thirdly, 'nonhuman primate societies and human groups vary in their response to individuals with serious disabilities'.[26] Berkson pointed out that in ancient Greece, even when the historiographically much-debated killing of individuals with disabilities occurred, this was limited to the neonatal period.[27] This is an important conjecture, since most cases of ID, and sensory impairments such as deafness, would be observable only weeks if not months after birth. While neonates with Down syndrome, or other developmental defects with concurrent physical discrepancies (foetal alcohol syndrome is one such), may be recognisable at birth, in other cases ID does not become apparent for many years, and thus at life-stages after which the neonate has acquired personhood. As documented for many cultures, both past and present, 'the neonatal child exists as a special category for whom "personhood is imminent but not assured" and infanticide is usually classified very differently to murder. Once a child is older however, no matter how "defective" they may be, killing them is impossible'.[28]

Some general observations from ethnology were summarised in a survey from the 1990s of more than twenty different cultures worldwide. The authors had looked at mental disabilities, primarily noting that in the understanding of many cultures the interpretation and differentiation of what modern Western society tends to call mental disability/learning difficulty would also include speech defects and psychiatric disorders, while allowing for lack of clarity in the ethnological terminology employed by Western observers. The cultural evaluation of mental disability in the majority of cultures was negative.[29] In contrast to the historiographical stereotype that 'primitive' cultures do not notice mental retardation, the authors observed that even mild disabilities would be recognised, something which they regarded as remarkable – so, ironically, subscribing to that historiographical view, otherwise why would this observation be remarkable. They refer to the Tamang, a people of Nepal, who regarded lack of verbal competence as a sign of mental disability, as well as difficulties with independent actions, and who distinguished between categories of persons as 'stupid' and 'half-stupid' (the latter implying mild mental weakness).[30] The anthropologist Edgerton, who had earlier conducted similar comparative studies, also noted that many cultures recognised even mild mental deficiencies and concluded from that: 'But I would be greatly surprised if even relatively slight degrees of retardation were not recognized and labeled in the great majority of the world's societies.'[31]

Recognition is one thing, reaction quite another. Some ethnic groups had extreme reactions to mentally disabled persons, such as the Araucanians of southern Chile, who killed newborns identified as mentally disabled – presumably this affected only such children whose difference would be visible at birth, such as children with Down syndrome.[32] If severe mental disability became apparent only some time after birth, then that did not negate extreme reactions, which in some ethnic groups could be justified by claiming such persons were totally useless or presented a (real or imagined) danger to others. In contrast, there are other ethnicities who expressly forbid the killing of mentally disabled persons. In just one ethnological study an isolating reaction was observed, where children with microcephaly were tied up in a hut to prevent them injuring others, whereas in the ethnographic literature overall the majority of reports cite help and assistance coupled with limited inclusion into the social life of a group, based on the extent of individual capabilities, as the main reaction towards the mentally disabled.[33] The authors summarise 'reactions' as follows: 'The degree of affection and consideration on the one hand, and restriction or discrimination on the other hand, could vary depending on the severity of disability but also as a consequence of individual decisions.'[34] Depending on such culturally specific variation, they therefore propose to speak of modified or restricted participation of mentally disabled persons in the socio-cultural life of a group. Most importantly, Neubert and Cloerkes concluded that social competence is regarded highly in all cultures, and that corresponding deficits entail marked disadvantages. The results of their survey permit the observation that while extreme reactions might be shown toward the severely mentally disabled, the majority of cultures display assistance and permit restricted participation, sometimes with clear indulgence of and special protection for the disabled.[35]

These generalised findings were borne out by a dedicated study. For a further ethnographic comparison it is worthwhile looking at the attitudes to and treatment of persons with ID among a traditional, non-Western, non-Christian ethnic group. A brief summary of the anthropological fieldwork conducted among the Semai (more commonly called the Semang) people of Malaysia was published in the 1960s. Overall, the Semai 'classify the dumb-ness of severe mental deficiency with the lack of verbal facility'.[36] People with mild mental deficiency were teased, but such teasing had to be interpreted within the wider social context, since the Semai teased anyone with a personal idiosyncrasy. Such persons with mild ID were not told to go away, although in times of scarcity they received inferior goods and food, as compared to the rest of the population. In general, 'normal' people recognised that 'mental incompetence excused behavior that would not be tolerable in other people'. If misdemeanours and/or accidents were caused by persons with ID, their fellow Semai would say, 'What can you do?' The culprit 'is dumb' is the reason given for such inappropriate behaviour. In summary, the anthropologist concluded that the Semai 'seem to find intellectual impairment a "problem" only when … it is associated with antisocial activities'. Most importantly, the Semai 'do not regard intellectual impairment as a disease that can lead to antisocial acts'. This attitude is in marked contrast to the modern Western way of thinking about ID. Additionally, the Semai were more concerned about 'making difficulties' for others than about levels of intellect. 'Therefore, inasmuch as intellectual impairment does not lead to "making difficulties for others", it remains socially acceptable in the sense that harmless idiosyncrasies are acceptable, although funny.' In the modern Western world, especially in the USA of the 1960s,' which the author was comparing with his ethnographic data, in contrast, 'intel-lectual impairment per se violates norms of behavior. The violation is serious, not something to laugh about.'[37] There is a lot going on here. On one level, the author was making an interesting and highly useful contrast between regard-ing ID as a disease, pathologising the condition, which the contemporary psychiatric and educational discourse still does, and the acceptance of lack of intellectual ability as something that 'just is'. On another level, the author was singing the praises of laughing at or about as a way of defusing concerns over 'difference' (what Dentan called idiosyncrasy). Ultimately, one reading of this study could be that if only modern Western people laughed (again) at people with ID – as allegedly medieval court fools were laughed at – they would stop pathologising harmless difference. And on yet another level, some of the descriptions given here very temptingly invite comparisons with medieval attitudes, especially the integration (not to be told to go away) into society of people with ID, yet at the same time the mockery (stereotype of the village idiot) and laughter such people may have been subject to.

DSM-5 considers IDs to be part of the broader category of mental disorder, so it is worth looking at what is defined as mental disorder: 'A mental disorder is a syndrome characterized by clinically significant disturbance in an individual's cognition, emotion regulation, or behavior that reflects a dysfunction in the psychological, biological, or developmental processes underlying mental functioning.'[38] The key phrase here is 'mental functioning', since at this point one may arguably insert the qualifier 'socially constructed' – different cultures at different time and place had differing concepts of mental functionality. The prime example is the irrelevance of being able to read or write in an illiterate society, in contrast to the DSM-5 definitions of specific learning disorders which become pathologies only in societies with universal expectations of literacy. Much of what DSM-5 pathologises will therefore simply not have been relevant to a pre-modern society. However, some of the diagnostic criteria appear to have cross-cultural relevance:

> Intellectual disability (intellectual developmental disorder) is characterized by deficits in general mental abilities, such as reasoning, problem solving, planning, abstract thinking, judgment, academic learning, and learning from experience. The deficits result in impairments of adaptive functioning, such that the individual fails to meet standards of personal independence and social responsibility in one or more aspects of daily life, including communication, social participation, academic or occupational functioning, and personal independence at home or in community settings.[39]

Although the specific definition, scope, range and therefore cultural diversity of expectations of what constitutes 'mental abilities' may vary inter-culturally, as ethnological studies have amply demonstrated, all cultures have expectations, and therefore observations of 'deficits', of mental functioning. The cultural and historical variance of mental functioning is the key investigative strand pursued here. Some of the symptomatology DSM-5 associates with ID is worth citing, to highlight not just how vague the symptoms might be, but how through this vagueness they can apply to many cultural/historical settings. IDs are sub-categorised as mild, moderate, severe or profound, each of which has different bearings on an individual's conceptual, social and practical domain. The stark differences between the behaviours of those with mild to moderate levels of ID and those in the severe to profound range have been a recurring theme since the 1960s. Thus, Clarke and Clarke already referred to ID (or 'mental deficiency' in the language of the day) as 'a socio-administrative rather than a scientific concept varying in different countries and within a given country at different times'.[40] For mild ID, DSM-5 cites impairment of money-management skills, a criterion already identified by fourteenth-century English legal records; the more general 'difficulties of regulating emotion and behavior in age-appropriate fashion', with such difficulties being 'noticed by peers in social situations',[41] can equally apply to a medieval (or any other cultural) setting. Similarly transcultural are these symptoms of moderate ID, which is characterised by a limitation in 'social judgment and decision-making abilities' so that 'caretakers must assist the person with life decisions'.[42] Substitute the term 'guardian' for caretaker, and again medieval legal and social concepts become apparent. From this one may surmise that while social expectations of 'mild' and 'moderate' ID may be inter-culturally similar, the definitions of conceptual and practical mental functionality are far more culturally specific. The symptomatological gap between the modern American culture of DSM-5 and the pre-modern period narrows much more when it comes to 'severe' and 'profound' ID. Persons characterised as having severe ID have conceptual domain problems with 'concepts involving numbers, quantity, time, and money',[43] which are inter-culturally relevant. To gave a basic example: in a pre-modern pastoralist society, the ability to count or otherwise have quantitative knowledge of one's herd of animals is highly important. And in cases of profound ID, with regard to the conceptual domain 'co-occurring motor and sensory impairments may prevent functional use of objects'.[44] Again, this is inter-culturally relevant; if, for instance an adult person has difficulties feeding themselves due to such motor or sensory impairments, it will have been regarded as problematic in all human societies, as will have been the impairment of verbal communication associated with profound ID in the social domain.

What is interesting, however, is that all these cross-cultural symptoms as defined by DSM-5 are from the social domain; none is from the conceptual or practical domain. When considering autism spectrum disorder (which is the new, consolidated label for what were previously regarded as the separate disorders of autism, Asperger's and pervasive developmental disorder[45]) the social aspects become even more important to diagnosis, so that levels of severity come to be 'based on social communication impairments and restricted, repetitive patterns of behavior'.[46] These diagnostic criteria are so culturally specific that it really brings to the fore the absurdity of retrospectively applying such labels to any pre-modern periods. Expectancies of the quality and quantity of 'social communication' vary inter-culturally, so that, for instance, the very behaviour that one society pathologises, another culture may value despite recognising strangeness or difference. (*DSM-5* itself tacitly acknowledges this: 'It remains unclear whether higher rates [of prevalence] reflect an expansion of the diagnostic criteria of DSM-IV to include subthreshold cases, increased awareness, differences in study methodology, or a true increase in the frequency of autism spectrum disorder.'[47]) A case in point would be the behaviour of medieval anchorites, people who voluntarily withdrew from the world, restricted their social interactions and indulged in some very regulated, if not repetitive, behaviours. A modern psychiatrist might be very tempted, in the absence of knowledge concerning culturally specific contexts, to diagnose such a medieval anchorite, or other member of a monastic, enclosed, regular (as in living according to a rule) community, as being on the autism spectrum.

Nevertheless, in general one may surmise that the more severely or profoundly a neurodevelopmental disorder, including ID, manifests, the less relevant inter-cultural variance becomes. Even *DSM-5* takes some account of socio-cultural factors in its generalised definition: 'The essential features of intellectual disability … are deficits in general mental abilities … and impairment in everyday adaptive functioning, in comparison to an individual's age-, gender-, and socioculturally matched peers.'[48] In this broad description, ID becomes something that manifests and can be identified in every human society, at all times and places, according to each society's own specific criteria, although in contemporary Western society it is a combined set of 'clinical assessment and standardized testing of intellectual and adaptive functions'[49] that determines diagnosis. While of course much of the modern diagnostic approach of *DSM-5* is simply not relevant to a study of pre-modern society, some of the descriptors are. For instance, *DSM-5* describes gullibility as an associated feature that can support diagnosis. 'Gullibility is often a feature, involving naiveté in social situations and a tendency for being easily led by others. Gullibility and lack of awareness of risk may result in exploitation by others,'[50] a facet of ID regrettably all too often encountered in the medieval (and earlier) sources, especially with regard to legal cases.

Idiocy, madness and historiography

But the historiographic inclination to read idiocy as something internal to an individual, and therefore to treat idiocy as an unchanging phenomenon present throughout time, actually becomes ahistorical. What one society calls 'idiocy' may not be the same for another society centuries later. And if it is not the same across time and/or place, we need to reflect on what the differences might be. 'We have no way of knowing for certain if someone called a "fool" in the sixteenth century would, if transported through time, be called "simple" in the eighteenth century, an "imbecile" in the 1890s, or "moderately or mildly retarded" in the 1960s; nor do we know if someone called an "idiot" in 1760 would still be one in 1860, or "severely retarded" in 1960.'[51] Questions such as how societies define(d) intelligence, and how the perceived divisions between congenital and acquired deviations from the 'norm' feed into such definitions, therefore remain pertinent to contemporary medical, bioethical and social experts and practitioners. Normative texts, such as medical, legal and natural-philosophical authorities, were the medieval equivalent of modern scientific experts with regard to defining, assessing and controlling notions of ID. We can then ask what the medical, legal and social implications of such concepts were. To find out more about how the names and words used to describe people also influenced the social and environmental treatment of them, this book will look at what the medieval equivalents to our modern scientific or psychiatric experts had to say about ID. It was medieval physicians, lawyers and the schoolmen of the emerging universities who wrote the texts where we can find their definitions of intellectual ability and its counterpart, disability. By studying such texts, which form part of our contemporary scientific and cultural heritage, we can gain a better understanding of which people were considered to be intellectually disabled back in the past, and how their participation and inclusion in society may have differed from the situation today.

What is meant by norms and normative texts? Anthropology and sociology have allowed us to recognise and describe models, standards or patterns of social behaviour and their concomitant attitudes as expressed by members of a group. If norms are stated explicitly ('Thou shalt not kill') one can also refer to them as rules. However, many rules exist only by implication, through the behaviour of individual people, which when taken in relationship to the behaviour of a given group becomes a behavioural pattern and hence a norm, or framework of norms that members of the group adhere to. Norms may not always be followed consciously, or described as norms, but if there is enough evidence that behaviour follows patterned ways, one may speak of norms, particularly in a historical context.[52] Since of course we cannot place a sociologist back in time amongst a certain group of medieval people to gather evidence from field work, we have to rely on the mainstay of historical research, written evidence, hence the concept of normative texts. Claims of authority by one group or individual over another group or individual, whether originally by oral declaration or later recorded in writing, are an explicit example of a norm. Normative texts therefore are invariably backed by authority, whether the authority of consensus among group members or the authority of a superior group imposing their normative order on a group perceived as inferior (for instance, self-appointed 'normal' people describing, categorising and labelling the abnormal).

In the late 1960s two books on madness appeared on either side of the Atlantic that could not have been more different in their approaches: Rosen's *Madness in Society* (1968) and Foucault's *History of Madness* (French 1961, first abridged English translation as *Madness and Civilization*, 1967). Their only common denominator was a similarly brief discussion of madness in the Middle Ages. Foucault's notion of the ship of fools as actual, real vessels that carried the insane from place to place was judiciously debunked by the Mahers' search through documentary evidence, failing to find that any such ships existed.[53] An example of how Foucault's fallacy found its way into subsequent literature may be gleaned from the work by Judge entitled *Civilization and Mental Retardation* – note the unfortunate juxtaposition of civilization and retardation – who treated the literary 'Ship of Fools' as a historical fact and asserted that medieval mariners were paid to put people on boats, to set them adrift or to dump them far away from the towns they came from, and whose work was in turn cited as historical reference point by Clapton in an article on 'Disability, inclusion and the Christian Church'.[54]

The already mentioned lack of interest of medical historians in mental disability (and even in disability more generally)[55] undoubtedly played a part in the paucity of literature on the history of ID. As a case in point, the monumental *Companion Encyclopedia of the History of Medicine* does not mention 'mental disability' as a term at all, but only briefly touches on John Langdon Down and his studies of feeble-minded children, leading straight on to the discovery in 1959 of a genetic basis for the eponymous syndrome; the only other mentions relate to the link between goitre and cretinism, as consequences of, respectively, nutritional deficiencies or endocrine disease.[56] Equally, the slightly less voluminous but more recent *Oxford Handbook of the History of Medicine* treats of 'mental disability' only in relation to a modern concern with child health and the rights of the child.[57]

After the linguistic turn in history we are now at the cognitive or neuroscientific turn in the humanities and arts: a phenomenon of recent academic growth, as increasing numbers of scholars (especially in literary studies) employ evidence from neuroscience in their research.[58] One provocative thesis on prehistory and human neurochemistry has been proposed by Smail, who in his assessment of the relationship between biology and culture critiques evolutionary psychology.[59] In essence, Smail argues for the abandonment of the idea of prehistory and posits that our brains are trans-historical. There is interaction between the humanities and the neuroscience literature on embodied cognition and embodied semantics, recognising perceptual simulation as part of social cognition, therefore cultural and social forces help to shape the meaning we construct from such neural response. Thus an increasing number of scholars from both the historical disciplines and the social sciences have argued lately that 'intelligence' and 'disability' do not describe natural, trans-historical realities, nor do they present self-evident certainties. Instead, paradigms shift and notions of health and illness change. For instance, concepts that were originally informed by classical and medieval socio-political and religious contexts of intellectual ability and disability subsequently became part of the modern, formal human science disciplines of psychology, medicine and biology. 'Intelligence' is not a constant, ahistorical, scientific entity, such as gas particles might be to a physicist, but a construction, value or perception, which makes it subject to cultural change: hence assessments, evaluations and measurements of 'intelligence' change(d) across time and place.

For years the only available histories of ID that had even hesitatingly alluded to the medieval period had been the books by Kanner and Scheerenberger on mental retardation, both works which traced the development of the professional treatment of people given these labels.[60] With the publication of Wright and Digby's historical survey, a seminal collection was made available, focusing rather on social and institutional than on psychiatric or biomedical history.[61] Goodey has emerged as the doyen of submitting the core concept of idiocy to historical analysis, often providing 'provocative and challenging analyses of the ideological development and application of idiocy and related concepts',[62] although his treatment of the Middle Ages has been rather sparse. He has been followed by Stainton, who is one of the few to take a closer, albeit slightly skewed, look at folly and disability in the medieval and early modern periods. McDonagh has joined them to form the triumvirate of Anglophone writers on the history of ID. Thus the research since the 1990s has begun to create a history of developmental disability, but has also generated further questions.

Myths of idiocy

McDonagh had highlighted one of the key assumptions when dealing with ID in the pre-modern past, namely that the 'idiot has been transformed into a resilient contrast group, a category of people against whom we rational modern (and post-modern) folk can identify ourselves, to affirm our intelligence and to assert our claims to respect and justice'.[63] Here we have one element of the mythology surrounding ID, that of modern rationality. As will be explained below, one thankfully now outmoded historiographic view treated the pre-modern past as infantile and irrational. We need to dispel some more modern myths: that all people with ID in the pre-modern past were badly treated; that their mortality rate was so high that most died anyway (which actually contradicts the first myth, since there would be hardly any children with ID reaching adulthood); and that if they did not die a natural death due to physical pathologies, then they died due to infanticide. For example, discussing the classical antecedents for medical views of mental illness, Dols bluntly stated in his otherwise magisterial volume:

> It is likely that mental incapacities generally were not as prevalent in antiquity as in modern times for a number of reasons, especially the high mortality of mentally impaired children. A priori, death would have resulted naturally from congenital illnesses that are associated with mental retardation in childhood. In addition, serious mental and physical anomalies would have been recognized in infants and young children and may often have led to their destruction by their parents.[64]

He based this unsubstantiated claim regarding the mortality rate on the equally unsubstantiated one by Heiberg,[65] which was obviously a claim coloured by the eugenicist thinking of the times (1920s). Dols also relied on the claims for infanticide of defective children sometimes alleged in classical texts, which have been grossly exaggerated by modern scholarship and are only starting to be refuted from the 1990s onward.[66] What is also exaggerated is the 'natural' death rate due to congenital illnesses. Even children with severe cases of Down syndrome and the concomitant physical diseases that sometimes ensue (e.g. heart problems) can quite readily survive to adulthood without any medical intervention whatsoever. Abandonment, as Dols goes on to mention,[67] and as was thoroughly discussed by Boswell,[68] was probably far more common than infanticide, and the 'preferred option', so to speak, for families and individuals to rid themselves of unwanted children; unwanted for a variety of reasons, including notions of physical or mental defectiveness, but more often than not economic distress.

Another myth, connected with modern arrogance, partly contradicts those just mentioned, namely that people in the past lived such less-demanding lives than we do anyway that they would not have noticed the presence of ID. This is the evolutionary, or developmental, view of civilisation, which believes that whole cultures move through phases, from lesser, infantile stages (i.e. any culture in the pre-modern past) via an adolescent stage (generally a couple of generations before the writer's own time) to the rational, adult phase (the writer's own contemporary culture). An example of the 'earlier equals more primitive' view can be found in both Huizinga's *Waning of the Middle Ages*, who imagined a Middle Ages filled with 'childish' emotions and Elias's *Civilizing Process*, who believed that it was not until the sixteenth century that people started to repress and control their emotive reactions.[69] If we follow these two authors, then the Middle Ages are the childhood or youth of humanity, and we now, in the modern present, have (finally?) reached adulthood. People in the medieval past would not have noticed ID so much, this myth alleges, because they themselves were still on a lower emotional and intellectual rung of the evolutionary/developmental ladder. Another view of primitivism is concerned with lack of technical or economic sophistication. Because medieval peasants did not need to be able to do sophisticated things like read or write, they would not have noticed mental deficiency, unless it was so severe, in which case they would label someone the village idiot who, however, because of the primitiveness of medieval agrarian society overall, could quite happily and easily be integrated into both economic and social structures of the peasant world. Or so that myth goes. And lastly there is the persistent myth that fools and jesters were the ubiquitous expressions of people with ID in the past. But if you called someone a fool in the Middle Ages, you may have described their occupation and not their alleged state of mind.

With regard to primitivism, one may note that at around the 1890s, the high point of scientific positivism, when Henry Wellcome was planning a book on the topic of animal substances as used in medicine, his approach of including even the treatment methods of 'the most primitive races' was unusual for the time. Non-Western, pre-industrial societies were deemed to be 'illogical, juvenile, and dim-witted' and their lack of technology was equated with lack of mental sophistication, hence it was believed so-called primitive people acted 'by habit and superstition rather than intelligence or reason'.[70]

The following historiographical exploration may shed light on why I refer to certain assumptions as myths, and warrants three citations from the early pioneers of the history of ID. Scheerenberger had (perhaps unwittingly) tried to set the agenda for social constructionism:

> Mental retardation is primarily a socioculturally determined phenomenon that undoubtedly has been apparent since the dawn of man. Any given society, including the earliest tribes, unquestionably contained members who were more capable and less capable than average. The impact of debility has, however, varied with the needs of society, its expectancies and social consciousness.[71]

This is actually not too implausible a summary, although it would have been improved by the additional statement that early tribes, or different cultures in general, were highly unlikely to have recognised, diagnosed or classified ID in the same ways, never mind according to the latest version of the DSM. Kanner, writing a generation before Scheerenberger, does deserve more credit than he is generally given by disability historians, since as early as 1949 he observed that there are socio-cultural factors differentiating attitudes to and treatment of people deemed mentally retarded, although he still had to couch this recognition in terms of the idea that in a simpler society simpler persons could more readily be accommodated:

> In less complex, less intellectually centered societies, the mentally retarded would have no trouble in obtaining and retaining a quality of realizable ambitions. Some might even be capable of gaining superiority by virtue of assets other than those measured by the intelligence test. They could make successful peasants, hunters, fishermen, tribal dancers. ... their principal shortcoming is a greater or lesser degree of inability to comply with the intellectual requirements of their society. In other respects, they may be as mature or immature, stable or unstable, secure or insecure, placid or moody, aggressive or submissive, as any other member of the human species. Their 'deficiency' is an ethnologically determined phenomena [sic] relative to the local standards and even within those standards, relative to the educational postulates, vocational ambitions, and family expectancies. They are 'subcultural' in our society but may not be even that in a different, less sophisticated setting.[72]

The crucial point is not, as Kanner would have it, that less sophisticated societies do not recognise and do not notice ID, but that the degree to which ID matters, or does not matter, is subject to the specific socio-cultural circumstances of each time and place. The notion of a pre-modern pastoral idyll that can accommodate the mentally less able must have appealed to the mid-twentieth-century psyche. Scheerenberger had summarised the pre-modern period thus:

> In most rural areas, mentally retarded persons probably toiled long hours alongside their parents, responding to the demands of their lord or nobleman to wage combat at varying intervals. Many undoubtedly died at an early age due to disease or pestilence. Some may have participated in the Crusades. The village idiot was common, and mentally retarded persons of mild temperament were allowed to roam the countryside unmolested, receiving aid and comfort from neighbors. Thus, on an individual basis, they became somewhat of a public responsibility.[73]

One need not restrict one's historiographical prejudices to ancient or medieval Europe. The authors of a study of ID in modern China and of the relationship between ID and technological societies have argued that mild mental retardation was not a problem in technologically less developed societies, as compared to the modern Western world, especially societies without writing and those lacking a formal education system.[74] This is blatant arrogance on the part of these authors vis-à-vis other cultures. It demonstrates the assumption that less technological societies are overall less mentally developed, and therefore individuals with mental deficiencies within such a society would not be noticed. However, as Neubert and Cloerkes pointed out in their survey of twenty-four cultures from around the globe, even minor mental deficiencies are undesirable, and social competence is evidently highly valued in all societies.[75]

When we turn to historiographies of the medieval period, we find frequent reiteration of such sentiments. The author of a social history of disability, Fandrey, subscribed to the view that less technology therefore meant less recognition of ID, so for peasant society he claimed that since the faculties of abstraction necessary to learn reading, writing and arithmetic were not part of the cultural norm, such societies did not know of 'learning disabilities'.[76] Or claimed that intelligence and education possessed a lower value in medieval society than they do today, due to the low practical importance of technology and science, so that therefore a person lacking intelligence was less of a social outlaw.[77] In general, Fandrey proposed for the Middle Ages less need for abstraction (because they were a less structured, time-driven, technological society) or for individual novelty (medieval popular culture liked repetition), and ultimately argued for greater acceptance of mental or behavioural difference. Withdrawal or flight from society, what might be branded as autism today, with radical reduction of interpersonal relations by retreating to church, cloister or hermitage, to be closer to God, were seen as acceptable, positive behavioural traits.[78] And Zijderveld's work on rationality and folly, for all its merits, falls into the category of those histories which take the view that people in the past were simpler, less rational and therefore themselves more childlike, and less developed, than us moderns. Although Zijderveld criticised Huizinga for his omission of fools and folly, he approvingly cited his *Homo Ludens* (1938), with its imagery of a Middle Ages 'brimful of play'[79] as an example of this earlier, traditional, less civilised and less rational culture. In our civilised modern world we have lost this, lamented Zijderveld, and instead 'we should compose ourselves when we feel the itch of folly because folly is "primitive", "childish", "irrational", "uncivilized"'.[80] He castigated the intellectualisation which hit medieval mentalities, singling out especially Aristotelianism, in its filtered version via Averroes, as a 'rationalistic strait-jacket of medieval minds', although he claimed that this 'intellectualization remained restricted to a relatively small elite, to wit the clergy and, within the clergy, to some specialists like the philosophically trained scholars'.[81] Like a number of other modern historians and sociologists, Stainton also subscribes to the view of life being easier in the past for people with ID, because their disabilities would, given the lower level of development of societal or technological structures, be less noticeable; for Roman antiquity, for instance, he stated: 'For people having what we might now label as mild intellectual impairments there was likely little actual disability in terms of functioning within the family and society.' [82] Also Goodey seems to take the 'primitivist' stance when he discusses medieval, or more generally pre-modern, social concepts, claiming that in that distant past the term 'idiot' held a precise meaning only when used 'in relation to that social group in which it would be an anomaly', meaning the educated upper classes. 'The peasant, by contrast, was already a born fool by social definition [...] He did not need a competence test to work in the fields.'[83] This betrays a repetition of the arrogance medieval writers themselves may be accused of, implying that agricultural activities are deemed so simple and intellectually undemanding tasks that even 'idiots' can do them. But, as evidence collected by social and economic historians like Clark demonstrates,[84] at the latest by the thirteenth century the mental competence of peasants was something that was of concern to their families and to their manorial ('feudal') lord; numerous manorial records survive from that time onward which relate cases where the land tenure and associated obligations are reshuffled within a manorial community because the previous peasant had become senile and therefore incapable of managing the land. Agricultural peasant activities required different but just as much planning, organisation and therefore mental competence as the higher-status occupations of craft production, trade or education.

'Idiocy involves interpretation'

'Idiocy involves interpretation, whether by physicians or psychologists performing a diagnosis, or historians and cultural analysts reading old documents. We ignore this process at our peril: we cannot pretend to understand the history of idiocy (or intellectual disability, or intelligence) if we forget to question and analyse what forces shape this concept and its precursors.'[85] In pursuit of idiocy there is good justification to be truly interdisciplinary, to look at the cultural, scientific (natural-philosophic), theological, philosophical, medical, legal and sociological aspects of the Middle Ages. Furthermore, the kind of study pursued here raises questions about historical periodisation. It may be possible to describe the distinguishing features of a topic, for instance idiocy, within a given period, but it is inadequate to describe why and how this happens within a period just by reference to the period itself. So to understand 'idiocy' in the context of the Middle Ages we need to both look back at antiquity, and forward to modern times. In some ways the (early) modern period is distinct from the preceding medieval, but in other ways it shares many continuities, and both medieval and (early) modern share many relations with classical antiquity.

My methodology employed a diachronic approach, in that one of the starting premises was that concepts of what is, or is not, ID, is situated in time and changes over time. One has only to think of the relatively recent shift in attitudes which underlies the change in words used to describe certain groups of people sharing a common condition (people with Down syndrome are no longer called 'Mongols', to give just one pertinent example). Nevertheless, to be able to describe a phenomenon one needs a terminological consensus, hence the medical model of disability does hold a (limited) methodological place. Significantly, as Berkson pointed out, 'although a generic concept of intellectual disability has been with us across history and different cultures, there has been continued refinement of the concept'.[86] This highlights a progressive development, meaning progressive not necessarily in a positivist sense, but simply implying movement or change, and is one of the reasons why historians of any flavour conduct research. It also highlights that as we move forward to the present day, the categorisation, subgrouping and ever more precise labelling and defining of mental states has become more of a preoccupation both with experts (first philosophers, then psychiatrists, now policy makers) and at a more diffused, broad cultural level.

ID is obviously not a conceptual category a medieval writer would have recognised or used. Therefore, for ancient or medieval sources I followed the terminology used in the source (such as, in translation, fool, idiot, simpleton) and tried best as possible to equate it with one of the modern terms. When medieval writers considered what we now label ID, or even call 'disability' more generally, their writings were spread across disciplines and types of texts we now classify as ethics, morals, theology, philosophy, jurisprudence and medicine. This disparity between modern and medieval definitions of what may (or may not) be the same phenomenon has forced modern researchers to engage with a wide variety of source material. It has occasionally been necessary to trawl through entire theological *summae* only to find a couple of lines on congenital 'idiocy', to peruse medical texts for a single mention of cognitive impairment or to scan Aristotelian commentaries on the soul for passages that speak, however indirectly, of what we now identify as ID. This has been necessarily an interdisciplinary, multi-textual approach, which the present author admits will contain many gaps and as-yet undiscovered sources. A further challenge for the historian of ID, having combed through what source material is available, then lies in assembling such varied and transdisciplinary material into a coherent narrative, all the while taking care not to impose modern assumptions on medieval categories. Medieval ideas about 'intellectual disability' were as contested as our ideas of the subject, so that one of the dangers inherent in anatomising the story of medieval 'idiocy' into its constituent texts and parts of texts is that when trying to recreate medieval contexts from the component parts we may sometimes confuse descriptive and argumentative writing. Perhaps all one can state with certainty is that medieval notions of ID were much less unified than the canons of medical history in general, and psychiatric history in particular, have suggested. ID was not simply described as a single state of being, but brought together a range of ideas (on what it meant to be human, on agency, culpability) which in turn informed social and behavioural actions.

Being aware of the usage of different types of sources means also being aware that although different texts may treat the same idea, they do not treat it in the same way. Theological, legal and even literary texts have all been mined for the present volume, but of course retain their distinctions as different kinds of writing, and retain their determinative effect on the ideas they are expressing and arguments they are making. I have tried to remain conscious of this fact, and as far as possible to draw the reader's attention to the bounded nature of texts, even if that meant more or less lengthy digressions and textual excursions.

Overview and structure of the book

The following chapter considers the semantics of ID by looking at the words and labels used across time and place for conditions that might be subsumed by the umbrella-term 'intellectual disability' in modern Western society. Lexemes from a range of languages are analysed, including the Semitic language family (Hebrew and Arabic), with Indo-European comparisons by way of trying to get at the linguistic roots of rationality and intellect, and a closer examination of ancient Greek and Latin, Old and Middle English, Old French, Old and Middle High German, concluding with a case study of the shifting meanings of the 'idiot'.

Chapter 3 moves on to concepts of ID in medieval natural science, that is, anatomical and medical texts; what we would now term the neurological foundations. Starting with a look at pathologies of the brain, which in turn allowed the formulation of medieval faculty theory (since then, as now, by looking at brain damage one can learn something about the functions of specific areas in the healthy brain) and anatomical ideas about the brain, the work of William of Conches in the early twelfth century is especially prominent;

the story continues with medieval attempts at the localisation of intelligence and a consideration of the developing brain from infancy through childhood to maturity, together with the implications of perceived childishness that this has for persons with ID. Aetiologies, and in particular the medieval emphasis on the materiality and physicality of 'idiocy' (with special reference to notions of ID as subject of wonder in texts by Gervase of Tilbury and Konrad of Megenberg), provide further context. The chapter concludes with a brief look at (the lack of) medieval institutions for people with ID and ponders the question of the absence of ID in medical texts.

Turning from the material aspects of neurology to the immateriality of psychology, Chapter 4 treats mind and soul in relation to ID. Starting with the question of rationality in the philosophy of antiquity, we move on to the importance of language for intellectual abilities, leading on to the connections between intellect and dominance. Medieval witnesses include Augustine on intellect and those treatises on the soul in the format of numerous tracts under the heading *De anima*; the scholastics such as John Blund on soul, intellect and the 'idiot'; and of course Albertus Magnus and Thomas Aquinas; in all which writings ID emerges as perpetual childishness. The chapter concludes with a brief look at the variant theologies surrounding the famous beatitude on 'the poor in spirit'.

The theme of childishness leads on to Chapter 5, which considers the legal position of persons with ID. Commencing with a glance at the antecedents in and comparisons with Judaic, Islamic and Roman law, one discovers a particularly rich source in the Old Irish legal texts; this is followed by medieval English laws, with particular reference to thirteenth-century sources such as the *Prerogativa Regis* and the writings of four more or less contemporary jurists (Bracton, *Fleta*, the *Mirror of Justices*, Britton), and German and French examples. The question of whether a legal case related to mental illness or ID is analysed, which may also be considered in relation to a number of samples from the English source known as the Patent Rolls. Thinking about legal agency returns to the themes of idiocy and infancy, thus rounding off this chapter.

Chapter 6 looks at the socio-cultural implications of ID through the lens of court fools, pets and entertainers. One theme is the ahistoricity of fools and idiots, in that a corpus of fictions and imaginings has stamped too strong an impression of the fool and jester onto discussions of medieval (and early modern) ID. An overview of the link between court fools, idiots and social theories of dominance leads on to classical antiquity and the origin of 'fools', with the fully fledged medieval court fools noticeable and remarkable for 'foolish' behaviour rather than medicalised traits. Foolish literature (pun intended), and especially the case of representations of the Psalm-fool, emerged to be misleading in the search for 'real' ID.

The book concludes with a chapter reconsidering some of the themes touched on above, especially in the light of notions of rationality, intelligence and human status. The thirteenth century emerges as something of a turning point in the discourse of ID, although antecedents must be kept in mind. Conspicuous by their (almost) complete absence are miracle healings of ID – this conundrum is pondered here also. In conclusion, it is worth remembering the fluidity of medieval norms and labels in contrast to modern fixations.

Notes

1 www.euro.who.int/en/what-we-do/health-topics/noncommunicable-diseases/mental-health/news/news/2010/15/childrens-right-to-family-life/definition-intellectual-disability (accessed 2 September 2014).

2 Christopher Goodey, *A History of Intelligence and 'Intellectual Disability': The Shaping of Psychology in Early Modern Europe* (Farnham: Ashgate, 2011), 219.

3 David Sprunger, 'Depicting the Insane: A Thirteenth-Century Case Study', in Timothy Jones and David Sprunger (eds), *Marvels, Monsters, and Miracles: Studies in the Medieval and Early Modern Imaginations* (Kalamazoo: Western Michigan University, 2002), 223–41, at 231.

4 J. Andrews, 'Begging the Question of Idiocy: The Definition and Socio-cultural Meaning of Idiocy in Early Modern Britain: Part I', *History of Psychiatry*, 9 (1998), 65–95, at 66.

5 Stephen Harper, 'The Subject of Madness: Insanity, Individuals and Society in Late-Medieval English Literature' (PhD thesis, University of Glasgow, 1997), 293 (available as PDF file from http://theses.gla.ac.uk/ [accessed 24 October 2013]); subsequently published as *Insanity, Individuals, and Society in Late-Medieval English Literature: The Subject of Madness* (Lewiston, Queenston, Lampeter: Edwin Mellen Press, 2003). There is of course the valid question of whether, and if so, to what degree, mental incapacity, mental impairment and mental illness are within one conceptual category; furthermore, if they constitute disabilities, a debate that is part of a very modern problem. For example, it has been argued that mental illness should be treated as a disability in the same way as physical impairments are; see Peter Beresford, 'What Have Madness and Psychiatric System Survivors Got to Do with Disability and Disability Studies?', *Disability and Society*, 15:1 (2000), 167–72.

6 R. Brooks, 'Official Madness: A Cross-cultural Study of Involuntary and Civil Confinement Based on "Mental Illness"', in Jane Hubert (ed.), *Madness, Disability and Social Exclusion: The Archaeology and Anthropology of 'Difference'* (London and New York: Routledge, 2000), 9–28.

7 Jonathan Andrews, 'Identifying and Providing for the Mentally Disabled in Early

Modern London', in David Wright and Anne Digby (eds), *From Idiocy to Mental Deficiency: Historical Perspectives on People with Learning Disabilities* (London: Routledge, 1996), 66. For the association of 'fool' with 'person with ID' see, most recently, Eliza Buhrer, '"But what is to be said of a fool?" Intellectual Disability in Medieval Thought and Culture', in Albrecht Classen (ed.), *Mental Health, Spirituality, and Religion in the Middle Ages and Early Modern Age* (Berlin: De Gruyter, 2014), 314–43.

8 Andrews, 'Identifying and Providing', 67.

9 Christopher Goodey, '"Foolishness" in Early Modern Medicine and the Concept of Intellectual Disability', *Medical History*, 48 (2004), 289–310, at 290.

10 *Diagnostic and Statistical Manual of Mental Disorders*, American Psychiatric Association (Washington, DC: American Psychiatric Association, 5th edition 2013) [hereafter *DSM-5*], 31, 38–9. See also Jacob A. Burack, Robert M. Hodapp, Grace Iarocci and Edward Zigler (eds), *The Oxford Handbook of Intellectual Disability and Development* (New York: Oxford University Press, 2012), xv, where the professed aim of the editors is 'to update developments in the field of developmental theory and research as they apply to the study of persons with intellectual disability (ID)'.

11 Alison Niccols, Karen Thomas and Louis A. Schmidt, 'Socioemotional and Brain Development in Children with Genetic Syndromes Associated with Developmental Delay', in J. A. Burack et al. (eds), *Oxford Handbook of Intellectual Disability*, 254–74, at 255.

12 David Wright, *Downs: The History of a Disability* (Oxford: Oxford University Press, 2011), 8.

13 Joanna Moss, Patricia Howlin and Chris Oliver, 'The Assessment and Presentation of Autism Spectrum Disorders and Associated Characteristics in Individuals with Severe Intellectual Disability and Genetic Syndromes', in J. A. Burack et al. (eds), *Oxford Handbook of Intellectual Disability*, 275–99, at 282.

14 Grace Iarocci and Stephen A. Petrill, 'Behavioral Genetics, Genomics, Intelligence, and Mental Retardation', in J. A. Burack et al. (eds), *Oxford Handbook of Intellectual Disability*, 13–29, at 13.

15 *DSM-5*, 31; also 38 for illnesses such as meningitis or encephalitis causing abrupt onset of IDs.

16 *DSM-5*, 39.

17 Ludmilla Jordanova, 'The Social Construction of Medical Knowledge', *Social History of Medicine*, 8:3 (1995), 361–81; David Harley, 'Rhetoric and the Social Construction of Sickness and Healing', *Social History of Medicine*, 12:3 (1999), 407–35; Paolo Palladino, 'And the Answer Is … 42', *Social History of Medicine*, 13:1 (2000), 147–52; Ivan Dalley Crozier, 'Social Construction in a Cold Climate: A Response to David Harley, "Rhetoric and the Social Construction of Sickness and Healing" and to Paolo Palladino's Comment on Harley', *Social History of Medicine*, 13:3 (2000), 535–46.

18 Ian Hacking, *The Social Construction of What?* (Cambridge, MA and London:

Harvard University Press, 1999), 100. I am grateful to my colleague at Swansea, Adam Mosley, for drawing attention to this.

19 Hacking, *The Social Construction of What?* 100.
20 Hacking, *The Social Construction of What?* 109.
21 Hacking, *The Social Construction of What?* 111.
22 Hacking, *The Social Construction of What?* 119.
23 Hacking, *The Social Construction of What?*119.
24 Hacking, *The Social Construction of What?* 122.
25 Deborah J. Fidler, 'Child Eliciting Effects in Families of Children with Intellectual Disability: Proximal and Distal Perspectives', in J. A. Burack et al. (eds), *Oxford Handbook of Intellectual Disability*, 366–79, at 372; cf. M. Daly and M. I. Wilson, 'A Sociobiological Analysis of Human Infanticide', in G. Hausfater and S. B. Hrdy (eds), *Infanticide: Comparative and Evolutionary Perspectives* (New York: Aldine Press, 1984), 487–502.
26 Gershon Berkson, 'Intellectual and Physical Disabilities in Prehistory and Early Civilization', *Mental Retardation*, 42 (2004), 195–208, at 195.
27 Berkson, 'Intellectual and Physical Disabilities', 204.
28 Laurence Brockliss and Heather Montgomery (eds), *Childhood and Violence in the Western Tradition* (Oxford and Oakville: Oxbow, 2010), 89, citing B. Conklin and L. Morgan, 'Babies, Bodies, and the Production of Personhood in North America and a Native Amazonian Society', *Ethos*, 24:4 (1996), 657–84, at 657–8.
29 Dieter Neubert and Günther Cloerkes, *Behinderung und Behinderte in verschiedenen Kulturen. Eine vergleichende Analyse ethnologischer Studien* (Heidelberg: Edition Schindele, 2nd, edn 1994), 44, and 109n9 cites the example of C. H. Hawes, *In the Uttermost East* (London: Harper, 1903), 250 who variously refers to one and the same individual as an idiot and as a madman.
30 Neubert and Cloerkes, *Behinderung und Behinderte*, 44; cf. L. G. Peters, 'Concepts of Mental Deficiency among the Tamang of Nepal', *American Journal of Mental Deficiency*, 84 (1980), 352–6.
31 R. B. Edgerton, 'Anthropology and Mental Retardation: A Plea for the Comparative Study of Incompetence', in H. Prehm, L. Mamerlynck and J. E. Crosson (eds), *Behavior Research in Mental Retardation* (Eugene: University of Oregon Press, 1968), 75–87, at 84.
32 Neubert and Cloerkes, *Behinderung und Behinderte*, 66 and 110n14.
33 Neubert and Cloerkes, *Behinderung und Behinderte*, 66.
34 Neubert and Cloerkes, *Behinderung und Behinderte*: 'Das Ausmaß an Zuneigung und Nachsicht einerseits und Restriktion bzw. Diskriminierung andererseits konnte in Abhängigkeit von der Schwere der Behinderung sowie auch als Folge individueller Entscheidungen variieren' (p. 66).
35 Neubert and Cloerkes, *Behinderung und Behinderte*, 68.
36 R. K. Dentan, 'The Response to Intellectual Impairment among the Semai', *American Journal of Mental Deficiency*, 71 (1967), 764–6, at 765.
37 Dentan, 'The Response to Intellectual Impairment among the Semai', 766.

38 *DSM-5*, 20.
39 *DSM-5*, 31.
40 A. D. B. Clarke and A. M. Clarke (eds), *Mental Deficiency: The Changing Outlook* (London: Methuen, 1st edn, 1958), xiv.
41 *DSM-5*, 34.
42 *DSM-5*, 35.
43 *DSM-5*, 36.
44 *DSM-5*, 36.
45 *DSM-5*, xlii.
46 *DSM-5*, 50.
47 *DSM-5*, 55.
48 *DSM-5*, 37.
49 *DSM-5*, 37.
50 *DSM-5*, 38.
51 Patrick McDonagh, *Idiocy: A Cultural History* (Liverpool: Liverpool University Press, 2008), 6.
52 See Neil MacCormick, *Institutions of Law: An Essay in Legal Theory* (Oxford: Oxford University Press, 2007), and Elizabeth Colson, *Tradition and Contract: The Problem of Order* (Chicago: Aldine Publishing, 1974).
53 Winifred Barbara Maher and Brendan Maher, '"The Ship of Fools": *Stultifera Navis* or *Ignis Fatuus?*', *American Psychologist*, 37:7 (1982), 756–61.
54 Cliff Judge, *Civilization and Mental Retardation: A History of the Care and Treatment of Mentally Retarded People* (Mulgrave, Australia: Cliff Judge, 1987); Jayne Clapton, 'Disability, Inclusion and the Christian Church: Practice, Paradox or Promise', *Disability and Rehabilitation*, 19:10 (1997), 420–6, at 422.
55 Discussed by Irina Metzler, *Disability in Medieval Europe: Thinking about Physical Impairment during the High Middle Ages, c.1100–1400* (London and New York: Routledge, 2006), 11–20.
56 W. F. Bynum and Roy Porter (eds), *Companion Encyclopedia of the History of Medicine*, 2 vols (London and New York: Routledge, 1993), Downs 429–30, goitre 480, endocrine 498.
57 Mark Jackson (ed.), *The Oxford Handbook of the History of Medicine* (Oxford: Oxford University Press, 2011), 323.
58 Warren S. Brown and Brad D. Strawn, *The Physical Nature of Christian Life: Neuroscience, Psychology, and the Church* (Cambridge: Cambridge University Press, 2012) study the implications of recent insights in modern neuroscience that attribute mental capacities, often ascribed to a soul, to physical brain function alone.
59 Daniel Lord Smail, *On Deep History and the Brain* (Oakland, CA: University of California Press, 2008).
60 Leo Kanner, *A History of the Care and Study of the Mentally Retarded* (Springfield, IL: Thomas, 1964) and Richard C. Scheerenberger, *A History of Mental Retardation* (Baltimore and London: Brookes, 1983).
61 David Wright and Anne Digby (eds), *From Idiocy to Mental Deficiency: Historical*

Perspectives on People with Learning Disabilities (London: Routledge, 1996); reviewed together with three other then recent books by J. A. Brockley, 'History of Mental Retardation: An Essay Review', *History of Psychology*, 2 (1999), 25–36.

62 In the description by McDonagh, *Idiocy*, 10; see Select Bibliography for Goodey's publications.

63 McDonagh, *Idiocy*, 2.

64 Michael W. Dols (ed. Diana E. Immisch), *Majnûn: The Madman in Medieval Islamic Society* (Oxford: Clarendon Press, 1992), 20.

65 J. L. Heiberg, 'Geisteskrankheiten im klassischen Altertum', *Allgemeine Zeitschrift für Psychiatrie*, 86 (1927), 1–44, at 10.

66 It goes beyond saying that a considerable number of disabled escaped the tests of parents or midwives; in the case of blind or hearing-impaired children, the disability is detected only after a certain period of time, and the same counts for certain forms of mental retardation. See Christian Laes, 'Learning from Silence: Disabled Children in Roman Antiquity', *Arctos*, 42 (2008), 85–122. The assertion that the ancients were crueller towards the mentally disabled, who would then have been exposed at a later age, does not come up in any ancient source. Hence, the assertion by W. V. Harris, 'Child Exposure in the Roman Empire', *Journal of Roman Studies*, 84 (1994), 1–22, at 12, that 'it is difficult to imagine that victims of congenital blindness were often allowed to survive' is uncalled-for and supposes that parents would kill their babies after some months. E. Eyben, 'Family Planning in Graeco-Roman Antiquity', *Ancient Society*, 11–12 (1980), 5–82, at 15 supposed that parents would dispose of a mentally disturbed child only once the disability was discovered (that is, even later than in the case of blind or deaf-mute children).

67 Dols, *Majnûn*, 21.

68 John Boswell, *The Kindness of Strangers: The Abandonment of Children in Western Europe from Late Antiquity to the Renaissance* (New York: Pantheon, 1988).

69 Johan Huizinga, *The Waning of the Middle Ages* (Garden City, NY: Doubleday and Company, 1954); Norbert Elias, *The Civilizing Process*, trans. Edmund Jephcott (New York: Urizen Books, 1978).

70 Frances Larson, *An Infinity of Things: How Sir Henry Wellcome Collected the World* (Oxford: Oxford University Press, 2009), 32–3; the statement by Wellcome is from a letter to Friedrich Hoffmann, 27 July 1896, Wellcome Foundation Archive WF/E/01/01/03.

71 Scheerenberger, *History of Mental Retardation*, 3.

72 Leo Kanner, *A Miniature Textbook of Feeblemindedness* (New York: Child Care Publications, 1949), 7.

73 Scheerenberger, *History of Mental Retardation*, 33.

74 N. M. Robinson, 'Mild Mental Retardation: Does It Exist in the People's Republic of China?', *Mental Retardation*, 16 (1978), 295–8, and E. Ginzberg, 'The Mentally Handicapped in a Technological Society', in S. Osler and R. Cooke (eds), *The Biosocial Bases of Mental Retardation* (Baltimore, MD: Johns Hopkins University Press, 1965), 7.

75 'Soziale Kompetenz wird ganz offenkundig in allen Gesellschaften hochgeschätzt.'
    Neubert and Cloerkes, *Behinderung und Behinderte*, 68.
76 'Abstraktionsfähigkeit für das Lernen von Lesen, Schreiben und Rechnen gehörte
    nicht zum kulturellen Standard, daher kannte man auch keine "Lernbehinderung".'
    Walter Fandrey, *Krüppel, Idioten, Irre. Zur Sozialgeschichte behinderter Menschen in
    Deutschland* (Stuttgart: Silberburg-Verlag, 1990), 12.
77 'Intelligenz und Bildung besaßen in der mittelalterlichen Gesellschaft aufgrund
    der geringen praktischen Bedeutung von Technik und Wissenschaft einen gerin-
    geren Stellenwert als heute – der Mangel an Intelligenz wurde wohl auch deshalb
    weniger sozial geächtet.' Fandrey, *Krüppel*, 22.
78 'Rückzug oder Flucht aus der Gesellschaft, radikale Reduzierung der zwischenmen-
    schlichen Kommunikation in Kirche, Kloster oder Einsiedelei – um Gott näher zu
    sein – erscheinen dem Mittelalter als akzeptable, positive Verhaltensweisen.'
    Fandrey, *Krüppel*, 14.
79 Anton C. Zijderveld, *Reality in a Looking Glass: Rationality through an Analysis of
    Traditional Folly* (London: Routledge and Kegan Paul, 1982), 58.
80 Zijderveld, *Reality in a Looking Glass*, 59.
81 Zijderveld, *Reality in a Looking Glass*, 43.
82 Tim Stainton, 'Reason, Grace and Charity: Augustine and the Impact of Church
    Doctrine on the Construction of Intellectual Disability', *Disability & Society*, 23:5
    (2008), 485–96, at 487.
83 Goodey, *History of Intelligence*, 145.
84 Elaine Clark, 'Some Aspects of Social Security in Medieval England', *Journal of
    Family History*, 7:4 (1982), 307–20; also discussion in Irina Metzler, *A Social
    History of Disability in the Middle Ages* (London: Routledge, 2013), 123–6 on
    maintenance contracts for impaired peasants.
85 McDonagh, *Idiocy*, 19.
86 Gershon Berkson, 'Mental Disabilities in Western Civilization from Ancient Rome
    to the Prerogativa Regis', *Mental Retardation*, 44:1 (2006), 28–40, at 29.

2

FROM *MORIO* TO FOOL: SEMANTICS
OF INTELLECTUAL DISABILITY

The terminology for what we now call *intellectual disability* has changed in
current times once or twice in each generation. In the last 50 years, *mental defect,
mental deficiency, mental retardation, developmental disability, mental handicap,*
and *mental subnormality* have been used in various times and countries.[1]

And this just covers the period since 1960. In his book-length history of ID,
Goodey supplied an even longer list of names as used from the mid-nineteenth
century to the start of the twenty-first, adding that the 'instability of names
surely points to a deeper conceptual problem and [...] to the absence of any
stable nature linking the people thus described'.[2] Today we speak of people
who are learning, intellectually or cognitively disabled, and we now recognise
the discrimination that until fairly recently used to be encountered in using
words like spastic or mongol. The change in words reflects a change in attitudes. But did similar words always mean similar attitudes in the past? If you
called someone a fool in the Middle Ages, you may have described their occupation and not their alleged state of mind. 'Idiocy, mental deficiency, folly,
mental retardation, intellectual disability and learning disability are not all the
same names for a trans-historically stable subject.'[3] The underlying ideas might
be related, but the individual manifestations varied across time and place, possibly with the exception of the universal 'folly' of late fifteenth- and sixteenth-
century literature ascribed to all post-lapsarian humanity. Which all points to
the importance of including the broader context of culture when considering
the discourse of idiocy.

Using politically correct language does not necessarily improve the social
position or contemporary civil rights of stigmatised groups, and the linguistic
terms used historically aid our understanding of past values and past social attitudes.[4] Some writers on ID therefore plead 'do not replace "idiocy" and its historical brethren with terms more harmonious to contemporary sensibilities,

such as "intellectual disability", because they are not the same thing, even if they are conceptually related'.[5] And Stainton and McDonagh programmatically stated that the 'inherently unstable concept' of ID enforced a wide range of terms, which, however, confuses historiography, because a tendency to retroproject modern contemporary terms onto the source material 'both distorts the history, for language is often a key to meaning, and assumes that we are talking about "the same thing" throughout history, which is far from certain'; furthermore, glossing over those words now deemed politically incorrect achieves nothing other than distortion of the historical record and presentation of 'a false trans-historical conceptual reality'.[6]

Following these useful methodological annotations, I also have chosen to leave terms in the original language(s), so as to encourage readers to observe the fluidity, malleability and subtlety of language; for the same reason McDonagh preferred 'idiocy' as a term because it has methodological utility in its ambiguity. The word 'idiot' as used in late antique and early medieval Latin just meant ignorant person, someone who does not have much knowledge, in the sense that 'country yokel' is used in modern English; *idiota* in medieval Latin generally meant someone who was ignorant of Latin letters. It is specifically in later medieval legal parlance that the idiot comes to mean a person with mental deficiencies. The chapter will therefore conclude with an overview of the semantic changes pertaining to 'idiot'.

Semitic languages

Since medieval concepts were much influenced by biblical and Graeco-Roman literature, it is appropriate to start with ID as presented in such texts. Lexemes for 'idiot' and 'fool' are found in many languages, such as in Akkadian (*lillu*) and Hebrew (*kesîl, petî, sotê*). In the Hebrew Old Testament the lexeme *petî* is mentioned approximately twenty times, and can convey a range of meanings, which in the Greek Septuaginta are translated with three different words: *aphron* meaning a deficit of intelligence, *akakos* meaning innocence and harmlessness [literally *a-*, 'not' + *kakos*, 'bad'] and *nepios* meaning childishness.[7] In the ancient Near East disability was connected with socio-economic states, so that 'words for physical disabilities such as *akû* and mental disabilities such as *lillu* can be used in cuneiform texts as synonyms for 'poor,' suggesting a close association between disability and impoverishment'.[8] Although lameness, blindness, missing limbs and other physical disabilities are classed as 'defects' (*mûmîm*) in the biblical context, neither deafness, muteness nor mental disability is classified as 'defect'. Therefore not all conditions modern Western society regards as disabilities were treated as such, with 'defects' being negatively constructed physical characteristics, while deafness, muteness and mental disability were excluded from the category 'defect'.[9] Note the emphasis on physical condition as defect, and further note that (most) mental disabilities have no physical, visible markers – Down syndrome being the obvious exception to ratify the rule. The problem with this analysis is that, as so often, the modern historian conflates mental disability with mental illness, so that the term 'mental disability' might more accurately be rendered 'psychiatric disorder which functionally renders the affected person disabled'. Mental disability is thus expanded from the narrower meaning of a congenital cognitive or intellectual disability (which is how I use the term) to a wider meaning of transient non-physical, non-sensory disability. With the actual lexemes scholars are on firmer ground. Olyan lists these as *kesîl, sakal, petî* and *'ewîl*, which are frequently found in biblical texts, and may be translated as 'fool' or 'simple-minded' person, together with the abstract nouns *kislah/kesîlût, sekel/siklût, petî/petayyût* and *'iwwelet*, which are usually rendered 'foolishness' or 'simplicity' and are share the same roots. The question remains, however, if such terms referred to persons with ID, since although many texts associated 'foolishness' with 'a lack of knowledge, understanding, discipline, prudence, and good judgment', the definitions are too vague.[10] This kind of foolishness, of making the wrong choices, is the metaphorical foolishness of people who could (and should) know better, therefore such biblical passages cover a wide range of behaviours and not just mental disability. As later in the medieval period, the accusation of foolishness is employed as a criticism for social or political purposes, used for people who have the ability to acquire knowledge and act prudently but who choose not to. However, some biblical passages may point more in the direction of mild forms of ID, such as the description of the 'simple minded' (*petî*) believing everything they are told or being unable to perform basic tasks (e.g. Proverbs 14:15; 22:3). 'Thus, terms typically translated "fool" or "simple minded" *might* sometimes refer to persons with mild forms of mental retardation, although this remains unclear.'[11] In Jewish culture, the Mishnah, compiled in its present form by the second century AD, groups three kinds of people among those who cannot fulfil the commandments, these being deaf-mutes, the mentally incompetent (*sotê*) and minors; these three groups are treated as a triple entity and are named over twenty times in the Mishnah, and in the Talmud even more frequently.[12]

In rabbinical literature too the distinctions between a person with mental disabilities, e.g. retardation, and a person with a mental illness, e.g. schizophrenia, are not made. The category *shoteh* does not just cover people with ID but also those who are merely foolish or morally misguided.[13] It appears that the Hebrew word *shoteh* is as problematic as the English words 'fool' or 'idiot':

'from the central meaning of the word *shoteh* – that is, one who has no *da'at* – one might find radiating out other meanings, as the word is applied to the mentally disabled, the mentally ill, an idolater (and, by extension, an ingrate), one who practices the sages' system poorly, and one who can't be interrogated'.[14] In simplified terms, *da'at* means knowledge, but possesses a further cluster of meanings related to cognitive ability, moral skills and purposeful action. The word *shoteh* may have a primary meaning, on top of which are loaded other conceptual categories. 'The prototype of the category *shoteh* is a person who is profoundly mentally ill, for example, schizophrenic, or a person who is mentally disabled, for example, of extremely low intelligence. Such persons are stigmatized, that is, discredited.'[15]

In the Bible, words for foolishness or idiocy become a trilingual confusion, if one takes the Hebrew together with Latin and English translations. For instance, take the famous Psalm 14[13]:1: 'The fool [*nabal*] hath said in his heart, there is no God' (*Dixit insipiens in corde suo non est Deus*). The Hebrew word *nabal* is rendered in the Vulgate as *insipiens*, which in the English of the King James version becomes 'fool'. Psalm 53[52]:1 repeats the same verse, but here the Vulgate reads *stultus* for the fool. So *insipiens* and *stultus* appear to be used interchangeably in Latin, while the Hebrew introduces yet a third term, *nabal*, for fool next to the more common *kesîl* and *petî*. *Petî* might correlate to 'simple-minded',[16] as in Psalm 116[114]:6: 'The Lord preserveth the simple [*petî*]', while Proverbs 17:21 employs both *kesîl* and *nabal*: 'He that begetteth a fool [*kesîl*] doeth it to his sorrow: And the father of a fool [*nabal*] hath no joy.' Kellenberger draws upon the Hebrew text, and points out that these two forms of 'fool' are differentiated: *kesîl* appears to mean the simpleton, the harmless innocent, while *nabal* refers to somebody more sinister, knowing what they are doing, so that the atheist, God-denying fool of Psalm 14 is a *nabal*.[17] That the words *kesîl* and *petî* are more likely to mean someone simple minded, that is, someone deemed to be intellectually disabled, might be seen in a further Old Testament passage. Ezekiel 45:20 concerns the need to purify the temple on the seventh day of the month 'for every one that erreth, and for him that is simple' (*pro unoquoque qui ignoravit et errore deceptus est*), i.e. if people either unwittingly and mistakenly polluted the temple, or were 'simple' (*petî* in the original Hebrew, i.e. mentally disabled), purification is necessary.[18] This might mean that people with ID may have been servants of the temple performing simple tasks (quasi unskilled workers), and because of the risk that they may unwittingly and by misadventure, clumsiness or such like pollute the sacred space, there is a requirement to purify the temple annually as a prophylactic measure. In any case, this passage refers to two distinct categories of potential pollutants: firstly, people of so-called 'normal' intelligence who may inadvertently make a mistake and thereby pollute the sacred, and secondly, those who are deemed 'simple'. Kellenberger's main argument with regard to Old Testament texts seems to be that people termed in Hebrew *petî* or *kesîl*, roughly meaning 'simple' (German *einfältig*), are characterised as ready to believe anything that is said to them unquestioningly, which can be both a negative (they are uncritical, thereby childishly trusting and foolish) and a positive (they believe God without scepticism).[19]

Staying with the Semitic language family for a moment, a brief excursion into Arabic brings us into the medieval period. It seems that medieval Islam had similar notions of the 'theological fool' as found in Psalms 13 and 52, as someone who ignores if not denies God. From a collection of characters called 'wise fools' by al-Naysâbûri (d. 1016), entitled *Kitâb 'Uqalâ' al-majânîn*, Dols listed a number of words used in Arabic to connote 'folly' in the widest sense, which are worth quoting here, since they demonstrate that medieval Islamic thought, like its Christian counterpart, had a range of differential terms for conditions that can loosely be equated with ID today: '*Ahmaq* was an imbecile or one who was dumb; *ma'tûh* was someone who was born *majnûn*; *akhrâq* was a person who was stupid or unable to manage his own affairs; *mâ'iq* was a fool; and *raqî'* was a fool who was illogical like the *balîd*, who was idiotic or stupid.'[20] The writings of six Sunni scholars in Cairo, Damascus and Mecca, whose work produced texts about so called 'blights' (*'âhât*) – 'a category that included individuals who were cognitively and physically different, disabled and ill'[21] – provides further examples. The Arabic term can refer to a 'blight' or 'damage' to crops, trees, animals as well as humans and encompasses not just 'disability' in the modern sense but, more widely, notions of aesthetic differences and character defects.[22]

Indo-European comparisons

Before we look at Greek, Latin and the medieval vernaculars, a comparative philological examination of linguistic evidence for the Indo-European language family provides suitable etymologies and terminologies. This sheds some light on the antiquity of semantic concepts. For instance, Latin *mens* 'mind' is derived from an Indo-European root *menos* 'power, craft, ability, skill', and Old English *dol* 'silly', related to Welsh *dwl* 'stupid', stems from the root-word *dhulos* 'dull, dim, numbstruck'. The concept of rationality, from Latin *ratio*, as in the faculty of reason, does not just exist since Aristotle allegedly claimed man was a rational animal, but goes back to an Indo-European root *rǝtos* (*râtos*) 'reasoning, calculation'.[23] If *ratis* may be treated as a reconstructed Proto-Indo-European word for reason, then this word is some six thousand years old – reasoning is certainly not just a modern preoccupation. Comparing living languages, or at least their nearest literary relatives, shows interesting similarities. A dictionary of synonyms in the main Indo-European languages provides too many entries for words relating to 'foolish' or 'stupid' to list in detail here, but notably among many others are these expressions: Greek *aphrôn, môros, blax, anoêtos, êlithios*; Latin *stultus, fatuus, stolidus*; Old English *dysig, stunt, dol, dwaes, sot*; Old High German *tumb, tol, tulisc, tusîc, gimeit*. 'Some of the words are merely etymological opposites ... of words for "wise", without necessarily being so mild as N[ew] E[nglish] *unwise*. The majority are based upon diverse notions, e.g. "soft, weak, stricken, stunned, dumb, wandering, confused", with specialized application to the mind.'[24] What the sheer number of words in many different languages does indicate, however, is that in all of these languages the notion of idiocy has been around for a considerable time, i.e. since the common ancestor of a given language family, and therefore it is cross-cultural. The diversity of notions displays on the one hand the verbal richness in these languages, and on the other hand the problems of delineating or categorising a phenomenon in the days before the advent of clinical psychiatry.

Ancient Greek

In ancient Greek there were two competing terms for 'fool': *salos* and *moros*. The word *salos* is usually translated as 'fool', but the word is of uncertain origin. The standard lexicon translates *salos* as an adjective meaning 'silly, imbecile'.[25] Discussing this term, Krueger pointed out that it is not to be confused with the similar Greek word *salos*, 'tossed' or 'agitated'.[26] And furthermore the word is unlikely to be a technical term referring to holy folly in hagiography, 'but rather it may have a slang quality to it, and abusive connotations',[27] as in a late fifth-century letter from Oxyrhynchus where someone is referred to as 'that imbecile' (*tou salou*).[28] A person described as *salos* should therefore not be equated with the holy fool often encountered in Byzantine texts. This contradicts what Dols had surmised concerning holy folly: '*Salos* became the usual designation in Greek for the "fool for Christ's sake" ... The New Testament term *moros* was not used.'[29] Dols had, however, relied on older literature, and was mainly concerned with Islamic concepts of madness, so that it is not surprising that he did not perform such a close reading of the hagiography as Krueger has. Remnants of the *salos*-concept can be found in the modern Russian word *blazhennyi*, which on the one hand means a form of sanctity, but on the other hand 'implies a kind of gentle imbecility, a feeble-minded person with a silly smile on his face (a "beatific" smile, as one might say), utterly unable to engage with the world.'[30]

When we look at the New Testament, the Vulgate translation into Latin, here from the Greek, introduces a new term for 'fool' besides *stultus* or *insipiens*: *moria*, a Latin concoction derived from the Greek. In 1 Cor. 1:18, 'For the preaching of the cross is to them that perish foolishness' (*verbum enim crucis pereuntibus quidem stultitia est*), some versions use the word *moria*, not *stultitia*.[31] To summarise, biblical Latin terminology includes *stultus* in many places for translations of the Old Testament, *fatuus* only in Proverbs (12:16; 13:16; 14:24; 15:2) and *insipiens* (as the inverse of *sapiens*) mainly in the Old Testament (Psalms, Proverbs, Ecclesiastes) and only twice in the New Testament (Luke 6:11 and 2 Peter 2:16).[32] Unlike *salos*, the noun *môros*, verb *môrainô*, is common in classical Greek and 'can be used, in a physiological context, of the slackness and fatigue of nerves', although it is most commonly used for psychological meaning, as for real insanity with confused understanding.[33]

Latin

Turning now to Romance and Germanic languages (i.e. Latin, French, English and German), a large number of lexemes for mental illness, disability and incapacity may be found, stretching from classical via medieval Latin and the vernaculars to modern usage. The following presents an overview of words for abnormal mental states. One of the rarer Latin words is *hebes*, which has the general meanings 'having a dull edge or point, blunt, dim, weak', but also dull of the senses; and of persons 'lacking in energy, sluggish, inert, dull-witted, stupid, dense, lacking (human) intelligence'.[34] This is not a common descriptor for mental states in medieval usage, but can be found particularly in writers who want to show off their knowledge of Latin vocabulary. Similarly, the more precisely used classical Latin term *morio* appears not to find its way into medieval texts, unless they are simply copies and transmissions of classical or late antique Latin (such as the writings of Augustine), this despite the fact that it is where the modern word 'moron', as one variant of mental retardation, comes from. There is an ambiguous term in *amentia*, which predominantly means 'mad, insane, senseless, demented'; but also sometimes folly. In pathology, *amentia* tends to refer to feeble-mindedness, either congenital or resulting from damage to the brain in early childhood.[35] Phrases such as *non compos mentis* or *non intellectum* are singularly unhelpful for ID, since they just generally mean not having full possession of mental faculties or being without understanding. The lack of perception they allude to could equally apply to the temporarily mentally ill as to the permanently intellectually disabled. The three already encountered

Latin terms *fatuus, insipiens* and *stultus*, which all commonly continue to be used in medieval texts, approximate more closely to meanings of ID. All three terms may mean in modern usage 'foolish, stupid, idiotic, imbecility' and 'silliness'. In a late fifteenth-century Latin–English dictionary, synonyms for *fonde* include among madness-types the idiocy-types *stultus, fatuus, stolidus, ineptus, insensis, simplex*.[36] The anglicised *insipience*, as lack of wisdom or foolishness, first appears in Middle English via Old French around 1422 in Hoccleve's *Tale of Jonathas*.[37] In patristic and medieval philosophical discussions there may be a conceptual difference between *stultus* and *insipiens*. The etymology of *in-sipiens*, implying the contrasting lack of, is obviously derived from *sapiens*, while *stultus* is connected with *stolidus* 'dull, obtuse'. 'The question whether there is a difference arose for Salvian from the Vulgate Psalm-text which says that both will perish: *simul insipiens et stultus peribunt* (Psalm 48.10). It could be argued that there is no difference. Both are damned.'[38]

No discussion of linguistics can avoid the *Etymologies* of Isidore of Seville (c. 560–636), which became one of the most influential books of the Middle Ages. Definitions of words and phrases are given in the vocabulary section (*De vocabulis*): The opposite of the wise (*sapiens*) person, for Isidore derived from taste (*sapor*), is the 'fool (*insipiens*), because he is without taste, and has no discretion or sense'.[39]

> A fool (*fatuus*) is thought to be so called because he understands neither what he says (*fari*, 3rd person *fatur*) himself nor what others say. Some think that the term 'fool' derives originally from admirers of Fatua, the prophesying wife of Faunus, and that they were first called *fatuus* because they were immoderately stupefied by her prophecies, to the point of madness.[40]
> (Fatuus ideo existimatur dictus, quia neque quod fatur ipse, neque quod alii dicunt intellegit. Fatuos origine duci quidam putant a miratoribus Fatuae, Fauni uxoris fatidicae, eosque primum fatuos appellatos, quod praeter modum obstupefacti sunt vaticiniis illius usque ad amentiam.)

For Isidore, idiot still has a meaning closer to the Greek origins of the term: 'Naive (*idiota*), "an inexperienced person"; the word is Greek (cf. *idiôtês*, "private person, ordinary person").' (*Idiota, inperitus, Graecum est.*)[41]

> Stolid (*stultus*), rather dull in spirit, as a certain writer says (Afranius, fragment 416): 'I consider myself to be stolid (*stultus*); I don't think myself a fool,' that is, with dulled wits, but not with none at all. A stolid person is one who in his stupor (*stupor*) is not moved by injustice, for he endures and does not avenge cruelty, and is not moved to grief by any dishonor. 247. Sluggish (*segnis*), that is, 'without fire' (*sine igni*), lacking native wit – for *se-* means 'without' (*sine*), as *sedulus, sine dolo*. ... 248. Stupefied (*stupidus*), 'rather often astounded (*stupere*)'.

(Stultus, hebetior corde, sicut quidam ait (Afran. 416): Ego me esse stultum existimo: fatuum esse non opino, id est obtunsis quidem sensibus, non tamen nullis. Stultus est qui per stuporem non movetur iniuria; saevitiam enim perfert nec ultus est, nec ulla ignominia commovetur dolore. 247 Segnis, id est sine igni, ingenio carens. 'Se' autem sine significat, ut sedulus sine dolo. ... 248 Stupidus, saepius stupens.)[42]

And contrary to the preconceptions of many modern writers on the history of psychology, medieval writers did distinguish quite clearly between mental illness and mental disability. Madness is yet again something different from folly in medieval philosophy: '*Dementia* goes beyond the foolishness of *stultitia*. *Dementia* is extreme. It is rashness. It is losing your mind: *si enim mentes non dementia pereretis*, says Augustine.'[43] It is just speculation on my part, but somewhere along the linguistic line in the Middle Ages a semantic difference between *stultus* and *fatuus* began, with *stultus* as meaning stupidity also implying philosophical stupidity, that is, doing something stupid despite having the capacity not to do so, as opposed to the natural fool, the *fatuus*, who is foolish because he cannot help himself. This difference will be explored more fully in Chapter 4 on philosophy. Suffice it to draw attention here to the distinction between natural and moral disability, the *fatuus* and the *stultus* respectively, which almost foreshadows the distinction between 'cannots' and 'will nots' in the terminology of modern 'education policy for pupils with emotional and behavioural difficulties'.[44]

Just in case the reader thinks this neat differentiation of *fatuus* from *stultus* points towards common linguistic ground with modern terminology, a note of caution is in order concerning seemingly identical words. The cautionary tale that the same word (phonologically) does not historically carry the same meaning (semantically), that a modern idiot is not the same as a medieval idiot, may also be found in the example of the 'imbecile'. In a miracle collection of the 1160s from southern Italy, a man, Teutonicus, was cured of *imbecillitatis clauditate* by the powers of the saints.[45] This does not mean he was cured of the lameness of intellectual weakness, as the association with modern 'imbecility' would suggest, but of the weakness of lameness. The Latin *imbecillitas*, meaning 'weakness, infirmity, feebleness, debility, impotence or incapacity', from which derives the modern English 'imbecile', is another one of the *idiot*-words, in that the modern meaning of intellectually disabled is misleading for medieval or classical texts. Therefore one should not equate the modern meaning of 'imbecile' as a mentally deficient person with Latin *imbecillitas*. A similar common misreading occurs with a German word, *gebrechen*. In modern German this is taken to mean to an illness, spuriously derived from the root-word for 'broken', so *ge* + *brechen* refers to something that has been broken. But as von Bernuth has commented with regard to a phrase in Konrad of Megenberg's *Buch der Natur* (c. 1350), *geprechen habent an der sêl werken* (having *gebrechen* in the workings of the soul), *gebrechen* in Middle High German 'does not refer to illness or malady but to need or want'.[46] Therefore one may go even further and equate *gebrechen* with Latin *impotens* as used in the medieval sense of powerlessness, hence dis-ability in a social, economic or political and not just somatic sense.

Old and Middle English

And so finally we can turn to English lexemes concerning ID. Old English has a particularly rich vocabulary for mental deficiency: *dwâês* 'dull, foolish, stupid'; *dwâêsian* 'to become stupid'; *dwâêslic* 'foolish'; *dwâêsnes* 'stupidity, foolish-ness'; *unwita* 'witless person, ignoramus'; *unmaga* 'needy person, dependent, orphan'; *ungerâêde* 'foolish'; *ungerâd* 'ignorant, foolish, unskilled, unfit'.[47] Lacking wisdom or sense, not guided by reason, being unreasonable, foolish or heedless can be expressed by further compounds of *wit*, such as *witléas*, also *gewitléas*. As the Latin *insipiens* is the 'not-sapiens', the Anglo-Saxon 'witless' person is the mentally deficient person who has no 'wit', a word originally meaning knowledge, wisdom. To these terms one may add *ungemynd* 'dement-edness' (literally 'no-mind') and *dysgung* 'foolishness.[48] In Old Irish someone is described 'as *óinmit* (modern Irish, *óinmhid*), which has been etymologized as **onment*, "lamb-witted".'[49] This is interesting, since *onment* appears similar to *amens/tis*, the Latin for lacking mind, and also to *unmagan*, the Old English for not being able to, which in modern German survives as *unmögen*. There is also *ungerâd*, Old English for 'ignorant, foolish', derived from the person who has no *rad*, no counsel – the famous cognomen of King Æthelred, 'the Unready', refers not to his lack of timing but his lack of wise counsel.

A 'simple' person is one, in the definition of the *Oxford English Dictionary* [*OED*], who in medieval usage (derived from Old French *simple*, then in English from the 1340s onward) is 'deficient in knowledge or learning; char-acterized by a certain lack of acuteness or quick apprehension', but only from 1604 is also defined as 'lacking in ordinary sense or intelligence; more or less foolish, silly, or stupid; also, mentally deficient, half-witted'.[50] The medieval term therefore retains some ambiguity in its generalising concept of the simple person as the down-to-earth, honestly behaving, uneducated person, but does not explicitly refer to a person with ID. With 'silly' we have another word, like imbecile or idiot, which changes meaning over time. Silly, from an older form *seely*, takes on the meaning of weak or deficient in intellect, feeble minded, imbecile or foolish only in the sixteenth century. The Middle English *seely* [*sele*] originally meant 'blessed, touched or favoured' by God, also 'innocent, harmless or helpless', which has transmuted to the modern English meaning of 'silly' and has become a word applied to the mentally disturbed – one may think of the modern usage of 'touched' when describing someone's odd behaviour.[51] It derived from Old English *sælig*, meaning 'happy, fortunate'.[52] By way of comparison, modern German, which has the same roots for *selig* (meaning blessed) knows only that sense of the word and makes no connection with foolishness. In another purely speculative mode I wonder whether the common ancestor of both Old English and Old High German, what historical linguists calls proto-Germanic, could be related to the Greek term *salos*, which as we have seen above was used to denote a fool, and possibly the 'holy fool'. That kind of 'folly' is exactly of the kind described by *selig*, especially the aspect of being touched by God. Since one of the earliest Greek hagiographies of a 'holy fool' dates from the 420s, it is not impossible that the word *salos* was taken to England by monks or clerics who may have come across the Greek idea of holy folly, and that linguistic vowel-shift changed *salos* to *sælig*.[53]

With the fool, we are on better-attested ground, at least linguistically if not necessarily semantically. Classical Latin had *follem*, *follis*, literally 'bellows', which in late popular Latin was employed in the sense of 'windbag', empty-headed person, hence fool. Both Middle English (*fōl*) and Old French (*fol*) used the word for one

> deficient in judgement or sense, one who acts or behaves stupidly, a silly person, a simpleton. (In Biblical use applied to vicious or impious persons.) The word has in modern English a much stronger sense than it had at an earlier period; it has now an implication of insulting contempt which does not in the same degree belong to any of its synonyms, or to the derivative *foolish*. Cf. French *sot*.[54]

Then there is the use of 'fool' as job description for one 'who professionally counterfeits folly for the entertainment of others, a jester, clown'.[55] Lastly, with regard to meanings related to ID, the *OED* cites a usage of 'fool' stemming from the 1540s as one 'who is deficient in, or destitute of reason or intellect; a weak-minded or idiotic person'.[56] Referring to a natural fool, or born fool, which implies a born idiot in modern usage, is, according to the *OED*, now rare and exclusively a term of abuse. How far social conditions and cultural concepts influence and define linguistic meanings is evidenced by the following interventionist statement which the normally sedate and laconic *OED* manages to interject: 'The "fool" in great households was often actually a harmless "lunatic" or a person of weak intellect, so that this sense and [the sense of ID] are often hard to distinguish.'[57] This is a topic that will be discussed further, and put to the test, in Chapter 6 on fools as entertainers.

French

The etymology of 'fool' takes us from English to French lexemes. In Anglo-Norman French the word *fol* related both to fools and madmen.[58] But according to a French study, in the fifteenth century the French *fol* was still equivalent in meaning to Latin *stultus*, and could in no way be construed as the semantic equivalent of insane or mad.[59] Another term approximating 'fool', the word *sot*, is equally problematic. The Old French *sot* is of unknown origin, but the medieval Latin *sottus* is recorded from about 800, which therefore seems to be the ancestor also of late Old English *sott*, Middle Dutch *sot* (*sod*), *zot* (*zod*; Dutch *zot*), Middle Low German and Low German *sot, sott*, and Middle High German *sot*.[60] In all these languages it meant a foolish or stupid person, a fool, blockhead, dolt. Linguistic ambiguity is present in the story of the expulsion from a French town in 1388 of a fool masquerading as a madman, 'un sot contrefaisant le dervé'. Welsford observed that while *sot* meant fool, *dervé* meant madman 'and the only way of interpreting this singular sentence seems to be to suppose that the *sot* was a more or less professional fool, who made himself objectionable by assuming the more violent form of imbecility'.[61] But it also shows the linguistic differentiation between mental disability (whether real or feigned) and mental illness that was already made in the later fourteenth century. In addition to and alongside 'idiot', the term 'simple' was also used in Old French, to suggest a negative, even dangerous, ignorance or stupidity, e.g. in Gautier de Coincy's *Miracles de la sainte Vierge* both terms were used as description (significantly given by the devil!) of a simple peasant, an idiot (*Un vilain simple, un ydïote*), and Henri de Mondeville, *Chirurgie*, complained 'there are some of these, like idiots, simple and ignorant ..., saying that they have the work of surgery' (*il est aucuns d'iceus, aussi comme ydiotes, simples et ignorans ..., disans que il ont l'oeuvre de cyrurgie*).[62] The latter quote still reflects the notion of the idiot as a layman, an unlearned person. Compared to other terms used to describe mental disturbance, terms for 'idiot' or 'simpleton' appear seldom in French letters of remission that Pfau has studied, a statistic also borne out by the English legal documents that Turner has examined. In Pfau's sample of 145 remission letters, only seven instances of 'idiot' are found. One letter in 1375 refers to someone as 'feeble-headed' (*affoible de teste*).[63] Another letter of 1405 describes someone as stunned in the head as well as an idiot, without sense or memory and as insensible (*estonna la teste, ydiot, perdi son sens et sa memoire* and *insensible*).[64]

German

We have already touched on some German etymologies in connection with Old English, but here are some of the main lexemes for what might today be described as ID. *Toll* 'mad, frantic' is one of those ambiguous words, as it stems from West Germanic **dula*, which in turn derived from Germanic **dwel-a*, 'to be confused', and hence carried a general meaning of mental deviation, which may just imply insanity but may also cover ID.[65] *Tor (Dor)* appears to be the equivalent of 'fool'. In its meaning of a mentally deficient person it is attested since the thirteenth century as Middle High German *tôr(e)*, derived from the Germanic **dauz*, via Old High German *tusîg* (related to Old English *dysig*) which survives in the modern German adjective *töricht* 'foolish, silly, unwise'. The *tor* is related to a verbal root *dösig* 'to be confused, benighted', which in turn is further related to *toll* 'mad', *taub* 'deaf, stunned' and *Dunst* 'haze, mist'.[66] Thus German *taub* from the Germanic **dauba* 'without hearing' equates to 'deaf', via the meaning of being senseless, out of one's wits, literally 'to be befogged [befuddled], confused', and *t(h)oub/taub* can also lead to the modern term *tobsüchtig* 'violently insane'. Since their Old High German usage, the words *tump* and *tumpheit* have retained meanings of a religiously influenced connotation with the opposite of wisdom, i.e. the Fool of the Psalms, with a wide range of associations from social inexperience and child-ishness to profound moral and ethical failings. Of course, *tump* also relates to a physical, rather than psychiatric, deficit, namely speech impairment, hence its relationship with the English word 'dumb'.[67] In similar fashion, the Middle High German *tôre*, according to a few sources of the early twelfth century, such as *St Trudperter Hohenlied*, originally connotes the deaf person, so that the consequences of a physical defect are seen to have an effect on psychological disposition as well. But, like *tump* and the other lexemes of senselessness dis-cussed so far, *tôre* has a spectrum of meanings rather than a single one, so that both the pathologically mad person and the one feigning madness are called *tôr*.[68] The loss of a sensory perception – deafness – and lack of mental powers are thus linguistically linked. Similarly, the madman was also named after the breakdown of the communicative medium between him and our world: the senses. Therefore the madman is the *insensatus*, the one without sense. His directional guidance is missing: his rationality has been taken away. That is why he is called *insipiens*: he has become like the fool who does not know what he is doing nor what he is saying, he is the outstanding *idiotus*. Further differen-tiation is between the *stolidus* and the *fatuus*: as *stolidus* his behaviour is brutal, while as *fatuus* he is acting shamelessly.[69]

Thus in courtly literature the *tôr* is the one naturally lacking human wit, a fool, madman, idiot, crazy person, whom one recognises by his inability to speak, also by his special clothes which indicate his position outside of normal society.[70] Another word for the court fool, *Geck*, is attested only from the fourteenth century on, so that it shares the same ambiguity as English 'fool' as being both the person with congenital ID and the courtly entertainer.[71]

Narr is the most common medieval German word for a fool, attested in eighth-century Old High German *narro*. But the word occurs only in German, or is borrowed from German, with an unknown origin.[72] The etymology of the word *Narr* is not sufficiently clear. Old High German *narro* can be found in collections of glossae dated between the eighth and eleventh centuries and is intended to render the Latin terms *brutus*, *narvus*, *stultus* and *murio*. In Middle High German, however, *narre* and *nerrischeit* are of little significance, occurring mainly as synonyms for *tôre* or in connection with the office and appearance of the court fool.[73] While *tôre* was imbued ever more during the late Middle Ages with ethical and religious concepts, *narre* did not experience such a semantic shift. Where it is not clearly synonymous with *tôr* or used for varieties of insanity, *narr* is hardly more than a coarse insult. From the fifteenth century onwards *narr* becomes more widely spread.[74]

Associated with terms for states of madness, derived via Isidore of Seville's *Etymologies*, in Old High German are a group of terms surrounding a state of not knowing (*unuuizzi*, *unuuistuom*), used by authors such as Otfried and Notker. Middle High German also used a range of lexemes derived from *un-sin* (without sense) which can, however, encompass the full range (idiocy, madness, possession, raging etc.) of mental afflictions. Further adjectives denoting states of intellectual deficiency, the absence of rationality and of intellectual faculties were *wan-witze* and *wan-witzic*.[75] In Old and Middle High German *wan-* is a prefix expressing lack of something, an emptiness, so that Old High German *wanawizzi* and Middle High German *wanwitze* mean a person without sense – the English *wit* is related. Etymologically, these words are the precursors to modern German *Wahnsinn* (madness, insanity, mental illness), but here the first syllable *Wahn*, meaning 'empty, insensible, deficient', hence delusion, is not semantically related, only homonymically similar.[76] *Wahnsinn* is *wahn* + *sinn*, so 'empty' + 'sense', therefore no sense, nonsense; similarly *unsinnigkeit/nit sinnig* equals senselessness, a word formation similar to the Latin *amentia* from *ā* away from + *ment-em* mind.

'Idiot': a case study

Last but not least, what about that most commonly used modern word, 'idiot'? Kanner had already sketched out the idiot's trajectory, commenting on the difficulty of pinning down the precise moment in time when 'idiot' acquired the present, modern sense, and had simply noted the derivations from and changes in meaning, starting with the 'private person' in Greek, via the concept of 'the common man', conceptually enhanced to denote 'the unsophisticated layman without professional knowledge', followed by the allusion to 'an ignorant, ill-informed individual'. 'Ultimately, quite a bit later than in the writings of the ancient Greeks, it was given the specific connotation of a mental defective.'[77] As always, the OED may provide a good starting-point. The English idiot found his way into the language via Old French and Anglo-Norman, ultimately derived from the ancient Greek *idiôtês* via classical Latin *idiôta*. The OED summarises the etymological development and gives abbreviated semantic and historical literary context:

> uneducated, ignorant person (1164), stupid person, mentally deficient person (c1374), (adjective) ignorant, uneducated (c1224), foolish, stupid, incapable of reasoning (c1300) [...] ordinary person, layman, amateur, private individual, in post-classical Latin also recent convert (Vulgate), ignorant, uneducated person (early 3rd cent. in Tertullian), professional fool or jester (12th cent. in a British source), stupid person, mentally deficient person (from 13th cent. in British sources), private person, person without professional knowledge, layman, ignorant, ill-informed person[78]

The modern meaning of idiot is used chiefly in legal and psychiatric practice and is defined by the OED thus:

> A person so profoundly disabled in mental function or intellect as to be incapable of ordinary acts of reasoning or rational conduct; *spec.* a person permanently so affected, as distinguished from one with a temporary severe mental illness. [...] By the older legal authorities in England an idiot was defined as a person congenitally deficient in reasoning powers, and this remained for a long time the common implication of the term.[79]

But where it gets interesting is at the semantic interstices, where the idiot shifts from one meaning to another. Tertullian (c. 160–c. 225) had used 'idiot' to describe someone as simple, rude, impolite and idiotic.[80] This still reflects the meaning of idiot as 'common man'. Similarly Bede (673–735) used *idiotas* to mean unlearned people.[81] But in the ninth century there is the first hint that the idiot might be someone with mental deviation, when Ermoald (Ermold the Black/Ermoldus Nigellus, active 824–30) equates the *idiota* with the person who is without sense (*demens*).[82] A specifically medieval meaning of *idiotae* is the technical term for new monks, novices or, in the case of the Cistercians, the lay brothers better known as *conversi*, which appears in the eleventh century, but does not equate the idiot with the mentally disabled, only with the uneducated, illiterate person.[83] However, it is around this time that the semantics of idiocy start gathering momentum. Archdeacon Gautier de Thérouanne (Gualterus Tarvanensis, 1090–1132) uses *insipiens, idiota* and *stultus* in the same context, all describing feigned behaviour.[84] In an anonymous twelfth-century *Life* of St Norbert, a catalogue of qualities is given, again relating to behaviour, here of the saint: 'he was illustrious among nobles, less than cultured among the ignoble, eloquent among the educated and foolish [*fatuus*] among the unlearned [*idiotas*]'.[85] A similar catalogue, but this time composed of opposites, is given in the religious autobiography of the convert Hermann the Jew (Hermannus Judaeus, c. 1108–c. 1181), who contrasted the wise with *idiotae*, the strong with the weak, the noble with the ignoble.[86] As yet this is not explicitly linking the *idiota* with what might equate to modern concepts of ID, but is it associating *idiotae* with modes of behaviour described by the more precise and well-known Latin terms (*fatuus, stultus*). With Arnold of Bonneval (Ernaldus Bonaevallis, d. 1156) the 'idiot' is shifted even more in the direction of mental deficiency, when he writes about those like idiots and the dim-witted (*idiotae et hebetes*) being struck by the [divine] word.[87] The twelfth century has been given the accolade of a renaissance, like a fair number of epochs before and after – to name but the Carolingian, Ottonian, Humanist renaissances – a title which generally denotes a revival of learning and intellectual culture. It may then come as no surprise that by the end of the twelfth century the 'idiot' was being analysed quasi-scientifically. Peter Comestor (d. 1178) commented on Acts 4:13 ('Now when they saw the boldness of Peter and John, and perceived that they were unlearned and ignorant men [*sine litteris et idiotae*], they marvelled')[88] by expounding on the alternative etymology of the word *idiota*. This other meaning Peter Comestor ascribed, whether correctly or falsely does not matter for the present argument, to Isidore of Seville, whose *Etymologies* he paraphrased;[89] here the *idiota* is alleged to be divided from the ears, which is to say the idiot, as if divided from understanding, is certainly the same as the fool (*fatuus*).[90] The association of mental disability with not having ears to hear, hence being deaf, hence not understanding conceptually, that was already found in the discussion of Germanic lexemes relating to *taub* is encountered here again. Peter Comestor does continue by citing the more common medieval meaning of 'idiot' as someone whose way of speaking defines them, who knows only one language, but by emphasising the alternative etymology Peter enables the notion of 'idiot' as an intellectually deficient person to gain hold. And around the same time Alan of Lille (Alanus de Insulis, c. 1116–1202) also described the *idiota* as the simple or foolish person (*simplex vel fatuus*), with the word again believed to be derived from being divided from one's ears.[91] By the early thirteenth century the explicit usage of *idiota* as intellectually less able, even disabled, appears to have found a firm place. One example stems from about 1220, in a work on synonyms by John of Garland. Here the established Latin terms *fatuus, insipiens* and *stultus* – which all mean foolish, stupid, and equate to the modern usage of 'idiot' – are listed as synonymous with *idiota*.[92] These words waver between expressing concepts of being socially intellectually inferior (due to lack of learning) and hence changeable, to concepts of innate (and hence unchangeable) characteristics, since *fatuus* has since classical Roman times implied a person born with intellectual deficiencies.

To sum up the semantic problems discussed above, French *sot* and German *narr* are of unknown origins, 'idiots' start off as private people, silly persons are, perhaps, derived from the Greek *salos*, originally the happily blessed, and none of the spuriously more precise terms (the Latin *stultus, fatuus* or *insipiens*) can truly and categorically be equated with modern understandings and definitions of ID. Nevertheless, words are all the historian has to go by, and it is precisely the differences in meanings, the changes in nuance, that make the search for pre-modern narratives of ID such an interesting if at times frustrating enterprise. One may conclude with Edward Sapir's general observation that 'vocabulary is a very sensitive index of the culture of a people and changes in meaning, loss of old words, the creation and borrowing of new ones are all dependent on the history of culture itself'.[93]

Notes

1 Gershon Berkson, 'Mental Disabilities in Western Civilization from Ancient Rome to the Prerogativa Regis', *Mental Retardation*, 44:1 (2006), 28–40, at 28.

2 Christopher Goodey, *A History of Intelligence and 'Intellectual Disability': The Shaping of Psychology in Early Modern Europe* (Farnham: Ashgate, 2011), 4.

3 Tim Stainton and Patrick McDonagh, 'Chasing Shadows: The Historical Construction of Developmental Disability', *Journal on Developmental Disabilities/ Le journal sur les handicaps du développement*, 8:2 (2001), ix–xvi, at xvi.

4 Anne Digby, 'Contexts and Perspectives', in David Wright and Anne Digby (eds), *From Idiocy to Mental Deficiency: Historical Perspectives on People with Learning Disabilities* (London: Routledge, 1996), 3.

5 Patrick McDonagh, *Idiocy: A Cultural History* (Liverpool: Liverpool University Press, 2008), 13.

6 Stainton and McDonagh, 'Chasing Shadows', xi.

7 Edgar Kellenberger, *Der Schutz der Einfältigen. Menschen mit einer geistigen Behinderung in der Bibel und in weiteren Quellen* (Zurich: Theologischer Verlag Zürich, 2011), 35; etymology of *lillu* 19–21.

8 Saul M. Olyan, *Disability in the Hebrew Bible: Interpreting Mental and Physical Differences* (Cambridge: Cambridge University Press, 2008), 7.

9   Olyan, *Disability in the Hebrew Bible*, 19, 30, 48–53; and Judith Z. Abrams, *Judaism and Disability: Portrayals in Ancient Texts from the Tanach through the Bavli* (Washington, DC: Gallaudet University Press, 1998), 23.

10 Olyan, *Disability in the Hebrew Bible*, 64; examples of such actions at 1 Sam 13:13, Jer 4:22, Ps 85:9 [8], Prov 22:15, Isa 44:25, Prov 15:7, Eccl 7:4, 5, 6; 10:2, 12 and Prov 1:4.

11 Olyan, *Disability in the Hebrew Bible*, 65.

12 Kellenberger, *Schutz der Einfältigen*, 68n38.

13 Abrams, *Judaism and Disability*, 139–44, 212n1.

14 Abrams, *Judaism and Disability*, 126.

15 Abrams, *Judaism and Disability*, 139.

16 See Kellenberger, *Schutz der Einfältigen*, 35.

17 Kellenberger, *Schutz der Einfältigen*, 120.

18 Kellenberger, *Schutz der Einfältigen*, 36–7 and 117.

19 Kellenberger, *Schutz der Einfältigen*, 35–8.

20 Michael W. Dols (ed. Diana E. Immisch), *Majnûn: The Madman in Medieval Islamic Society* (Oxford: Clarendon Press, 1992), 352.

21 Kristina L. Richardson, *Difference and Disability in the Medieval Islamic World: Blighted Bodies* (Edinburgh: Edinburgh University Press, 2012), 5. However, this definition of cognitive difference is restricted to mental illness, where arguably cognitive functioning is impaired, but has not a single mention of cases we would now identify as persons with ID, despite other authors' references to fools in Islamic culture.

22 Richardson, *Difference and Disability in the Medieval Islamic World*, 36.

23 Stuart E. Mann, *An Indo-European Comparative Dictionary* (Hamburg: Helmut Buske, 1984), s.v. *menos, dhulos, rƏtos*.

24 Carl Darling Buck, *A Dictionary of Selected Synonyms in the Principal Indo-European Languages* (Chicago: University of Chicago Press, 1949), 1215.

25 Henry George Liddell and Robert Scott, *A Greek–English Lexicon*, revised and augmented throughout by Sir Henry Stuart Jones with the assistance of Roderick McKenzie (Oxford: Clarendon Press, 1940).

26 Derek Krueger, *Symeon the Holy Fool: Leontius's 'Life' and the Late Antique City* (Berkeley: University of California Press, 1996), 63–6.

27 Krueger, *Symeon the Holy Fool*, 64.

28 Oxyrhynchus papyrus *POxy* LVI 3865, line 57 [at http://perseus.mpiwg-berlin.mpg.de/ (accessed 10 February 2013)].

29 Dols, *Majnûn*, 372.

30 Sergey A. Ivanov, *Holy Fools in Byzantium and Beyond*, trans. Simon Franklin (Oxford: Oxford University Press, 2006), vi; at 31–8 also explaination of word *salos*, etymology deemed unclear.

31 See John Saward, *Perfect Fools: Folly for Christ's Sake in Catholic and Orthodox Spirituality* (Oxford: Oxford University Press, 1980), 5 for use of *moria* in the New Testament.

32 See the tabulation in Aleksandra Nicole Pfau, 'Madness in the Realm: Narratives of Mental Illness in Late Medieval France' (PhD diss., University of Michigan, 2008), 14.

33 Saward, *Perfect Fools*, 5.

34 P. G. W. Glare (ed.), *Oxford Latin Dictionary* (Oxford: Clarendon Press, 1992), s.v. *hebes*.

35 *Oxford English Dictionary* [hereafter *OED*] s.v. *amentia*.

36 Sidney J. H. Herrtage (ed.), *Catholicon Anglicum*, Early English Text Society, os 75 (London, 1881), 137.

37 *OED* s.v. *insipience*.

38 G. R. Evans, *Getting It Wrong: The Medieval Epistemology of Error* (Leiden: Brill, 1998), 156. Salvian, *Adversus avaritiam*, *Patrologiae cursus completus, series latina*, ed. J. P. Migne, 221 vols (Paris, 1841–64) [hereafter *PL*], vol. 53, col. 21: 'Quid inter stultum sit et insipientem, non est nunc disserendi locus; nec sane interest quae inter eos meritorum sit differentia, quorum est una perditio. Quod causae itaque sufficit, cum dixisset simul insipientem et stultum esse perituros; videamus quid vel ad causam vel ad cumulum perditionis adjecerit.'

39 Book X.S.240, *The Etymologies of Isidore of Seville*, trans. and intro. Stephen A. Barney, W. J. Lewis, J. A. Beach and Oliver Berghof (Cambridge: Cambridge University Press, 2010), 228; 'Cuius contrarius est insipiens, quod sit sine sapore, nec alicuius discretionis vel sensus.' This and the following Latin citations of Isidore are from http://penelope.uchicago.edu/Thayer/E/Roman/texts/Isidore/home.html (accessed 21 January 2013).

40 Book X.F.103, *Etymologies*, 219.

41 Book X.I.143, *Etymologies*, 222.

42 Book X.S.246–248, *Etymologies*, 228–9.

43 Evans, *Getting It Wrong*, 160. See Augustine, *Contra epistulam Parmeniani*, I.ii.3.1, in ed. *Corpus Scriptorum Ecclesiasticorum Latinorum* (Vienna, 1866) [hereafter *CSEL*], vol. 51; Augustine, *Contra Faustum*, XXII.45, in ed. *CSEL* vol. 25; Augustine, *Contra Gaudentium*, I.xxvii.30, in ed. *CSEL* vol. 53.

44 C. F. Goodey, 'The Psychopolitics of Learning and Disability in Seventeenth-century Thought', in David Wright and Anne Digby (eds), *From Idiocy to Mental Deficiency: Historical Perspectives on People with Learning Disabilities* (London: Routledge, 1996), 93–117, at 115n8.

45 *Inventio, translationes et miracula ss. Mauri, Pantaleonis et Sergii* in *Acta Sanctorum*, July VI, 359–71 (at 370 lect. iii); Amy Devenney kindly provided the reference.

46 Konrad von Megenberg, *Buch der Natur*, ed. Franz Pfeiffer (Stuttgart, 1861), 488; Ruth von Bernuth, 'From Marvels of Nature to Inmates of Asylums: Imaginations of Natural Folly', *Disability Studies Quarterly*, 26:2 (2006), no pagination, online publication at www.dsq-sds.org (accessed 1 August 2014).

47 Arthur R. Borden, *A Comprehensive Old-English Dictionary* (Washington, DC: University Press of America, 1982), s.v. *dwǽs* etc.

48　Wilfred Bonser, *The Medical Background of Anglo-Saxon England* (London: Wellcome Historical Medical Library, 1963), 262.

49　Saward, *Perfect Fools*, 225n34.

50　*OED*, s.v. *simple*.

51　C. Corèdon and A. Williams, *A Dictionary of Medieval Terms and Phrases* (Cambridge: D. S. Brewer, 2004), s.v. *seely*. The word was also applied to lepers.

52　*Middle English Dictionary*, at http://quod.lib.umich.edu/m/med/med_ent_search.html (accessed 16 January 2010), s.v. *seli*.

53　All of which begs the even more speculative question if there is a common Indo-European root for *salos/sælig*, something that refers to divine inspiration or similar, which I must leave to the linguists to pursue.

54　*OED*, s.v. *fool*.

55　*OED*, s.v. *fool*.

56　*OED*, s.v. *fool*.

57　*OED*, s.v. *fool*.

58　Judith Weiss, 'The Metaphor of Madness in the Anglo-Norman Lives of St Mary the Egyptian', in Erich Poppe and Bianca Ross (eds), *The Legend of Mary of Egypt in Medieval Insular Hagiography* (Dublin: Four Courts Press, 1996), 161–74, at 162.

59　Joel Lefebvre, *Les fols et la folie* (Paris: Klincksieck, 1968), cited by Angelika Groß, *'La Folie'. Wahnsinn und Narrheit im spätmittelalterlichen Text und Bild* (Heidelberg: Carl Winter Universitätsverlag, 1990), 10.

60　*OED*, s.v. *sot*.

61　Enid Welsford, *The Fool: His Social and Literary History* (London: Faber & Faber, 1935, rpt 1968), 121.

62　Pfau, 'Madness in the Realm', 21.

63　Pfau, 'Madness in the Realm', 26; Paris, Archives Nationales series JJ book 107, fol. 193v, no. 377.

64　Pfau, 'Madness in the Realm', 26; Paris, Archives Nationales series JJ book 160 fol. 70v, no. 91.

65　E. Seebold (ed.), *Kluge. Etymologisches Wörterbuch der deutschen Sprache* (Berlin/Boston: De Gruyter, 25th edn, 2011), s.v. *Toll*. The Old English *dwǽs* derives from the same Germanic root *dwel-a*.

66　'Mit *dösig, Dusel* zu einer Verbalwurzel, die "verwirrt sein, umnebelt sein" bedeutet (hierzu weiter entfernt auch *toll, taub* u.a.) und mit *Dunst* verwandt ist.' Seebold, *Kluge. Etymologisches Wörterbuch der deutschen Sprache*, s.v. *Tor, Taub*.

67　Dirk Matejovski, *Das Motiv des Wahnsinns in der mittelalterlichen Dichtung* (Frankfurt-a-M.: Suhrkamp, 1996), 27 and 313n36.

68　Matejovski, *Motiv des Wahnsinns*, 27.

69　'Men noemt hem ook naar het uitvallen van het communicatiemedium tussen hem en de wereld van ons: de zinnen. ... Het richtinggevend stuur ontbreekt hem: zijn ratio is hem ontnomen. ... Men noemt hem insipiens. Hij is geworden tot de dwaas, die niet weet wat hij doet, noch wat hij zegt. Hij is de idiotus bij uitstek. ... Als stolidus is hij de brutale, als fatuus de smadelijk handelende.' H. H. Beek,

Waanzin in de Middeleeuwen: Beeld van de Gestoorde en Bemoeienis met de Zieke (Haarlem: De Toorts/Nijkerk: G. F. Callenbach, 1969), 7.

70 'tôr ist der, dem witze als ein allen Menschen zukommendes naturale fehlt, ein Narr, ein Irrer, ein Blödsinniger, Verrückter; man erkennt ihn daran, daß er nicht sprechen kann, auch trägt er ein besonderes Kleid, welches anzeigt, daß er außerhalb der Gesellschaft normaler Menschen steht.' Jost Trier, *Der deutsche Wortschatz im Sinnbezirk des Verstandes. Die Geschichte eines sprachlichen Feldes, Bd. 1. Von den Anfängen bis zum Beginn des 13. Jahrhunderts* (Germanische Bibliothek. Zweite Abteilung. Untersuchungen und Texte Bd 31) (Heidelberg, 1931), 268, cited by Matejovski, *Motiv des Wahnsinns*, 27.

71 Kluge. *Etymologisches Wörterbuch*, s.v. *Geck.*

72 'Das Wort ist nur Deutsch (oder aus dem Deutschen entlehnt). Herkunft unklar.' Seebold, Kluge. *Etymologisches Wörterbuch*, s.v. *Narr.*

73 Matejovski, *Motiv des Wahnsinns*, 29.

74 'Während "tore" im Laufe des Spätmittelalters immer mehr mit ethisch-religiösen Inhalten aufgeladen wurde, vollzog »narre« eine solche Bedeutungsverschiebung nicht. "Narr" ist da, wo es nicht eindeutig als Synonym für "tôr" oder als Bezeichnung für Spielarten der Verrücktheit gebraucht wird, kaum mehr als ein "grobes Schimpfwort". Vom fünfzehnten Jahrhundert an ist eine größere Verbreitung des Wortes "Narr" zu verzeichnen.' Matejovski, *Motiv des Wahnsinns*, 30.

75 'Als weitere Adjektive, die sich auf Zustände intellektueller Defizienz, auf die Abwesenheit von Rationalität und Verstandeskraft beziehen, wären "wan-witze" und »wan-witzic« zu nennen.' Matejovski, *Motiv des Wahnsinns*, 26.

76 Seebold, *Kluge. Etymologisches Wörterbuch*, s.v. *Wahnsinn.*

77 Leo Kanner, *A History of the Care and Study of the Mentally Retarded* (Springfield, IL: Thomas, 1964), 5.

78 *OED*, s.v. *idiot.*

79 *OED*, s.v. *idiot.*

80 'Te simplicem et rudem et impolitam, et idioticam compello', *De testimonio animae Liber adversus Gentes, PL*, vol. 1, col. 610B.

81 'se idiotas ac propheticae lectionis ignaros temporum cursum probare non posse causarentur', *In Lucae evangelium expositio*, IV, cap. 12, *PL*, vol. 92, col. 501C.

82 'Quis nam idiota ferat demens', *Carminis in honorem Ludovici christianissimi Caesaris Augusti*, Lib. IV, *PL*, vol. 105, col. 638A.

83 Saward, *Perfect Fools*, 65, noting that here the emphasis is on the lack of sophistication and on simplicity, 'rather than on any psychological inadequacy'. See also William of Hirsau (c.1030–91), *Constitutiones Hirsaugienses*, Lib. I, Cap. I: De diversitate novitiorum, *PL*, vol. 150, col. 932D for novices described as idiots.

84 'et alii quidem calumniabuntur insipientem, alii subsannabunt praesumptorem, alii idiotam judicabunt, nonnulli quoque stultum merito inclamabunt.' *Vita prior auctore Gualtero archidiacono ecclesiae Morinorum*, epilogue, *PL*, vol. 166, col. 942C.

85 'Inter nobilis illustris, et inter ignobiles rusticanus; inter peritos disertus, et inter idiotas tanquam fatuus', *Vita S. Norberti auctore canonico Praemonstratensi coaevo*, cap. 1, *PL*, vol. 170, col. 1259A.

86 'Sed cum indifferenter ibi prudentes et idiotae fortes et invalidi, nobiles et ignobiles', *Opusculum de sua conversione*, cap. VI, *PL*, vol. 170, col. 816A.

87 'Nec jam quasi idiotae et hebetes huic verbo applaudebant carnaliter', *Liber de cardinalibus operibus Christi usque ad ascensum ejus ad patrem ad Adrianum IV pontificem maximum*, XI De ascensione Christi, *PL*, vol. 189, col. 1668B.

88 Vulgate: 'videntes autem Petri constantiam et Iohannis conperto quod homines essent sine litteris et idiotae admirabantur'.

89 Although the modern critical edition by W. M. Lindsay (Oxford: Oxford University Press, 1911) does not include this passage.

90 'Nota quod aliam hic habemus etymologiam hujus nominis idiota, quam ab Isidoro. Nam secundum Isidorum, idiota dicitur quasi divisus ab auribus, idi, enim, *divisio*, ota *auris* interpretatur, ut dicatur, idiota, quasi divisus ab intellectu, scilicet fatuus. Sed secundum etymologiam, quam hic ponitur dicitur idiota, quasi ab idiomate. Dicti sunt ergo idiotae, quasi contenti solo idiomatae linguae suae Hebraeae quam satis noverant, et nihil aliud.' *Historia Scholastica*, Historia libri actuum Apostolorum, cap. 20, *PL*, vol. 198, col. 1657C-D.

91 '*Idiota*, proprie, simplex vel fatuus, quasi iduatus, id est divisus, a *iota*, vel quasi habens iduatas otas, id est *divisas aures*.' *Liber in distinctionibus dictionum theologicalium*, s.v. B, I, *PL*, vol. 210, col. 814D.

92 Joannes de Garlandia, *Opus synonymorum*, *PL*, vol. 150, col. 1589C-D. The full list of terms is: 'Est fatuus, stolidus, erroneus, insipiensque, /Inscius, et brutus, simplex, idiotaque, stultus /Indoctus, simul insipidus conjungitur illis, / Inconsultus, et eligius cui verba negantur.'

93 Edward Sapir, *Selected Writings of Edward Sapir in Language, Culture, and Personality*, ed. David G. Mandelbaum (Berkeley: University of California Press, 1949), 27.

3

COLD COMPLEXIONS AND MOIST HUMORS: NATURAL SCIENCE AND INTELLECTUAL DISABILITY

Idiocy, an important social phenomenon, merited little attention in the medical texts, since it was designated both by law and by medicine as a permanent, hereditary state which was, consequently, intractable.[1]

Medical texts are relatively reticent when it comes to describing diagnoses, let alone advocating treatment, mainly of course for similar reasons as already encountered with regard to physical disability, connected with the permanence and incurability of ID, in that physicians tended to steer clear of intractable, incurable conditions. We should perhaps suppose the existence of an antique notion of a specific but hardly articulated knowledge of the incurability of IDs, since attempts at healing are conspicuous by their absence, featuring neither in the magical literature of the ancient Near East or of antiquity, nor in antique medical texts, nor for that matter in medieval miracle healings. Where they do say anything on ID, medical texts seem to be heavily influenced by two types of other texts – theological-philosophical texts on human intelligence and reason, and legal texts on the treatment of people deemed judicially incapable. While head wounds that could lead on to impairment of mental and/or cognitive functions, sustained, for example, by a knight during battle, might be treated surgically, as the many *Cirurgia*-type texts of the period attempted to describe, the 'natural fool' was just that: a 'natural' case. Nevertheless, a study of the available medieval medical literature is valuable, if just to prove the assumption being stated here; furthermore, medical texts provide incidental statements regarding ID that can inform our understanding of one particular element in the cultural package of medieval constructions of what is and what is not deemed mental health.

Back in the 1970s Clarke had made some educated guesses as to the incidence of mental illness in general and ID in particular for medieval England.

He took as his statistical starting-point an estimate for an overall population of three million around 1300, and came up with a figure of almost 11,000 cases of ID; his suggested rates of 3.6 per 1000 for ID were based on statistics derived from a 1962 article in the *British Medical Journal*, but convincingly assumed similar genetics between the medieval and modern population. 'Handicaps restricting development and normal life and likely to be taken in practice as evidence of mental subnormality would swell this figure' – presumably Clarke was thinking of conditions like congenital deafness – 'while early mortality of the genuinely intellectually subnormal would tend to reduce it.' Medieval medical categories need not be precisely identical to modern medical categories, more a case of varying degrees of overlap, generally based on functionality rather than aetiology. Therefore, Clarke surmised, not just persons with what we now call ID would have been classed as *fatui naturales*, but also 'numerous cases of congenital deafness, poor vision (not then corrigible), speech defects, spasticity and other physical handicaps, some epilepsies and some schizophrenic withdrawals and other eccentricities'; the argument being that in the absence of modern educational, rehabilitative or other therapeutic interventions these conditions, whether in isolation or in combination, 'would preclude adequate social learning and participation'.[2]

Already Aristotle alleged that congenital deafness affected mental functioning. In *De sensu* he asserted that hearing is the superior sense over sight, which is more commonly regarded as such when it comes to learning: 'Incidentally, however, it is hearing that contributes most to the growth of intelligence. For rational discourse is a cause of instruction in virtue of its being audible, which it is not in its own right, but incidentally; since it is composed of words, and each word is a symbol. Accordingly, of persons destitute from birth of either sense, the blind are more intelligent than the deaf and dumb.'[3] This was repeated in *De proprietatibus rerum* by Bartholomaeus Anglicus, written probably during his time at the Dominican convent in Magdeburg during the 1240s, which was the first modern-style encyclopaedia, with alphabetical entries, and a perennial best seller not just during the later medieval period, but also well into the early modern. The original Latin was translated into Middle English by John Trevisa in 1397 as *On the Properties of Things*. Hearing is the essential sense for learning, as Bartholomaeus says, since according to Aristotle 'þe lyme of herynge is ful of kynde spirit, for as þe kynde spirit makeþ þe meuynge of puls in þe veynes, so he makeþ in þe eere þe vertu of heringe; and þat þerfore men lerneþ by þe wit of heringe'.[4] Thus congenital hearing loss would have entailed functional loss of communication, and with that the perception of someone with the sensory disability of deafness as also being intellectually disabled. There were a few dissenting voices. On the confusion between congenital deafness and mental retardation, Origen (c. 185–c. 254) stated that speech is independent of voice (*Patr. Grec.* 11,91), because while speech manifests the thoughts of the mind, voice just articulates them, plus in developmental terms voice is earlier (e.g. there is voice in children before they can speak). Nemesius of Emesa (in *On the Nature of Man*, around 400) said people who are mute from birth are rational, as are those who are mute from accident or injury. This is so because utterance is not a prerequisite for reasoning. And Gregory of Nyssa (d. 395), *On the Making of Man*, believed that the seat of reason is not in the brain, but all over the body; the soul is diffused throughout the body; a speech defect is therefore not a mental defect.[5]

The confusing and overlapping medieval medical terminology of madness, mental illness and mental disability may partly be explained by the main categorisations of the various medical schools and authorities a writer followed, e.g. Galenic or Hippocratic.[6] For instance, the above-mentioned thirteenth-century encyclopaedia described mental illness in Book VII, where Bartholomaeus discusses *frenesis, amentia* and *stupore et litargia*, respectively. Frenzy, the first mental illness mentioned, is a kind of madness that is typified by loss of sense (*witte*) and of mind (*mynde*), stemming from sickness of the brain and accompanied by wakefulness and raving, thirst, anguish, rolling eyes and lots of other bodily movements. The second, *amentia* and *mania*, are one, again caused by an infection of the brain with privation of imagination, but here also linked with melancholia ('melancolia is infeccioun of þe myddel celle of þe heed wiþ priuacioun of resoun');[7] the behaviour is described to be as diverse as the causes for the disease are diverse, some patients being active and violent, others withdrawn and hiding themselves away. The third mental illness is called *stupor*: 'And *stupor* is iclepid a disese of þe soule; as Constantinus [*Viaticum* I.16] seiþ, *stupor* is blindenes of resoun, and he is as it were slepe wiþ i3en iclosed. And so for defaute of spiritis þe soule demeþ nou3t of þing[es] þat ben iseyne'.[8] The causes are 'perturbacioun of resoun', a blockage in the paths of the spirits (or neurological damage in modern parlance) and humoral imbalance mainly due to excessive cold. Stupor is also associated with forgetfulness, affecting the hind cell of the brain, and sleepiness (hence *letargia*), wherefore it is mainly a disease of the elderly. However, none of these three disease descriptions is in any way comparable to ID, and all are considered treatable.

In general, the interstices between different discursive terrains, which are extremely difficult to reconstruct, and the processes of exchange and influence between medicine, literature and theology, plus the concurrent models of rational-scientific and magical explanations, all point to conceptual reasons why the medieval structuring of knowledge concerning mental pathologies cannot be forced into the schema of modern positivistic natural sciences.[9] One common element in both mental illness and mental disability, however, was the medieval emphasis on physicality. The attitude demonstrated in medieval medical texts differs from the modern approach of separating between mental and behavioural disorders, on the one hand, and physical, on the other, in that medieval texts appear not to have distinguished mental and physical disorders, and, crucially, 'almost all kinds of mental disorder were attributed to, or at least believed to be mediated by, the breakdown of some physiological process'.[10] This will become obvious below, in a more detailed look at late antique and medieval theories on the brain, its anatomy and functions. John Philoponus (John the Grammarian), a Christian Neoplatonist working in Alexandria in the sixth century and commentator on a number of Aristotle's works, set the tone. Parts of his commentary on Aristotle's *De anima*, which survives in the form of lecture notes based on seminars of his teacher Ammonius, were translated into Latin in the thirteenth century by William of Moerbeke and thus may have in turn influenced Thomas Aquinas' *Expositio in libros de anima*. Philoponus ascribed degrees of intelligence to physical composition or mixture. 'In general, people turn out to be better talented [*euphuês*] and more sharp-witted or, on the contrary, dull-witted, according to the corresponding mixture. This, then, is the ground for the doctors' saying that the faculties of the soul follow the mixtures of the body.' However, 'talented' (*euphuês*) could also be translated as 'more intelligent'.[11]

Pathologies of the brain

Learning disabilities are comparatively neglected in medieval medical and philosophical discourse, in contrast to modern psychology, which treats learning ability as a fundamentally desirable skill. Thomas Aquinas considered a few of the themes related to modern theories of learning in his account of dispositions, placing what we now call psychological dispositions under the rubric 'acts of will', for instance courageous behaviour or being able to speak and understand a foreign language.[12] 'Like modern behavioral repertoires they are generally acquired gradually and strengthened by repeated actions as the passive potentialities are acted on by active elements, and may be lost or extinguished through lack of use.'[13] The keyword for ID is 'passive potentialities', since if these are not fully there or fully developed, then no amount of active elements can influence the dispositions.

With regard to ID ascribed to people who have a sensory impairment, mainly congenital deafness, Kellenberger mentioned the semantics of the Akkadian word *sakku* meaning 'blocked, deaf, stupid'. Furthermore, Greek and Jewish authors noted that epilepsy sometimes went hand in hand with ID, such as Aretaios (second century AD), who claimed that this illness damages *dianoia* and affects a *môrainein*; and Pseudoaristotle, *Problemata XXX*, wine makes people stupid (*moros*) like those who are epileptics from childhood; cerebral palsy can be the cause of further ID, something hinted at in descriptions in Mesopotamian medical texts of children who have spastic convulsions and who can neither get up out of bed, nor chew bread nor speak.[14]

Galen's *De locis affectis*, composed after AD 192, dealt with general pathology and systematic description of diseases of the different physiological systems of the body, hence including the brain and nervous system. In Book III, chapter 5 Galen treated the location of 'intelligence' in the modern sense. In his *Commentaries on the dogmas of Hippocrates and Plato* Galen had written what he summarised here, 'that everyone is convinced that the reasoning soul is located in the brain, that courage and emotions reside in the heart, and desires in the liver. One can learn this every day by listening to those who speak about it, also in regard to [the idea that] the stupid people have no brain, and that knaves and cowards have no heart.'[15] Overall, as to be expected, Galen said next to nothing on ID, other than the lapidary remarks that stupid people have no brain, or that melancholics are like children and uneducated adults. Memory loss he described a bit more distinctly, but then that is a progressive disease, whereas ID is by definition congenital. In *De locis affectis*, III, 11 Galen cited *morosis, mania, lethargos, phrenetis, paraphrosyne, apoche* and *melagcholia*, but the criteria for differentiation are unclear; more often than not the people denoted by these terms are acting foolishly but are otherwise of normal intelligence, although it might also refer specifically to 'born fools' (*physei moroi, naturaliter fatui*).[16] Galen categorised cognitive decline as dullness (*morosis, dementia*) or foolishness (*moria*), both due to diminishing powers of reasoning (*ellipes tes dianotikes energeias; intellectus perditio*), in which understanding and memory were severely impaired; more serious was *anoia* (*amentia*; the privative *a*, and *nous*, mind), which Galen also termed a *paralysis* of the thinking faculties and which could be due to senility, excessive coldness of the brain or humoral damage of mental faculties, but also the result of severe phrenitis, lethargus or melancholy.[17] Hence Galen was concerned only with acquired cognitive disability or, rather, mental illness, and not with congenital ID or developmental disorders. Galen believed that health was a sort of harmony, but that physical and mental patterns of this harmony differed according to the individual's constitution. Minor variations were physiological, not pathological, so that something was a disease only if 'the normal equilibrium of the humors was severely disturbed'.[18] And most importantly, 'weakness of function' was not, strictly speaking, considered to be a sign of disease,[19] presumably because a weakness is just that, a diminution of something, but not something contrary to nature. Following this line of argument, Galenic views would entail that mental disability, being a weakness of function rather than a severe imbalance like insanity, would not be pathological and therefore would not be a disease. And if something was not a disease, what was the point of treatment? In a mocking tone Galen, *De locis affectis* III, 7 related that his colleague Archigenes treated a *môrôtheis*, which Siegel translates as: 'Archigenes applies remedies to the heads of persons suffering from memory defects, and he will administer everything to the head in the attempt to cure some moron.'[20] In this connection Goodey declared: 'Greek doctors explicitly denied that intellectual inferiority was the province of medicine; their mythical patron Asclepios made the blind see and the lame walk but, it was said, could not make a fool wise.'[21]

Medieval faculty theory

The main feature of medieval concepts of the brain was the localisation of mental faculties in the ventricles. 'In its basic form, the faculties of the mind (derived from Aristotle) were distributed among the spaces within the brain (the ventricles described by Galen).'[22] The 'common sense', which integrated physical sensory inputs such as sight, sound or smell, supplied information to the first ventricle, where images, and also fantasies, were generated; this information was then transferred to the second or middle cell, which, due to its central location, was not only warmer but held what we now call cognitive processes, that is, reasoning, judgement and thought; finally, the third cell was devoted to memory, hence information storage. This basic scheme remained unchanged for centuries, with just minor refinements, for instance by the tenth century 'the original static localization shifted to a more dynamic process analogous to digestion',[23] with a kind of 'cooking' or masticating action taking place in the warmer, second cell. Poseidonius, a Byzantine in the fourth century, appeared to have been the first to describe in detail the effects of brain damage to specific areas, pointing out that damage to the front of the brain impaired imagination, damage to the back impaired memory, but damage to the middle resulted in diminished reasoning. Kemp explained and summarised medieval theories of cognition as the inner senses or inward wits, which 'were psychological faculties that, throughout the Middle Ages, were assumed to be located in the ventricles of the brain'; in their activities of remembrance or imagination, brain ventricles functioned like other sensory organs (such as eyes or ears), and hence embodied the materiality of medieval psychology. Ventricular theory 'was created by assigning the various perceptual and cognitive facilities identified by Aristotle in his *De Anima* to the spirit-filled cerebral ventricles described by Galen in his discussion of the anatomy of the brain'.[24] The ancient authors never combined these theories, but late antique or early medieval ones did: 'Precisely who was responsible for formulating the theory is unclear but the basic idea of ascribing different faculties to the ventricles is contained in the writings of both Augustine and Nemesius.'[25] Nemesius, late fourth-century bishop of Emesa in Syria and author of a treatise *De natura hominis* (c. 400), was translated into Latin by Alfanus of Salerno in the second half of the eleventh century and again by Burgundino of Pisa c. 1165. In this work Nemesius discusses the place of humans in the cosmic order, moving on to the relationship of soul and body, then discussing more general physiology, psychology and the emotions. Having taken on board Galenic medical theories, Nemesius also considered the psychic functions of the brain, which was divided into three ventricles with different functions. In section 13 [69.15] of his tract, Nemesius gave a brief description of how the three faculties of the soul operate together: 'the faculty of imagination hands on things imagined to the faculty of thought, while thought or reasoning, when it has received and judged them, passes them on to the faculty of memory'.[26] The locations are therefore from front to back, going from imagination to intellect in the middle, with memory to the rear. 'In the Middle Ages, belief in something like Nemesius' version of the theory was practically universal among both scholars and physicians, although there was some debate about the details.'[27] Nemesius then uses the examples of damage to one or other of these three parts to demonstrate the workings of the parts.

> If the frontal cavities are damaged in any way the senses are impaired but thought remains unharmed. If the central cavity alone suffers thought is overthrown but the sense-organs continue to preserve their natural [power of] sensation. If both the frontal and the central cavities suffer, reason is damaged together with the senses. But if the cerebellum suffers, memory alone is lost together with it without sensation and thought being harmed in any way. But if the posterior suffers together with the frontal and central ones, sense, reason and memory also are destroyed, in addition to the whole creature being in danger of perishing.[28]

Thus for Nemesius the evidence for the localisation of faculties of the soul is derived from various psychological dysfunctions, depending on which part of the brain is damaged.[29]

William of Auvergne (1180/90–1249) wrote *De immortalite anime* in the 1220s or 1230s, in which he set out to use philosophical arguments to counter the theologically erroneous beliefs that the human soul is mortal. His interest lay in proving that the intellective power is immortal and not hindered or failed by physical things, since certain observations of the physical world present problems for the notion that the intellective power is immaterial. William therefore also referred to brain damage:

> Moreover, it is clear that this [intellective] power does not have in the body an organ for its operation. Although from an injury to the middle compartment of the head the operation of this power seems to be impeded or completely destroyed, still it is clear that this impedes or destroys only the operation it has from below, that is, from the side of sensible things. For its representation of the sensible forms is like another book, a book that the imaginative power offers or presents to it. Since, then, it cannot abstract or strip these forms from particular conditions because of the disturbance or injury of the middle compartment of the head, into which they pass from the imaginative power, though more stripped and abstracted from matter, this noble power is prevented from seeing and reading them. This is due to the fact that the middle compartment, which <through the imaginative power> ought to become like a book for it by means of such an inscription as we mentioned, is by reason of injury from an infection or from a wound unsuited to be inscribed by the imaginative power. Hence, this power is prevented from the reading <that it would do in such a book,> that is, it is prevented from understanding and from reasoning about sensible things which come to it in no other way.[30]

Medieval theories of brain function also found a physiological or materialist explanation for perceived differences in intelligence, such as those of Costa ben Luca (864–923): the refined brain substance or *spiritus* found in more intelligent people, and the slower, thicker one found in women, children and, by implication, in 'idiots'. Costa ben Luca wrote a short treatise in Arabic, translated into Latin during the twelfth century by Johannes Hispalensis as *De animae et spiritus discrimine,* and often falsely attributed by medieval authorities to Constantinus Africanus.[31] In the original work the three ventricles of the brain are said to be linked by *vermis,* a substance of the brain which functions somewhat like a valve between the different chambers and ensures that only the most rarefied spirit reaches the posterior third ventricle. Costa ben Luca stated 'that a man's rational powers depend on the quality of the animal spirit in the middle ventricle. The rational and thoughtful have subtle clear spirit, whereas the mindless and irrational, the light-minded and foolish, have the opposite kind of spirit.'[32]

These ideas on the brain were picked up and reiterated by Robert Kilwardby. Kilwardby taught grammar and logic at Paris around 1237–45, then moved to Oxford, where he was a regent master in arts c. 1256, became archbishop of Canterbury in 1272 and died as a cardinal at Viterbo in 1279. Kilwardby stated with regard to imagination: 'Aristotle says in the *Posterior Analytics,* namely, that if the sense is defective then knowledge based on that sense is also defective.'[33] *De differentia animae et spiritus* by Costa ben Luca is quoted extensively by Kilwardby in his tract on imagination, in particular those passages which describe the structure of the brain. Costa ben Luca had written: 'Understanding, thinking, and practical reasoning are carried out by means of the soul which is in the ventricle shared by the two ventricles at the front of the brain.'[34] This passage is quoted almost verbatim by Kilwardby when he explains that 'it is taught that in the front of the brain there are two ventricles in which the common sense and the imagination work. And many pairs of nerves lead from there, so that one pair leads to the eyes so that there should be a seeing in them, and another pair leads to the ears so that there should be a hearing in them, and so on.'[35] Kilwardby expands on this a little later on:

> Since therefore present things are, as it were, right before us, God has rightly arranged the chamber of common sense with its imagination in the fore part of the brain, since sensible grasp of present things is in the fore part. And perhaps for that reason two chambers are placed in the fore part of the brain, one to serve common sense, the other to serve imagination. And since past things have, as it were, been sent to the back, God rightly arranged that the chamber to which the intention to remember would make its way should be in the rear part of the brain. For that intention, as it were, makes its way to things put behind one, when it recollects past things. And since the rational mind reasons about, and judges, both present things and past ones, and also considers both sorts of things, God rightly arranged the chamber called the 'rational chamber' in the middle of the brain as an aid to thought and to rational consideration. For this should draw from each of the extremes and should adjudicate about all the things which each extreme contains.[36]
>
> (Quia igitur presentia quasi coram sunt, ideo in anteriori parte cerebri recte ordinauit Deus cellula<m> sensus communis cum sua ymaginacione, quia ad ante est sensibilis apprehensio [et] presentium. Et forte ideo ponuntur due cellule in anteriori parte cerebri ut una sensui communi deseruiat et altera ymaginacioni. Et quia preterita quasi a tergo dimissa sunt, recte ordinauit in posteriori parte cellulam ad quam recurreret intencio in recordando. Quasi enim ad post tergum dimissa recurrit intencio, dum recordatur preteritorum. Et quia de utrisque, scilicet presentibus et preteritis, racionatur mens racionalis et iudicat et utraque considerat, recte ordinauit cellulam in medio cerebri in adiutorium cogitacionis et racionalis consideracionis, que uocatur 'cellula racionalis'. Hec enim debet haurire ab utroque extremorum et de omnibus diiudicare que utraque extremitas continet.)[37]

As an interesting aside, one may point out that as late as 1672, when Thomas Willis worked out his doctrine of mental deficiency, the causation for dullness of intellect, stupidity or foolishness was given as being a mechanical defect in the relationship between imagination and memory, both of which were called by Willis 'forekindred' centres and thus, like in Costa ben Luca, were situated at the front of the brain.[38] Thus one should emphatically acknowledge the lasting influence of Costa ben Luca, stretching across from the tenth to the seventeenth centuries at least.

Anatomies of the brain

More anatomical considerations of the brain are given in Kilwardby's tractate on imagination, in a passage taken directly from the Pseudo-Galenic *Anatomia vivorum*.[39] 'The brain is harder in its rear part both on account of the nerves which produce motion and which arise there (for those nerves have to be harder than the nerves which can sense), and also on account of the part in which the store of memory and the repository of forms are situated.'[40] This provides an interesting materialistic perspective on the brain, since it could allow a medieval anatomist to explain damage to the cognitive parts of the brain, damage of which could lead to congenital idiocy, in all sorts of physical ways: the relevant parts of the brain might be too hard, too soft, nerves might not connect correctly, and so on. I am not aware that any medieval medical or philosophical text that I have examined states such causes explicitly, but by treating the brain and nerves, in other words what modern terminology calls neurology, in strictly material terms, the door is opened for a perfectly 'natural' causation of congenital idiocy. During foetal development things can go wrong in the neurological matter in the same way as things can go wrong with bodily development, thus both physical congenital disability (the birth of blind, crippled or 'monstrous' children) and mental congenital disability can in these medieval explanations be placed theoretically on the same epistemological scale – one is not 'worse' than the other.

The popular encyclopaedia of Bartholomaeus Anglicus also described human anatomy, the brain and the mind/soul dichotomy. On the anatomy of the brain he wrote:

> Good disposicioun of þe brayne and yuel is iknowe by worchinge and dedis; for 3if þe substaunce of þe brayne is neissche, þinne, and clere, it fongiþ li3tliche þe formynge and þe prentinge of schappes and liknes of þinges. He þat haþ such a brayne is swifte and good of disciplyne an lore. Whanne it is a3enwarde, þat þe brayne is notte neissche, oþir 3if it is troubly, he þat haþ suche a brayne fongiþ slowliche þe felinge and prentinge of þinges. But noþeles whanne he haþ ifonge and resceyued hem, a kepiþ hem longe in mynde; and þat is signe and tokene of drynes, as superfluite and for3etinge is token of moisture, as Haly seiþ.[41]

He also included a discussion on spirits, which are subtle and airy substances that incite the virtues of the body, the purest form of which is, according to the physicians, called the vital spirit originating in the heart; part of the vital spirit goes to the brain, where it is refined even more and changed into the animal spirit in the foremost chamber of the brain. The foremost brain chamber also holds the common sense and the imaginative virtue. Then the spirit moves into the middle chamber which is called '*logica* to make þe intellect and vndirstondinge parfite'.[42] Afterwards, the spirit passes on to the third chamber, memory. Bartholomaeus Anglicus explains 'þan for diuers office in diuers lymes þe same spirit haþ many names and hatte *spiritus corporeus, subtilis, aereus*. Also for by worchinge of þe lyuour he hatte *spiritus naturalis*, in þe herte *vitalis*, and in þe heed *animalis*.'[43] The spirit is, however, not the reasonable soul, but following Augustine it is the instrument of the soul, which joins the soul to the body. Thus this 'material' spirit is subject to injury, just as the 'grey matter' of the brain might be damaged. 'And þerfore 3if þis spirit[is] ben apeired and ihurt and ilette of here worchinge in eny maner worchinge, þe acord of þe body and soule is resolued, [and] þe resonable spirit is ilette of alle his werkes in body, as it is isene [in] a mased [amazed], madde man and frenetik and in oþir þat ofte leseþ vse of resoun.'[44]

Kemp asked what advantages might be garnered from adopting the theory of the inner senses, since by that 'the rational soul had many of its psychological functions stripped from it', which posed theological problems, such as the question of how an immortal, immaterial soul might remember anything from the impressions gained during life, if the inner sense was defunct; the answer seems to be that the inner sense 'produced an explanation for two facts that were otherwise difficult to explain: that human psychological disorders often follow head injury and that the behavior of animals suggests some sort of information processing capacity on their part'.[45] An interesting comparison of the three cells of the brain with the function of the spatial arrangement of the classical law courts was made by a twelfth-century anatomical text, the *Anatomia Nicolai Physici*, 'derived from an Islamic synthesis of Nemesius and Poseidonus with Greek humoral and pneumatic physiology'.[46] The interplay between legal and medical, or even the forensic character of physiological description, is what is striking enough to warrant citation in full:

> On the account of the three divisions of the brain the ancient philosophers called it the temple of the spirit, for the ancients had three chambers in their temples: first the vestibulum, then the consistorium, finally the apotheca. In the first, the declarations were made in law-cases; in the second, the statements were sifted; in the third, final sentence was laid down. The ancients said that the same processes occur in the temple of the spirit, that is, the brain. First, we gather ideas into the cellular phantisca, in the second cell, we think them over, in the third, we lay down our thought, that is, we commit to memory.[47]

Memory was valuable – memory defined what we now term identity or personhood – so the patristic writers picked up on the Galenic notion of the firmer posterior cell of the brain as a more suitable location for safe storage than the softer, more pliant middle or anterior regions.

In his 'Long Commentary' on Aristotle's *De anima*, Averroes (1126–98) situated memory in the back of the brain, the cogitative faculty in the middle ventricle of the brain, while the imaginative faculty was located in the front of the brain, all of which made these faculties (on which material intellect depended), as well as the brain in which they reside, 'generated-destructible',[48] that is, materialist and liable to damage or defect. A materialist concept of intellect allows for the possibility that intellect might be 'defective' if the brain or the senses are 'defective', thus opening up the path for the kind of medical-anatomical aetiologies of 'intellectual disability' that Goodey postulated only for the post-Cartesian era. Averroes' 'Long Commentary' was the only one of his seven texts on intellect that was available in a Latin translation of around 1230 to the Western Christian schools and universities. During the second half of the thirteenth century Averroes' 'theory of material intellect propounded in the Long Commentary achieved notoriety',[49] but for reasons to do with critique of the materialist conceptions that are only tangential to my discussion of the implications of theories on intelligence.

William of Conches on the brain

William of Conches (c. 1080–c. 1150) wrote two works which mention functioning of the brain: *Philosophia mundi* (also titled *Dragmaticon* of c. 1147–49) and *Philosophia seu Summa philosophiae* (written 1136x41). The *Dragmaticon* was composed in the dialogue tradition, between a Philosopher (William himself) and a Duke (Geoffrey the Fair). Both texts introduced the ventricular doctrine into Western medicine, although William speaks of cells within the brain, rather than of ventricles. The anatomy was derived by William in part from Constantinus Africanus' *Pantegni*. He located mental disorders in the brain, stating that a dull wit, soggy memory and imperfect speech are due to humoral influences on the brain, with the rational faculty situated in the middle (ventricle) of the brain.[50] In *Dragmaticon* (Book VI, part two, chapter 18.7) William says physicians had noted that when one of three brain cells is wounded and thereby damaged, the patient loses the faculty that resided there, but retains the mental virtues located in the other two brain cells (or ventricles or cavities). Since none of the writers antedating William appears to have assigned qualities to individual ventricles of the brain 'it may be suggested that William's idea of distinctive qualities for each of the cerebral cavities was a new concept which represented a significant elaboration on the basic theory of ventricular localisation'.[51] This is important because, yet again, it nudged toward a kind of materialism, placing psychological functioning within the physiological principles of the time. William's innovative statement was that all the nerves in the human body originated from the cerebral membranes, which is why he called these latter 'mothers'. The schema was further refined by associating the origin of the nerves of sensation with the pia, and those of voluntary motion with the dura mater. Nerves of sensation 'stretched towards the anterior portion of the head, and thus reached the "window of senses", while the latter grew towards the occiput and extended from there to the members of voluntary motion'.[52] Thus William combined humoral physiology with ventricular localisation to expound what would in the next century develop into Scholastic psychology. Since the *Dragmaticon* is therefore a landmark text, it is worth taking a closer look at those sections that are pertinent to medieval notions of ID.

Having written, among other, on how a defective, paralysed infant can grow into a fully formed, rationally minded adult in the discussion on birth and infancy, the dialogue asks how that is possible: 'Since, as you state, the first age enjoys sensation but lacks reason and intellect, say what sensation [*sensus*] is and why it is present at this first age; say also what reason and intelligence are, and why the first age lacks them.'[53] The Philosopher responds that this answer will require a long discussion, and elaborates first on the senses, plus the definition of reason and intelligence, before returning to provide the answer: 'Since reason and intelligence are faculties of the soul, why is it that infancy and childhood lack these faculties, although infants and children have a soul?'[54] The Philosopher explains that this is all due to corruption, with the corrupt body oppressing the otherwise perfect soul, which may retain the potential 'power and faculty to discern and understand'[55] but cannot do so straight away without learning by exercise and experience. Then a physiological, i.e. humoral, explanation is given.

> The first age [of infancy] neither has any previous practical experience nor can it be suitable for learning. For since infancy is warm and moist, the child digests food at once and seeks more, so that it stands in need of a frequent intake and excretion, and a thick and continuous vapor is produced that, making for the brain, in which the soul exercises its faculty of discerning and understanding, upsets the soul.[56]

Bodily functions distract from intellectual pursuits, an age-old paradigm, and by implication, then, the ideal intellectual is an ascetic.

The physiology of the brain is discussed by William, using the tripartite scheme of cells or ventricles, with imagination in the front, rational thought [*logistica*] in the middle and memory at the rear. The humors exert an influence on neurological and cognitive functionality:

> If the said qualities of the brain are changed, they impair these functions. For if someone has a moist brain in his rear cell, because moistness flows in different directions and alters shapes and colors, that person has a bad memory. For this reason some authors call a bad memory damp [*madida*]. If someone's middle cell brain is utterly distemperate, that person is mad, without reason; if it is only a little distemperate, one's reason is impaired; and the more it is distemperate, the less reason one has; the less distemperate the brain, the more reason one has. Similarly for the front cell: if its brain is extremely cold, one is stupid and without any talent. And the colder one is, the slower one's talent; the less cold one is, the sharper one's mind.[57]

The faculties of the soul are described and placed into hierarchical categories, with intellect, not surprisingly, coming out on top. Noteworthy here is the almost modern emphasis on speed, with people who are 'quicker on the uptake', as it were, being held to be more intelligent than 'slow thinkers':

> There is ingenuity, there is opinion, there is reason, there is intelligence, there is memory. Ingenuity or talent [*ingenium*] is a certain faculty implanted in the soul and dominant [over other faculties] on account of its own strength. Alternatively, ingenuity [or intellect] is the natural faculty of the soul to understand something quickly. Thus, people who quickly understand what they hear are said to be of good and sharp intellect; those who do so slowly, of dense and doltish intellect.[58]

William explains the interaction between reason and intelligence thus: 'Intelligence is born of reason not because reason becomes intelligence, but because it is the cause for it.'[59] The first people were led by reason in their philosophising about the material word, the nature of bodies, from which they concluded that certain actions could not come from bodies and hence their agent had to be incorporeal; these first people formed opinions about what they considered, some of which were true, some false. 'They eliminated the false opinions by long and laborious efforts and confirmed the true ones by necessary arguments. And so, under the guidance of reason, intelligence was born.'[60] These arguments are based on William's gloss on what he knew of Plato's work,[61] not on Aristotelianist explanations.

The assumption is made that reason is one thing, intelligence another, which puts the interlocutor in the dialogue in the position of asking, then, if God only has either reason or intelligence, so that if He had no reason, He would not be rational. To this the Philosopher replies:

It is one thing to know the literal meanings [*proprietates*] of words, another their usages and figurative meanings [*translationes*]. You have heard about the proper meaning of the noun *reason*. Now hear about its usage. Sometimes every true and certain judgment about a particular thing is called reason, and in this sense it is said that in God there is reason. Sometimes [we call reason] whatever is reasonable, as when we say, 'It stands to reason that we should love God.' Sometimes [reason means] computation or account, as in the [Gospel] passage, 'Account for your administration of my estate.' [Luke 16:2] Sometimes it means the order of doing things, by which we know what should be done or said in what place. It is in these and many other accepted meanings that one and same word *reason* occurs.[62]

From which it follows that the varied uses of reason are not just confusing for modern readers, but presumably also for William's contemporaries, since he felt compelled to explain himself. Nevertheless, it becomes clear from the above that whichever way one looks at it, according to William's philosophy, people with ID would not have possessed the full measure of reason.

The locus of intelligence?

William of Conches also applied theories of nutritional qualities to the cells of the brain, which of course conforms to the tenets of humoral theory, presenting a type of *regimen sanitatis* of material for the brain. If (brain) cells require certain nutritional qualities, then this puts, yet again, a material basis on intelligence. If the input, i.e. nutritional substances taken in by the body and carried to the brain cells, goes wrong, so does the output, i.e. the faculties, including the rational faculty/intelligence, of the brain get disturbed and become defective. Aquinas in *Summa theologiae* also stated that the intellect has no organ, but nevertheless 'the exercise of intellect may be impeded by injury to the organs of the imagination (as in a seizure) or of memory (as in a coma). Such brain damage prevents not only the acquisition of new knowledge, but also the utilization of previously acquired knowledge.'[63] For Thomas Aquinas, intellect was inseparable from the body and the inner senses, since the action of thought was impossible without the formation of images, without imagination, so that the inner senses were essential for both the acquisition of new knowledge and the processing of previous knowledge. Because head injury or coma impairs understanding, it is evident that thought and knowledge have a physiological basis. Learning empirically about new things is how understanding worked for Aquinas, 'not by in some way reminding ourselves of what is already present in our minds'.[64] Islamic scholars also emphasised the materiality of cognitive functions. Avicenna (980–1037), in the *Canon*, not only located the reasoning faculty in the central compartment of the brain, but also differentiated between damage and deficiency.

> Concerning frivolity [ru'ûna] and stupidity [humq], Ibn Sînâ states that the distinction between them and confusion of the mind is that, while they are all injuries of the reason and the cause of them may be located in the middle part of the brain, confusion of the mind is an injury to the thinking function depending on the changed nature of the thought process, and frivolity and stupidity are the result of deficiency or nullity. The latter are similar to the conditions of the senile and the child.[65]

According to this description, then, ID would have been regarded as a lack or a deficiency, but not a disease. However, we need to be careful with medieval medical terminology. For Bernard de Gordon, *Lilium medicinae* (c. 1305), '*stupor* was a partial sensory or motor loss', so that the term *stupidi* 'refers to this condition, not to low intelligence'.[66] Which helpfully goes to show that one should not let oneself be guided by etymological guesswork alone. Words that sound similar to modern ones may have had quite different meanings during the medieval period, even such apparently obvious ones like stupidity (*stoliditas infantilis*). According to Arnald de Villanova (c. 1240–1311), damage to the imaginative faculty in the brain which reduced it led to conditions described as *hebetudo* and *stupor*, while corruption of that faculty led to *fatuitas*, and if the faculty of *scientia*, i.e. of knowledge and understanding, was damaged, this led to *stoliditas* or *amentia*.[67] In *De parte operativa*, Arnald of Villanova wrote concerning *stultitia* that it was a deprivation of both fantasy and imagination; furthermore, people who had fallen into *stupida laetitia* would laugh without obvious cause.[68]

Childishness and child development

In cases of reduced or completely removed *scientia* we encounter the diagnostic pictures of *amentia* and *stoliditas*; these patients demand to be like children, they laugh about the things they do, and like children they can be corrected only with much effort; they become lazy and make buildings out of mud and sticks.[69] Although the imagery of patients playing around with what were evidently children's toys of mud and sticks is fascinating in its own right, the problem is, as so often, that although the pattern of inappropriate childish behaviour demonstrated by adults is tempting to ascribe to ID, there is no indication that this could not be symptomatic of acquired mental aberration or mental illness. Beek cited Valascus de Taranta (d. 1418), one of the physicians from the school at Montpellier, who related that he once had such a patient who laughed incessantly, especially on a full stomach, whom he cured by phle-botomy and purging, so that when he got a nosebleed he became better.[70] This shows just how fluid the terms *stoliditas* or *amentia* could be: the symptoms they describe could derive both from congenital and acquired causes, thus one cannot say with certainty whether people termed *stolidus* in medical texts could be equated with the modern label of ID. Johannes Michael Savonarola (1382–1462) a physician trained at Bologna, also compared various mental afflictions with childishness:

> *Amentia* for *ablatio, stoliditas* for *diminutio*. Other names are *fatuitas* or *infantili-tas*. The sick are like children who have no capacity for thinking, apart from what is present by nature, so that [symptoms are] closing of the eyes and touching of the eyeball, the stretching out of arms and hands so as not to fall and to seek support. Let others quarrel more over names, this is not suited to *medici*.[71]

Again, while it is tempting to see the description of symptoms as childlike as an indicator of ID, these behaviours of *amentia* and *stoliditas* could just as readily be due to acquired mental illness. Unless the source text mentions the pres-ence from birth of a condition, the symptoms are too ambiguous.

Having touched on the topic of childishness, it is appropriate to turn to medieval child physiology and the psychology of irrationality. With regard to cognition and the brain, the scholastic authorities argued that the causality for the unintelligence or nescience of human infants was identical to that for their physical debility, based in the humoral complexion, which in the infant was still immature, so that a baby's brain was simply not ready to support intellectual cognition. In brief, the complexion of infants is too humid, too fluid, too wet to function properly yet. Both the external and internal senses are too immature to enable intellectual understanding. Like Hugh of St Victor, Thomas Aquinas 'argues that the infants of Eden would not have been *ignorant* but only *nesci-ent*, since ignorance is lack of such knowledge as one ought to have at a given time of life'.[72] Albertus Magnus, in *Physica*, described how the senses perceive universals, in this context to back up his statement that unified things (*unita*) are better known to sensory perception than distinct things (*distincta*). The example he gave was of how children perceive and categorise things:

> This shows itself in the understanding of children, since through their senses they grasp the general concept (*commune*) earlier than the particular. That is why in the beginning they call all men 'father' and all women 'mother', and later, with successive years, they discern him who really is the father from other men, and her who really is the mother from other women.
> (Apparet autem hoc in apprehensionibus puerorum, quia illi prius per appre-hensionem sensibilem accipiunt commune quam particulare. Unde in principio

omnes viros vocant patres et omnes feminas vocant matres et posterius confor-
tata aetate discernunt eum qui vere pater est, a viris aliis et eam quae vere mater
est, a feminis aliis.)[73]

A little further along in the same chapter, Albertus provides the physiological
reason as to why this should be the case:

> For these [infants] do not perceive the differences of the sensible as long as
> because of the liquidity of the brain they do not have a united (*adunatam*) cogni-
> tion, and therefore their indistinct cognition remains with the general concept
> (*communi*). But when the brain slowly becomes drier, cognition is unified, and
> the specifics of the sensible remain in them by which is distinguished what is
> known through the senses, and then their cognitions are determined.
> (Hi enim quamdiu propter fluxum cerebri cognitionem non habent adunatam,
> non percipiunt differentias sensibilium, et ideo stat eorum cognitio in communi
> indistincta. Cum autem paulatim siccatur cerebrum, adunatur cognitio, et rema-
> nent in eis sensibilia propria, per quae distinguuntur cognita per sensum, et tunc
> determinantur cognitiones eorum.)[74]

If medieval theories of cognition seem somewhat suspect by modern standards, then equally so should modern retrospective diagnosis. Two cases may
illustrate the problem. For ID in the Bible, the chief witness is the story of
David feigning mental incapacity to avoid being harmed by the Philistines in 1
Sam. 21:11–16 [10–15]. Two behavioural traits acted out by David – allowing
spittle to run down his beard and, according to the Septuagint reading, drumming on the doors of the gate (the Masoretic texts refers to making marks on
the doors) – are identified by Olyan as being representative of mental disability. He argued that drooling is characteristic of people who have lost muscle
control to their face, often the result of a stroke, which may also cause various
degrees of mental retardation, while drumming is 'a repetitive and frequently
attention-seeking behavior often associated with severe mental retardation
and autism. ... If David is indeed drumming while drooling, he is portrayed
as acting in ways indicative of severe mental retardation in a most public place
– at the city or palace gate.'[75] We are perhaps on slightly firmer ground with
Katharine (1253–57), the daughter of Henry III and Eleanor of Provence,
who may have been developmentally retarded. She died young and had apparently been a sickly child (on one occasion in 1256, Henry had a silver votive
image placed on a shrine). Matthew Paris described her as 'mute and useless
though a most beautiful face' (*muta et inutilis, sed facie pulcherrima*).[76] Howell
suggested that Katharine might have been affected by a degenerative disorder
which would have been symptomless from birth until signs begin emerging
several months afterwards, with such a disease pattern perhaps resulting from

an infection or the late effects of brain damage at parturition. The likely candidate is Rett syndrome, a rare disease which affects only girls, and which is marked by the onset of developmental retardation (such as inability to speak) after apparently normal development in the first year.[77]

Aetiologies

'They are always congenital idiots, and never result from accidents after uterine life,'[78] wrote Langdon Down in an essay which appeared in 1866 and is generally credited as being the first clinical description of what he called 'mongoloid idiocy'. His views were elaborated in the book *Mental Affections of Children and Youth* (London: Churchill, 1887). Down observed what medieval physicians, lawyers and theologians could also readily have observed, namely that, by definition, ID was present from or near birth. The topic of neonatal illnesses and the impacts of the maternal condition on the foetus during pregnancy was of importance for medieval notions of the conception – in both senses of the word – of the mentally disabled.[79]

Albertus Magnus noted that some planetary conjunctions are recognised as particularly malicious, and pointed out that conception and birth should be avoided at such times. Specific problems might arise with regard to children born under a new moon, as they might be defective in sense and discretion.[80] An early fifteenth-century book of homilies has the full catalogue of birth defects arising out of parental malpractice (wrong kind of intercourse, wrong time): 'That is when her husband knows she has the evil women have at certain times of the month [i.e. menstruation] … at such time are begotten lepers, maimed, unshapely, witless, crooked, blind, lame, dumb, deaf and many other mischiefs.'[81] To avoid this, medieval prospective parents might take preventive action: keeping a book, a sacred text, as a talisman to ensure the birth of a healthy child. In one of the Old English *Lives of St Margaret*, chapter 19 states that in a house where the book of her martyrdom is kept, no unwell child shall be born, no cripple, no dumb, no deaf, no blind nor witless child – so here is an allusion to the 'witless' child, the child with IDs, as well as to the more usual list of physical impairments.[82]

Another aetiology of mental retardation was supplied by Avicenna, *Canon of Medicine*, namely that in medical treatments one should be cautious about applying cupping-glasses to the forehead because this practice might affect the intellectual abilities of any children born to a patient treated in such a way. Concerning application to the forehead, 'most people have a horror of applying cupping-glasses here, as they believe that the senses and intellect will suffer thereby'. And:

There is a danger of transmitting forgetfulness, for as some say, the posterior part of the brain has to do with the preservation of memory, and the cupping enfeebles this faculty, and the offspring will suffer. Some say that cupping over the occiput and top of the head is beneficial for insanity, vertigo, and for preventing the hair from going grey. But we must take it that this effect on the hair applies only to feeble-minded people and not to other types of person, for in most cases the use of cupping in this situation brings premature greyness, and also dulls the intellect. ... It impairs the activity of the intellect, making the offspring dull and forgetful, with poor reasoning powers, and permanent infirmity.[83]

The physicality of ID according to ancient and medieval notions has already been alluded to, in contrast to modern concepts. *Physiognomonika*, a text attributed to Aristotle until the sixteenth century, but probably compiled or composed around 300 BC, has a passage where the physiognomic 'type' of the person without full sense, that is, the mentally disabled, is described. The insensible 'stupid' person, literally without sense of feeling [*anaisthêtou sêmeia*], has these physical characteristics: firm and healthy flesh; fleshy, stiff and firm nape of the neck and legs; squat hips, hunched up shoulder blades; a large, round and fleshy brow, pale and blunt eyes; the calves around the ankles thick, fleshy and squat; large and fleshy jaws; disproportional distances between nape and sternum and to navel; compressed area around the clavicles; fat nose, rounded forehead and small head.[84]

The Byzantine physician Michael Psellos (1018–78) wrote a tract on the origin and causes of human intelligence and retardation, roughly translated entitled as 'How in humans intelligent and moronic (*môroí*) ones come about'.[85] Psellos used philosophical arguments for the different levels of intelligence in humans, and finished with the example of a youth of about 20 called Eudokimos, whose mental development and shape of his head varied somewhat from the norm. Eudokimos had a massively enlarged head almost 'like that of cattle' (*tou boos*) with a very long forehead; he had a 'languid' mind and a weak and 'effeminate' soul, in contradiction to which Psellos described him as having a 'wild look' (*tôn ommatôn agrion*) about him yet preferring to occupy himself with feminine tasks.[86] Kellenberger pointed out that the Greek phrase *tôn ommatôn agrion* can mean not just a wild look, but could also refer to a rigid, inflexible, staring look.[87] And one may cite the Arabic Galenist, Ibn Ridwan (c. 988–c. 1061, commentator on the *Tegni, or Ars Parva*, which via the twelfth-century translation by Gerard of Cremona found its way into the Latin tradition), who wrote that 'smallness [of the head] is the essential sign of a bad brain composition' because it 'constricts the channels and ventricles ... [and] the soul spirits do not have enough space in the brain to let them move on freely to complete their operations'.[88]

Physicality of idiocy: minds, bodies and wonders

The theme of a physiognomy of stupidity was popularised by Konrad of Megenberg (1309–74), whose *Buch der Natur*, original title *Daz puch von den naturleichen dingen*, written 1348/50 contained two sections of interest to us. Book I, on human nature and condition (*Von dem menschen in seiner gemainen natur*), was made by Konrad as a free translation of Thomas of Cantimpré's *Liber de natura rerum* (1233–40). Konrad omitted the section on *De anima*, which Thomas had dealt with in Book II of his work, but instead added the physiognomics of Rhases, *Liber Almansoris*. In Book VIII, 2 and 3, respectively 'Von den wunder menschen' and 'Von den wunderleichen laeuten', Konrad discussed wonders, with a final section on wondrous people. Konrad here also drew heavily on the *Liber de natura rerum* by Thomas of Cantimpré, writing about the category of monstrous individuals, in which he put not just the usual physical aberrants but also included the 'natural fools', i.e. those we would now consider to be mentally retarded.

This is where natural fools are functionally different from normal humans. According to the logic of Konrad's *Book of Nature* there is a causal relationship between exterior and interior; the deviant anatomy of a brain is therefore also recognisable in the head shape of the natural fool.[89] Thus Konrad refers to marked differences in the shape of the cranium in fools, basing this on physiognomic theories of the time. In his section 'von den zaichen der naturleichen siten' [on the signs of natural demeanour] (Book I,49), with subsections on physiognomy he discusses how the form of a person and of their limbs delineates for us their natural demeanour. All the constituent characteristics are put together as follows in Book I,49.27 'Wer stumpfs synns sey' [who is of blunted sense, i.e. stupid]:

> The person of a stupid nature is either very pale or coloured very dark, has a fat belly and bent fingers. His face is round and very fleshy. But also he is stupid whose neck and feet, in fact whose whole body, is very fleshy. His belly is round and protruding. His shoulders drawn up towards the head. His forehead is round as a ball, humped and fleshy. His jaws are strongly developed and his legs long. His face is long and the neck thick.
>
> (Der ist einr stumpfen natur, der gar weiss ist oder gar praun vnd hat einen groezzen pauch vnd chrump vinger. Sein antluetz ist gar sinbel vnd hat vil flaisches auf den wangen. Der ist auch stumpf, der vol fleisches ist auf dem hals vnd auf den fuezzen vnd an den stucken dez leibes, die da zwischen sint. Sein pauch ist sinbel vnd pauzzt her fuer. Sein ahseln sint erhebt gegen dem haupt. Sein stirn ist sinbel geleich einem pallen, fam ob si hofrot sei, vnd hat vil flaisch. Sein chinbacken sint grozz vnd seinew pain lanck. Sein antluetz ist lank vnd der hals grozz.)[90]

Konrad here wants to demonstrate the teaching of Rhases according to his book on medicine.[91] Putting all this together, Konrad states that one may recognise natural fools because they have unseemly heads, either too large or too small.[92] But really and more accurately natural fools can be identified by their actions, because they do not act according to the actions of ensouled people but yet have a human soul like children do.[93] Thus the rational soul of natural fools (*naturleichen torn*) is only as evident as it is in children – Konrad is here repeating the long-established notion of the cognitively disabled as perpetual children – but a closer description of what brain damage or neurological defects might cause a disruption to the powers of the soul is not to be found in the *Buch der Natur*. 'The mental difference of natural fools is only explicable from a congenitally deviant brain structure, which is not to be understood as an illness. Their deviance is rather to be seen as a unique extraordinary appearance and therefore justifies their inclusion in the section on wondrous peoples.'[94] One may add to the medieval observations of Konrad that such notions were still alive and well in the early modern period, so that the discourse of idiocy sometimes characterised people with mental disabilities as also having physical differences, such as a deformed appearance, mainly due to decreased height (stunted, dwarfish or crooked).[95]

Konrad of Megenberg also describes people who are marvels of nature, which he categorises as being of two sorts: one sort had a human soul even if their body did not appear very human, while the other sort may have the appearance of humans but did not have a human soul (the latter may be an allusion to so-called 'wild children' or to apes). Amongst the marvellous people with a human soul, Konrad distinguished further between those with a bodily defect and those with mental defects, although Konrad is eager to point out that both kinds derived from Adam, stating that without Adam's original sin all persons would be born without defects. Those marvellous people who were born with defects Konrad termed the natural fools who in Latin are called *moriones* ('natürleichen tôren, die ze latein muriones haizent'),[96] and whose head was 'unseemly' (*ungeschicket*), that is, too large or too small. Those marvellous people who had acquired defects were those who had grown up in the woods far away from sensible people and living like the beasts ('in den wäldern erzogen werdent vern von den vernünftigen läuten und lebent samt daz vieh').[97] These passages are given from Book VIII,2 and 3 are worth citing in full.

On monstrous races:

> There are two kind of wondrous people, those with souls and those without. To the former I count those who have a human soul, but who suffer an infirmity. The

unsouled however remind on the outside somewhat of the human form but they do not posses a soul. The ensouled wondrous people in turn fall into two groups, those with bodily and those with mental defects. Both are descended from Adam and his sins, since I believe that, had the first man not sinned, all people would be born without infirmity.

(Es giebt der Wundermenschen zwei Arten, die einen sind beseelt, die anderen nicht. Zu den ersteren rechne ich die, die eine menschliche Seele haben, aber mit Gebrechen behaftet sind. Die Unbeseelten dagegen erinnern zwar äusserlich einigermassen an die menschliche Gestalt, haben aber keine Seele. Die beseelten Wundermenschen zerfallen ihrerseits wieder in zwei Gruppen, solche mit körperlichen und solche mit seelischen Mängeln. Beide stammen von Adam und seinen Sünden ab, denn ich glaube, das, hätte der erste Mensch nicht gesündigt, alle Menschen ohne Gebrechen geboren würden.)[98]

On natural versus artificial fools:

Of the ensouled wondrous people who have mental defects, there are two kinds. Some are like this since birth, others by habit. Those born with mental infirmities are the naturally mentally disabled, who in Latin are called muriones [*recte moriones*]. In them the place for mental faculties within the skull is not properly developed. One can recognise them by their unseemly, too large or too small heads. They do not act according to the impulse of a human soul, although they do possess a soul, just like children. Those who have mental infirmities by habit are those who have grown up far away from sensible people in the woods and live like beasts. All these wondrous peoples are descended from Adam.

(Der beseelten Wundermenschen, die seelische Mängel haben, giebt es zwei Arten. Einige sind von Geburt an, andere durch Gewohnheit so geschaffen. Die mit dem seelischen Gebrechen Geborenen sind die natürlichen Geisteskranken, die lateinisch Muriones heissen. Bei ihnen ist der Raum für die seelischen Kräfte im Schädel nicht richtig entwickelt. Man erkennt diese daran, dass sie unförmliche, zu grosse oder zu kleine Köpfe haben. Sie handeln nicht nach den Impulsen der Menschenseele, trotzdem sie eine Seele besitzen, grade wie die Kinder. Diejenigen, die durch Gewohnheit seelische Gebrechen haben, sind die, welche ferne von den vernünftigen Menschen in den Wäldern aufgewachsen sind und wie das Vieh dahinleben. Alle diese Wundermenschen stammen von Adam ab.)[99]

Konrad's distinction between *wunder menschen* and *wunderleichen laüten* follows the wider distinction between *miraculi* and *mirabilia*, based on Thomas of Cantimpré, whereby wondrous things are distinguished according to their causality. Thus *mirabilia* are still subject to the divine order and are wondrous only because they are preternatural, whereas *miracula* come about through the complete revocation of natural laws by direct divine interference.[100] Exotic species are part of the *mirabilia*, but individuals are part of *miracula*. Therefore, for Konrad, *wunder menschen* are the monstrous individuals and thus *miracula*, to which he reckons natural fools, whereas exotic other human (we would say ethnic) groups, the *wunderleichen laeut*, are only *mirabilia*. One needs to add that Konrad was not just drawing on Thomas of Cantimpré, but on the earlier *Otia imperialia* (c. 1210/15) of Gervase of Tilbury.[101] Gervase had discussed the novelty value of the extraordinary – and incidentally, thereby perhaps had given a reason for the keeping of fools and jesters at court – except that he had to avoid calling novelty something done out of inquisitiveness or curiosity (*curiositas*), which would have been censured, as ever since Augustine[102] theoretical curiosity, that is, what we now call science, was suspect. Investigating into phenomena ran the danger of interfering with divine creation.[103] The third book of the *Otia imperialia* consists of 143 chapters on miracles and marvels, while the first two books had been more of a traditional description of the world in the footsteps of Isidore's *Etymologiae* or the *Imago mundi* (written in various redactions between 1107 and 1139) of Honorius Augustodunensis.[104] Gervase wrote in his preface to the third book:

> And since the appetite of the human mind is always keen to hear and lap up novelties, the oldest things will have to be presented as new, natural things as miraculous, and things familiar to us all, as strange. For we reckon that things are adjudged novelties on four criteria: for their originality, or their recentness, or their rarity, or their strangeness. So, anything that is newly created gives pleasure by reason of the working of nature. Anything that has only just happened causes excitement, less if it happens often, more if it is rare. When anything strange is observed we seize on it, partly because of the inversion of the natural order which surprises us, partly because of our ignorance of the cause, whose working is a mystery to us; and partly because of seeing our expectation cheated in unfamiliar circumstances of which we lack a proper understanding. From these causes arise two things, miracles and marvels, though they both result in wonderment. Now we generally call those things miracles which, being preternatural, we ascribe to divine power, as when a virgin gives birth, when Lazarus is raised from the dead, or when diseased limbs are made whole again; while we call those things marvels which are beyond our comprehension, even though they are natural; in fact the inability to explain why a thing is so constitutes a marvel.
>
> (Et quoniam humane mentis auiditas ad audiendas ac hauriendas nouitates semper accuitur, antiquissima commutari necesse erit in noua, naturalia in mirabilia, apud plerosque usitata in inaudita. Censemus enim noua quadruplici ratione iudicari: aut creatione, aut euentu, aut raritate, aut inauditu. Que ergo noua creantur delectant ex nature motu. Que nuper eueniunt, si frequentia minus, si rara plus habent admirationis. Que inaudita percipiuntur amplectimur, tum ex mutatione cursus naturalis quam admiramur, tum ex ignorancia cause cuius ratio nobis est imperscrutabilis, tum ex assuetudine nostra quam in aliis

uariari sine cognitione iudicii iusti cernimus. Ex hiis, duo proueniunt: miracula et mirabilia, cum utrorumque finis sit admiratio. Porro miracula dicimus usitatius que preter naturam diuine uirtuti ascribimus, ut cum uirgo parit, cum Lazarus resurgit, cum lapsa membra reintegrantur. Mirabilia uero dicimus que nostre cognicioni non subiacent, etiam cum sunt naturalia; sed et mirabilia constituit ignorantia reddende rationis quare sic sit.)[105]

Gervase here emphasised 'customary experience' as the crucial litmus test, so that marvels and miracles became relative to the observer. What was novel to one person might be mundane to another and its mystique might be lost through the acquisition of better information (which is also what the modern notion of 'scientific progress' is supposedly meant to be about). Banks and Binns note in their edition that 'Gervase was not the first to define a marvel as something natural but unexplained',[106] as William of Newburgh (*Historia rerum Anglicarum*, i.28) has already done so, but the distinction between marvel and miracle became a commonplace henceforth.[107] Curious or novel things are therefore fine, as long as they are defined as divinely influenced (*miracula*) or as those astonishing things which have not been explained (*mirabilia*). From the mid-twelfth through the mid-fifteenth centuries textual witnesses regarded wonders as something generally positive, since embodying the marvellous, divine creation wonders were to elicit both awe and pleasure, and by virtue of their miraculous nature elevated the experience of wonder. 'The contemporary natural philosophical tradition, however, presented wonder with more ambivalence.'[108] In the latter, wonder was seen as springing from ignorance of the natural causes; superstition, confusion and intellectual backwardness prevent the understanding of 'the natural order as a complicated and semi-autonomous chain of secondary causes that depended distantly, but only distantly, on the First Cause, God'.[109] It is therefore tempting to equate the scholastic medieval, essentially Aristotelian, notion of a body of universal and knowable 'truths' with the modern notion of 'science'. But science (a word used in its present sense only since the nineteenth century) includes much that medieval philosophers 'would have rejected as lowly and fallible guesswork, while it excludes theology, which they considered to be the model of *scientia*, since it dealt with the immutable realm of the divine'.[110]

As we have seen, in the second section of Book VIII Konrad turned to the individual wonders, for which modern research has not been able to identify a source.[111] This is possibly Konrad's personal contribution to the knowledge of his times, and he developed his own classification and aetiology of human wonders. Some human wonders possessed souls, others did not, but natural fools were firmly located into the ensouled category. Konrad argued that different structures of the brain in such individual wondrous people were the cause for natural fools. He believed, following established theories of brain cells and ventricles, that the *fantastica* of the first chamber formed the common sense, where sensory input from all five senses came together, before this information was imparted to the second chamber, the seat of reason (Book I,1). Note that Groß had interpreted the presence of congenital defect as implying only physical defect, and treated the acquired defects as the purely psychological ones, seemingly confusing congenital with physical and acquired with psychological/psychiatric. Groß (mis)read Konrad's statements on congenital versus acquired defects as equating physical versus mental.[112] Rather, for me, Konrad of Megenberg seems to quite accurately describe the difference between on the one hand people with some form of ID, something ingrained and natural, and on the other hand the cultural phenomenon of developmental deficiencies due to lack of socialisation, both descriptions quite neatly tying in with the more conventional medieval differentiation between natural and artificial fools. Of interest also is his mention of too large a head (hydrocephalus?) or too small a head (microcephalic?) as physical phenomena, something the strictly medical tracts discussed above had not considered worth noting.

Nicole Oresme (c. 1320/25–82) in *De causis mirabilium* also treated of miracles. He touched on the uncertainty of whether the child or the foetus is a man (i.e. human), and argued for the importance of mental and sensory defects in determining human status:

> Thus we see that it is always uncertain whether the child or the fetus is a man until the point where it can be determined whether or not it is capable of reason; and if not, it seems to me that it ought more to be determined that way that it is not a man, rather than doing so at the moment of birth because of bodily appearance and suchlike, for in human nature it is a greater monstrosity to be defective in sense organs and in those of the mind than in other bodily members.
> (Ideo videtur quon semper esset dubitandum utrum puer vel fetus sit homo usquequo videatur si possit uti ratione; quod si non, videtur michi quod magis deberet credi in casibus positis quod non sit homo, quam in principio nativitatis propter diversam figuram et cetera, quia in natura humana est maior monstruositas defectus in membris sensuum et sedibus seu organis anime quam in aliis membris.)[113]

Therefore mental faculties are deemed more important than physical appearance overall, or the shape and form of the body in general. One can read Oresme in sympathy with Augustine, who in the *City of God* 16:8 emphatically places so-called monsters with the human, no matter how physically deformed they are, provided they are a rational and mortal being – hence privileging reason above all other criteria for what it is that makes a creature human. 'If anything, the transformation of body seems less threatening than that of mind, given that the possession of a rational faculty is often cited as the fundamental defining trait of a human being.'[114]

John Metham wrote in the mid-fifteenth century, his work surviving in a unique manuscript containing a romance, together with treatises on palmistry, physiognomy and the days of the moon. He called himself a 'sympyl scoler of philosophye',[115] making mediocre translations and compilations from standard Latin texts for a probably equally mediocre patron, a member of the middling nobility of Norfolk. Metham may be credited with noting that 'rounded ears, excessively narrow nasal passages and tapering shoulders (all characteristic of trisomy-21) signified foolishness and 'a man dysposyd to no kunnyng'.[116] Samples of the sort of phrases Metham compiled are as follows: 'A scort scapyn hed ys with-owte wytt and wysdam. ... A gret hed, with a gret forhed and a gret face, betokynnyth slowthe, mekenes, and hard to be taught.' Also, an uneven head, or a crooked-shaped head, demonstrate 'foltyschnes' (foolishness). 'Gret erys, thei sygnyfye foltyschnes. ... Erys the qwych be round off schap, thei sygnyfe onabylte off lernyng. ... Sstreyt nosethyrlys and round and very smale, thei sygnyffye foltyschnes. ... They the qwche haue passyng fulle nekkys, grete and fatte and schort, thei be hasty and hard to be taught. ... Feette, qwan thei be flat with a lowe instep and fulle off flesch, thei sygnyfye a foltysch persone.'[117]

Beek cited a case from the medical observations of Pieter Van Foreest (1521–97), a physician working in Alkmaar and Delft, who, although a sixteenth-century doctor, still encapsulated the medieval approach to patient histories. The borderline between medieval and Renaissance is not a straight line, but one with peaks and troughs that sometimes reach far into the Renaissance, then again recede deep back into the Middle Ages.[118] This concerns Cornelius Nicolaas of Alkmaar, whom the children nicknamed Kesius, who stammered and spoke badly since his early youth.

> He was feeble-minded and a fool, although he was very stubborn ... From nose and mouth a thin trickle of phlegmatic fluid flowed, especially when he spoke. This came from his cold cerebrum, as I presumed. A surgeon tried unsuccessfully to cure him from this. These patients always have these deviations from the cradle onwards [i.e. congenitally]. Furthermore he had a misshapen, small and pointed head ... When this feeble-minded person had reached adulthood he stayed in the town of Naarden. This town was taken by the Spanish and even this unfortunate man was, although innocent, slaughtered with all the other men of the town. How awful is that war, which does not even spare the silly innocents. (Hij was een zwakzinnige en een dwaas, hoewel hij zeer eigenzinnig was ... Uit neus en mond vloeide gedurig een dun flegmatisch vocht af, vooral als hij sprak. Dit kwam voort uit zijn koude cerebrum, zoals ik veronderstel. Een chirurg poog

detevergeefs hem hiervan te genezen. Deze patiënten hebben immers van de wieg af deze afwijking. Voorts had hij een vervormd, klein en puntig hoofd ... Toen deze zwakzinnige tot volwassenheit gekomen was, verbleef hij in de stad Naarden. Deze stad werd ingenomen door de Spanjaarden en ook deze ongelukkige werd, hoewel onschuldig, afgeslacht met alle andere mannen uit die stad. Hoe afschuwelijk is de oorlog, die zelfs de onschuldige onnozelen niet spaart.)[119]

In this admittedly slightly off-period case – Naarden was taken by the Spanish in 1572, which event dates Cornelius Nicolaas' death – we nevertheless encounter all the features of physicality that medieval physicians in general and Konrad of Megenberg in particular had catalogued: the cold complexion of the cerebrum, the moist humor emanating from phlegm, the intractable nature of the condition, congenital origin, unusual head shape, and regarded as 'innocent' – a topic that will be more fully explored in the following chapters.

With advances in the understanding of genetics, of DNA and of molecular biology, modern science is, in a circuitous way, returning to the physicality of medieval medical theory. Thus Neaman surmised that recognition of the importance of such physical causes and an increasing conceptual shift in modern biomedical science toward an interdependence of body and mind is a sea-change that would have strongly appealed to medieval medicine and physiology. Despite many differences between modern psychiatry and medieval medicine and natural philosophy, there are also similarities. 'Our "primitive precursors" arrived at many of the same conclusions we have, but their reasons for reaching them were different from ours. From the present-minded point of view, we are bound to say that medieval physicians had the right ideas for the wrong reasons.'[120]

Medieval institutions: treatment or confinement?

Some historiographic controversy has been caused by the late-medieval German custom of allegedly confining mentally ill or disabled people in purpose-built structures variously referred to as *Narrenhäuser* or *Dollkisten*. Bertram made the interesting observation that the evaluation of the term *Narrenhaus* requires caution, since it had a different meaning in the past to today, due to the custom of confining people who disturbed the peace (e.g. through drunken behaviour) in see-through cells so that they could be mocked and ridiculed, reminiscent of the stocks; such houses were termed *Narrenhäuser* because their inmates were to be *genarrt*, to be made fools of.[121] Thus the *Narrenhäuser* were not originally intended to house mentally ill (or mentally disabled) people; however, the *Narrenkisten* or *Dollkisten* were, as in the *dorden Kisten* instituted by the council of Lübeck and first recorded in

1471, or the *cista stolidorum* (mentioned 1376) at Hamburg. Scheerenberger was probably carried away by the use of the term *stolidorum*, since he asserted, without evidence, that it was the mentally retarded who were confined to a tower in the city wall which he translated as 'Idiot's Cage'.[122] This exemplifies the dangers of transposing modern meanings of a translation (Latin *stolidus* into modern English 'idiot') onto medieval meanings of the same lexeme; just because a word is formed of the same letters does not entail that it actually *means* the same.

The Lübeck *dorden Kisten* were situated just outside two of the town gates, with windows facing the road – presumably so that inmates could receive alms from passers-by, since the provisions were scanty and insufficient. Wealthier burghers of Lübeck therefore petitioned the council that their relatives who had been declared 'insane' were to be housed in a room in one of the prison towers instead, at costs carried by the family, as documents from the years 1465 to 1478 testify.[123] But in the 1470s the court scribe Peter Monnik and three other Lübeck burghers pledged to personally care for and provide for 'the poor imbeciles and senseless people' (*armen Dullen und afsinnige Lude*), with the council naming them preceptors (*Vorständer*) of the *Narrenkisten*. Their philanthropic example was followed in 1479 by Gerd Sunderbeck, who bequeathed 700 Lübeck marks to the 'poor witless people, who sit in front of the gates and portals in the mad-chests'.[124] In summary, in the German regions medieval 'care' of the mentally ill existed only in so far as those people deemed dangerous or disturbing were confined, in the interests of public order and protection of the 'public good', while those deemed harmless – which more often than not meant the intellectually disabled – were allowed to wander about or to work under supervision. Relatives were responsible in the first instance, failing which the mentally ill were confined in the hospitals of prisons.[125] In all this there is no mention of medical treatment.

The question of the presence of people with ID in medieval hospitals was echoed by the authors of a dedicated history of Bethlem Hospital, who concluded that if the medieval period 'operated a form of "care in the community", it was ... very much a *laissez-faire*, reactive system'.[126] Stainton's main findings, based on literature analysis, were that some people with ID were found in the medieval equivalent of 'institutions' in the modern sense, mainly hospitals and alms-houses, but that their presence should not be interpreted as institutionalisation in a twentieth-century sense, but rather as support provided to people who primarily had fallen into poverty and only secondarily happened to be intellectually disabled. For medieval English hospitals, Stainton found doubtful evidence for only one hospital, out of around 1,100 institutions, that specifically mentioned ID.[127] This is the hospital of St John the Baptist in

Chester, founded 'for the sustentation of poor and silly persons' by the Earl of Chester and Richmond who died in 1232, but no further details are given.[128] This absence of hard evidence also frustrated Clarke, who had to rely on older, second-hand information, stating that 'there was a hospital at Chester for poor silly people before the time of Henry III, that is before 1216', and admitting that 'little seems known'.[129] Other than this lone example, Stainton had no medieval evidence, or even presumed evidence, since his next mention of the presence of 'idiots' or similar people in an English hospital comes from the late sixteenth century, at St James and St Mary Magdalene of Chichester, by then an alms-house.[130] In fact there was one English institution just at the end of the Middle Ages which did cater for people with ID: in 1514 the statutes of Wyggeston's Hospital, Leicester, provided for twelve unmarried men who should be 'blind, decrepit, paralytic, or maimed in their limbs, and idiots wanting in their natural senses, so that they be peaceable, not disturbing'.[131] The emphasis on 'peaceable' behaviour as a characteristic of 'idiots' is what distinguished the person with ID from the person with mental illness, the *furiosus* or *freneticus*, in medieval medical thinking.

For the medieval precursor to a modern institutional setting we need to look to a Spanish example. The foundation charter of the Valencia hospital, issued in 1410 by Martin I, King of Aragon, appears to mention people with ID, the 'innocents':

> As it is an Institution of Mercifulness and very pious deed to care for those who are in need, not only in corpus due to weakness or fault of members of infirmity but more if the need is due to weakness of understanding or discretion, by innocence, madness of insanity, as such people cannot and do not know how to subvene to their life, even in the case of being bodily strong and robust, as they are constituted in such innocence of madness, their free communication with other people results in damage, dangers and other inconveniences.[132]

The foundation myth alleges that Father Jofré was motivated by a key experience on 24 February 1409, since while out and about on the streets he witnessed some children teasing and maltreating a madman, which prompted him that same day to address his audience at the cathedral with this sermon:

> there is still outstanding a big need, such as is a hospital or house where the poor innocents and frantics may be sheltered; as there are a lot of poor innocents and frantics going astray through this town, enduring hard rebuffs, hunger, cold and injuries. As such, on account of their innocence and madness can not neither earn or request what they necessarily need for their own sustenance, for which reason they sleep in the streets in peril through famine and cold; wicked persons, who not having God before the eyes of their conscience, sorely injure and hurt

them; most particularly whenever they find them sleeping, they vex them, bring-
ing shame on some females. The poor frantics as well, cause damage to many
persons who go through the streets. ... it would be a saintly thing and a very
saintly doing, if in Valencia were built a lodging or hospital where such insanes
and innocents stayed in such a way that they neither go through the city or could
harm anybody or be themselves harmed.[133]

This is an important passage, since it covers a number of issues in relation to
ID. Firstly, the consistent juxtaposition of innocents with insane/frantics/
madmen indicates that the innocents were seen as separate and distinct from
other forms of mental disorders; secondly, some of the social consequences
of ID are mentioned, in that the poor innocents, that is probably those economically too poor to be supported by a kinship group, were left wandering
by themselves and hence easy pickings for verbal and physical abuse; which,
thirdly, also mentions specifically the sexual abuse of female 'innocents', a
topic even rarely touched on in modern discussions of ID and all the less in
medieval texts. The poverty of mentally ill and disabled persons, due partly
to an inability to beg effectively, is also highlighted for northern German
towns. Such people are mentally incapable of the elaborated technique of
begging and, more importantly, are unable to fulfil their part of the reciprocal
arrangement of begging – unlike the blind, crippled, leprous – whereby the
recipient of charitable alms is duty bound to say a prayer for the soul of the
donor.[134]

When it comes to therapies for ID, not surprisingly, due to the permanent
and intractable nature of the condition, there is next to nothing in pre-modern
sources. For late antiquity, harsh treatment, not to say shock therapy, is
attested in the case of the mentally retarded, being 'treated' with whips or
clubs.[135] As so often, modern authors have confused treatment for mental
illness with treatment for mental disability. Walker cited the tenth-century
Anglo-Saxon scribe Cild and his recipes, some of which concern herbal con-
coctions to be drunk, sometimes out of special vessels such as church bells,
with similar remedies for the 'feeble-minded'.[136] Drinking out of a church bell
is in Bald's Leechbook, but is applied for a demoniac and not an idiot as Walker
had erroneously claimed.[137] Another recipe by Bald appears to be more prom-
ising: 'Against mental vacancy [*ungemynde*] and against folly [*dysgunge*]; put
into ale bishopwort, lupins, betony, the southern or Italian fennel, nepte, water
agrimony, cockle, marche, then let the man drink. For idiotcy [*ungemynde*]
and folly [*disgunge*], put into ale, cassia, and lupins, bishopwort, alexanders,
githrife, fieldmore, and holy water; then let him drink.'[138] But the word
ungemynde can also mean 'forgetful, heedless', and although *dysgung* possibly
means mentally retarded it can also imply general madness.[139]

Absence of ID in medieval medical texts?

On the almost materialist approach to mental illness (i.e. humoral causality, treatments by what we would call chemical measures) by medieval physicians, Harvey noted that 'the doctors were led to the treatment of disordered reason almost as though it were a purely physical function; whereas the philosophers insisted that reason as such fell outside of medical control'.[140] This is one possible reason for why medical texts say next to nothing about ID, but theological-philosophical texts do. In the former sort ID is regarded as an intractable permanent state that defies treatment, whereas in the latter there is no interest in treatment, but in the very presence of ID, which poses interesting academic problems for analyses of what it is to be human, and how deviations from the norm can be explained as part of divine creation. Clarke provided another reason why ID rarely features in medical texts which, interestingly, is rather different from the more frequently encountered one of the incurability and intractable nature of ID. 'One relatively numerous group of people with whom the populace at large probably had more familiarity, and more practical wisdom in handling, was that of the mental defectives, those of low native capacity. The extent of "community care" in their management was such that they did not really become a medical textbook topic.'[141]

Medieval medical texts tended to focus on three types of mental disorder (phrenitis, melancholia and mania) that had already been described in classical and late antique texts. The nearest thing to mental disability ever mentioned in such medical texts might be 'lethargy', which, like congenital idiocy, was associated with too much cold and moisture. Lethargy 'is representative of a group of disorders which involved extreme somnolence or stupor and were conceived of as cold diseases, calling for remedies to warm and stimulate the patient and to thin and disperse an accumulation of phlegm'.[142] On the rare occasions where medical texts say anything at all on congenital idiots, this is as far as it goes. Humoral reasons concerned with wet and cold are the main aetiologies, and the few therapeutics attempted tended to reflect the 'warming' actions.

Jackson made the interesting point that most of what we now call madness was considered a disorder of the brain by classical and late antique physicians, while conditions like lethargy were grouped with disorders of the soul. Disorders of the soul were regarded as 'strictly psychological ... a disorder of the soul being conceived of without underlying physiological dysfunction rather than as a disorder of the *soul-and-brain*'.[143] This differentiation may be overly simplistic, but for speculation as to why there were no medical cures, never mind miracle healings, of fools and idiots, this may be leading in the right direction. All the conditions cured by miracle (deaf, blind, dumb, crip-ples) are somatic, since even the sensory impairments have a physiological basis. And the miracle cures of insanity would actually nicely fit the antique/medieval medical model, which regarded certain types of mental disorder as firmly anchored in humoral pathology, and hence somatic in nature. By further extension, mental illness lay within the domain of the curable, by either medical or miraculous means. But disorders of the soul seem to fall outside that. The basic distinction is between God-determined and unchangeable, on the one hand, and temporary and curable (whether by pills or prayer), on the other hand. The soul is God's alone: perhaps that is why even the appeal to miracle fails with regard to idiots.

According to medieval notions, the human is part of both the external material world and the higher immaterial world. 'The inward wits stand at the point of communication between these two worlds in man, between the body and the soul, the realm of sense, and the realm of intellect. They fill a gap in the medieval scheme of things.'[144] The inward wits can also be collectively referred to as the spirit. 'The spirit is the border between body and soul, the middle term linking the two extremes of immaterial and material. It mediates between animal perception and angelic reason, as man himself is the middle term between the beasts and the angels.'[145] But not all theologians/philosophers agreed with this description. Aristotelians like Albertus Magnus and Thomas Aquinas preferred to regard spirit as an instrument, rather than a medium between soul and body.[146] For Aquinas, a person was not just defined by soul but was an entity composed of both body and soul (homo non est anima tantum, sed est aliquid compositum ex anima et corpore).[147] 'Aquinas's insist-ence on man's composite nature, rather than on his intellect in isolation, leads to a momentous change of emphasis: a re-assertion of the debt intellect owes to sensation.'[148] What this means for people with ID is that in philosophical – and medical – terms a more materialist explanation of ID can be postulated, in that if some aspect of the sensory input is damaged (through illness, accident or what we now call genetic mutation), then insufficient or none of the infor-mation needed for the intellect to process it actually reaches the intellect, and then that alone may explain why some people appear mentally disabled.

The 'chain of being', in which authors like Nemesius placed humans, 'may be regarded in two ways: as a progress from the material to the immaterial, and from the insentient to the intelligent'.[149] The transition from material to immaterial is at that location where the animal spirit, or the inward wits, reside. The point of intersection might be difficult (or impossible) to define, but that stopped neither medieval philosophers nor physicians from trying. Natural philosophers approached the question of reason, rationality and knowledge by asking about the soul, how sensory and physical information (hence acquired through the body) impacted on the soul. Medieval physicians looked to the same question of what is reason or knowledge by examining how physiological trauma, bodily injury and corporal defects affected the soul. 'Both medicine and philosophy contributed to the final formulation of the idea of the inward wits; but the idea developed differently in the two disciplines.'[150] Now that we have looked at the material, in modern terms 'neurological', basis of ID in medieval texts, these remarks now lead in to the following chapter, on the intangible 'psychology' of mind and soul.

Notes

1   Judith S. Neaman, *Suggestion of the Devil: Insanity in the Middle Ages and the Twentieth Century* (New York: Octagon Books, 1978), 14.

2   Basil Clarke, *Mental Disorder in Earlier Britain: Exploratory Studies* (Cardiff: University of Wales Press, 1975), 64.

3   Aristotle, *De sensu*, 437a10–16, English by J. I. Beare (trans.), 'Sense and Sensibilia', in Jonathan Barnes (ed.), *The Complete Works of Aristotle: The Revised Oxford Translation* (Princeton: Princeton University Press, 1984), 694.

4   Book V.xii, *On the Properties of Things: John Trevisa's Translation of* Bartholomæus Anglicus De proprietatibus Rerum. *A Critical Text*, Vol. I, eds M. C. Seymour and Colleagues (Oxford: Clarendon Press, 1975), 191.

5   Ynez Violé O'Neill, *Speech and Speech Disorders in Western thought Before 1600* (Westport, CT and London, 1980), 71, 72, 73–4.

6   Dirk Matejovski, *Das Motiv des Wahnsinns in der mittelalterlichen Dichtung* (Frankfurt-a-M.: Suhrkamp, 1996), 318n39.

7   Book VII.vi, *On the Properties of Things*, 349.

8   Book VII.vii, *On the Properties of Things*, 350.

9   Matejovski, *Motiv des Wahnsinns*, 61–2.

10 Simon Kemp, *Medieval Psychology* (New York: Greenwood Press, 1990), 114.

11 Passage 51,12–14, Philoponus, *On Aristotle's 'On the Soul 1.1–2'*, trans. Philip J. van der Eijk (Ithaca: Cornell University Press, 2005), 68, 134n375. On memory and physiology cf. Aristotle, *On Memory and Recollection*, 449b7–8 and 450a31.

12 Thomas Aquinas, *Summa theologiae* [hereafter *ST*], I, question 2, article 54, 4; I, question 2, article 51, 4.

13 Kemp, *Medieval Psychology*, 157–8, with *ST*, I, question 2, articles 50–3.

14 Edgar Kellenberger, *Der Schutz der Einfältigen. Menschen mit einer geistigen Behinderung in der Bibel und in weiteren Quellen* (Zurich: Theologischer Verlag Zürich, 2011), 59–60.

15 Rudolph E. Siegel, *Galen on the Affected Parts: Translation from the Greek Text with Explanatory Notes* (Basel et al.: S. Karger, 1976), 80.

16 Edgar Kellenberger, 'Augustin und die Menschen mit einer geistigen Behinderung.

Der Theologe als Beobachter und Herausgeforderter', *Theologische Zeitschrift*, 67 (2011), 56–66, at 57.

17   Rudolph E. Siegel, *Galen on Psychology, Psychopathology and Function and Diseases of the Nervous System* (Basel: Karger, 1973), 274–5.

18   Siegel, *Galen on Psychology*, 26.

19   Siegel, *Galen on Psychology*, 27.

20   Siegel, *Galen on the Affected Parts*, 84.

21   Christopher Goodey, *A History of Intelligence and 'Intellectual Disability': The Shaping of Psychology in Early Modern Europe* (Farnham: Ashgate, 2011), 212.

22   Charles G. Gross, 'From Imhotep to Hubel and Wiesel: The Story of Visual Cortex', in Kathleen S. Rockland, Jon H. Kaas, Alan Peters (eds), *Extrastriate Cortex in Primates* (Cerebral Cortex Volume 12) (New York: Springer, 1997), 1–58, at 31.

23   Gross, 'From Imhotep to Hubel and Wiesel', 31 and 34.

24   Kemp, *Medieval Psychology*, 53; cf. Aristotle, *De anima*, 3.2–8; Galen, *On the Usefulness of the Parts of the Body*, ed. and trans. M. T. May (Ithaca, NY: Cornell University Press, 1968), 413–32. Note that the complete text of the latter was not fully translated until 1317, by Niccolò da Reggio, a bilingual doctor in the kingdom of Naples; cf. Lawrence I. Conrad, Michael Neve, Vivian Nutton, Roy Porter and Andrew Wear, *The Western Medical Tradition 800 BC to AD 1800* (Cambridge: Cambridge University Press, 1995), 177.

25   Kemp, *Medieval Psychology*, 54; cf. Augustine, *The Literal Meaning of Genesis*, *CSEL* 28.1, 7.18.24.

26   *Nemesius: On the Nature of Man*, trans. with intro. and notes R. W. Sharples and P. J. van der Eijk (Liverpool: Liverpool University Press, 2008), 121.

27   Kemp, *Medieval Psychology*, 54.

28   *Nemesius*, 122.

29   Simo Knuuttila, *Emotions in Ancient and Medieval Philosophy* (Oxford: Clarendon Press, 2004), 106.

30   William of Auvergne, *The Immortality of the Soul [De immortalitate animae]*, trans. and intro. Roland J. Teske (Milwaukee, WI: Marquette University Press, 1991), 41–2.

31   Therefore printed in Constantinus Africanus, *Opera* (Basel, 1539), 308–17; a more modern edition of Latin as *Costa-ben-Lucae, De differentia animae et spiritus Liber*, ed. C. S. Barach (Bibliotheca Philosophorum Mediae Aetatis) (1878).

32   E. Ruth Harvey, *The Inward Wits: Psychological Theory in the Middle Ages and the Renaissance* (London: Warburg Institute, University of London, 1975), 38.

33   *Robert Kilwardby O.P.: On Time and Imagination. Part 2: Introduction and Translation* by Alexander Broadie (Oxford: Oxford University Press, 1993), 88. 'Prima proposicio patet per uerba Aristotilis in 1 *Posteriorum*, quod deficiente sensu, deficit scientia secundum illum sensum', *Robert Kilwardby O.P.: On Time and Imagination: De Tempore. De Spiritu Fantastico*, ed. by P. Osmund Lewry O.P. (Oxford: Oxford University Press, 1987), 71; cf. *Analytica Posteriora*, trans.

Iacobi, ed. L. Minio-Paluello and B. G. Dod, *Aristoteles latinus*, 4, 1–4 (Leiden, 1968), i, 18 (81a38–40).

34 *Costa-ben-Lucae, De differentia animae et spiritus*, 2, ed. C. S. Barach (Bibliotheca philosophorum Mediae Aetatis 2) (Innsbruck, 1878), 126.

35 *Robert Kilwardby*, trans. Broadie, 113. Latin: 'docetur quod in anteriori parte cerebri sunt ventriculo duo in quibus operatur sensus communis et ymaginacio. Et inde procedunt multa paria neruorum, ita quod vnum par ad oculos ut in illis uideatur, et aliud ad aures ut in illis audiatur', *Robert Kilwardby*, ed. Lewry, 94.

36 *Robert Kilwardby*, trans. Broadie, 122–3.

37 *Robert Kilwardby*, ed. Lewry, 103.

38 Robert S. Kinsman, 'Folly, Melancholy, and Madness: A Study in Shifting Styles of Medical Analysis and Treatment, 1450–1675', in R. S. Kinsman (ed.), *The Darker Vision of the Renaissance: Beyond the Fields of Reason* (Berkeley: University of California Press, 1974), 273–320, at 298. The influential chapter 'Stupidity or Foolishness' is included in Thomas Willis' *De anima brutorum*, first published 1672, chapter reprinted *in toto* in J. J. Manget, *Bibliotheca medico-practica* (Geneva: Chouet, 1698); cf. Paul F. Cranefield, 'A Seventeenth Century View of Mental Deficiency and Schizophrenia: Thomas Willis on "Stupidity or Foolishness"', *Bulletin of the History of Medicine*, 35 (1961), 291–361.

39 *Anatomia vivorum*, 41; the text is published as *Anatomia Ricardi Anglici*, ed. R. von Töply (Vienna, 1902), 28, whose attribution to Ricardus Anglicus was disproved by K. Sudhoff, *Archiv für Geschichte der Medizin*, 8 (1914), 71–2.

40 *Robert Kilwardby*, trans. Broadie, 121; Latin: 'cerebrum in posteriori parte sui durius est propter neruos motiuos inde orientes, quia duriores habent esse quam nerui sensibiles. Et propter illam partem in qua est thesaurus memorie et repositio formarum.' *Robert Kilwardby*, ed. Lewry, 102.

41 Book V.iii, *On the Properties of Things*, 176; reference to Haly means the *Articella*.

42 Book III.xxii, *On the Properties of Things*, 122; 'ad cellulam logisticam, ad perficien-dum intellectum', Bartholomaeus Anglicus, *On the Properties of Soul and Body. De proprietatibus rerum libri III et IV*, ed. R. James Long (Toronto: PIMS, 1979), 55.

43 Book III.xxii, *On the Properties of Things*, 123; 'Vnus igitur et idem spiritus corpo-reus, subtilis tamen et aereus propter diuersa officia, in diuersis membris diuersis nominibus est vocatus. Nam spiritus naturalis est in epate; spiritus vero vitalis in corde; sed spiritus dicitur animalis prout in capite operatur.' Bartholomaeus Anglicus, *On the Properties of Soul and Body*, 56.

44 Book III.xxii, *On the Properties of Things*, 123; 'Vnde illis spiritibus lesis et in suis effectibus qualitercumque impeditis, resoluta corporis et anime [et] armonia, rationalis spiritus cunctis suis operationibus in corpore impeditur, vt patet in maniacis et in freneticis et aliis in quibus vsus rationis sepius non habet locum. Bartholomaeus Anglicus, *On the Properties of Soul and Body*, 56.

45 Kemp, *Medieval Psychology*, 58–9.

46 Gross, 'From Imhotep to Hubel and Wiesel', 35.

47 George Corner, *Anatomical Texts of the Earlier Middle Ages: A Study in the*

Transmission of Culture (Washington, DC: Carnegie Institution of Washington, 1927), 72; 67–86 gives full translation of *Anatomia Nicolai Physici*.

48 A term Averroes used for perishable entities; see Herbert A. Davidson, *Alfarabi, Avicenna, and Averroes, on Intellect: Their Cosmologies, Theories of the Active Intellect, and Theories of Human Intellect* (New York and Oxford: Oxford University Press, 1992), 336.

49 Davidson, *Alfarabi, Avicenna, and Averroes*, 300.

50 O'Neill, *Speech and Speech Disorders*, 128–9. See also Ynez V. O'Neill, 'William of Conches and the Cerebral Membranes', *Clio Medica*, 2 (1967), 13–21; T. Silverstein, 'Guillaume de Conches and Nemesius of Emessa: On the Sources of the "New Science" of the Twelfth Century', in *Harry Austryn Wolfson Jubilee Volume* (Jerusalem: American Academy for Jewish Research, 1965), vol. 2, 719–34.

51 Ynez Violé O'Neill, 'William of Conches' Description of the Brain', *Clio Medica*, 3 (1968), 203–23, at 207.

52 O'Neill, 'William of Conches' Description', 210.

53 *William of Conches: A Dialogue on Natural Philosophy (Dragmaticon Philosophiae)*, trans. Italo Ronca and Matthew Curr (Notre Dame, IN: University of Notre Dame Press, 1997), 141, Book VI, part two, 11.1.

54 *William of Conches*, trans. Ronca and Curr, 172, Book VI, part two, 26.8; based on Latin critical edition *Guillelmi de Conchis Dragmaticon*, ed. Italo Ronca (Guillelmi de Conchis opera omnia vol. I), *Corpus Christianorum Continuatio Mediaevalis*, 152 (Turnhout: Brepols, 1997).

55 *William of Conches*, trans. Ronca and Curr, 172, Book VI, part two, 26.9.

56 *William of Conches*, trans. Ronca and Curr, 173, Book VI, part two, 26.10.

57 *William of Conches*, trans. Ronca and Curr, 155, Book VI, part two, 18.6.

58 *William of Conches*, trans. Ronca and Curr, 170–1, Book VI, part two, chapter 26.1.

59 *William of Conches*, trans. Ronca and Curr, 171, Book VI, part two, chapter 26.4.

60 *William of Conches*, trans. Ronca and Curr, 171, Book VI, part two, chapter 26.4.

61 See *Guillaume de Conches, 'Glosae super Platonem'*, ed. E. Jeauneau (Paris: J. Vrin, 1965), 173, 284.

62 *William of Conches*, trans. Ronca and Curr, 172, Book VI, part two, chapter 26.7.

63 Anthony Kenny, *Aquinas on Mind* (London and New York: Routledge, 1993), 94–5, on *ST*, I, question 84, article 7.

64 Kemp, *Medieval Psychology*, 65–6; cf. Aquinas, *ST*, I, question 84, article 7 and I, question 85, article 5.

65 Avicenna, *Canon*, Part 3, chapter 4, as explained by Michael W. Dols (ed. Diana E. Immisch), *Majnûn: The Madman in Medieval Islamic Society* (Oxford: Clarendon Press, 1992), 78.

66 Clarke, *Mental Disorder in Earlier Britain*, 96.

67 H. H. Beek, *Waanzin in de Middeleeuwen: Beeld van de Gestoorde en Bemoeienis met de Zieke* (Haarlem: De Toorts/Nijkerk: G.F. Callenbach, 1969), 94, refering

to Arnaldus de Villanvoa, *Opera omnia* (Venice, 1514), fols 269–81: De parte operativa.

68 'Species alienationis simplicis alienatio, in quasi phantasiae vel imaginationis pravitas'; 'stultitia dicitur, quasi stupida laetitia, quoniam tales in extasi velut rapti laetantur, et rident sine causa exterius manifesta', *De parte operativa*, in *Arnaldi Villanovani philosophi* ..., 1585 (Hereford Cathedral Library M.6.1), 270.

69 Beek, *Waanzin in de Middeleeuwen*, 95: 'Een verminderde en opgeheven scientia treffen wij bij het ziektebeeld van de amentia en stoliditas aan. Deze patiënten verlangen ernaar als kinderen te zijn; zij lachen om dingen die zij doen; zij kunnen, gelijk kinderen, moeilijk gecorrigeerd worden. Zij worden lui en maken bouwwerken uit klei en stokken.'

70 'Valascus kreeg zulk een patiënt te behandelen die voortdurend lachte, vooral bij volle maan. Hij deed hem aderlaten en purgeren. Hij kreeg een neusbloeding en genas zo.' Beek, *Waanzin in de Middeleeuwen*, refering to Valascus de Taranta, *Philonium aureum ac perutile opus medicine* (Lyon, 1535), fol. 27v.

71 'Amentia voor ablatio, stoliditas voor diminutio. Anderen noemen het fatuitas of infantilitas. De zieken zijn als kinderen, die geen denkvermogen hebben, behalve wat er van nature is, zoals het sluiten van de ogen op het aanraken van de oogbol, het uitstreken van armen en handen om niet te vallen en steun te zoeken. Laat anderen maar over namen twisten, medici past dit niet.' Beek, *Waanzin in de Middeleeuwen*, 95–7, citing Johannes Michael Savonarola, *Practica major ... omnia morborum genera a capite usque ad pedes mortalibus advenientia curans* (Venice, 1547), fol. 66r.

72 Philip L. Reynolds, 'The Infants of Eden: Scholastic Theologians on Early Childhood and Cognitive Development', *Mediaeval Studies*, 68 (2006), 116; cf. Thomas Aquinas, *De veritate* 18.7 ad 3, and *ST* I, question 101, article 1, ad 2.

73 Albertus Magnus, *Physica*, pars I, liber 1, tr. 1, cap. 6, in Albertus-Magnus-Institut (ed.), *Albertus Magnus und sein System der Wissenschaften. Schlüsseltexte in Übersetzung Lateinisch-Deutsch* (Münster: Aschendorff, 2011), 136–7.

74 Albertus Magnus, *Physica*, pars I, liber 1, tr. 1, cap. 6, in *Albertus Magnus und sein System der Wissenschaften*, 144–5.

75 Saul M. Olyan, *Disability in the Hebrew Bible: Interpreting Mental and Physical Differences* (Cambridge: Cambridge University Press, 2008), 68.

76 H. R. Luard (ed.), *Matthaei Parisiensis, Monachi Sancti Albani, Chronica Majora*, vol. 2, *A.D. 1067 to A.D. 1216*, Rolls Series 57 (London, 1872), 1964, v. 632, 643.

77 Margaret Howell, 'The Children of King Henry III and Eleanor of Provence', *Thirteenth Century England*, vol. 4 (Proceedings of the Newcastle upon Tyne Conference 1991), ed. Peter R. Coss and Simon D. Lloyd (Woodbridge: Boydell, 1992), 57–72, at 63–4, esp. 64n48.

78 J. Langdon H. Down, 'Observations on an Ethnic Classification of Idiots', *London Hospital Reports*, 3 (1866), 259–62, at 261.

79 William F. MacLehose, *'A Tender Age': Cultural Anxieties over the Child in the Twelfth and Thirteenth Centuries* (New York: Columbia University Press, 2008),

1–31, chapter 'Nurturing Danger'. Cranefield, 'A Seventeenth-Century View of Mental Deficiency', 311, listed physical insults to the body which could affect fetal development so that parents engendered imbecilic children.

80 Albertus Magnus, *De natura boni*, tr.2, p.3, c.2, 2, 3, A, 1, 1. Albertus is here following the ideas of Firmicus Maternus, *Matheseos*, IV, c1, n.10; cited by B. B. Price, 'The Physical Astronomy and Astrology of Albertus Magnus', in *Albertus Magnus and the Sciences*, ed. J. A. Weisheipl (Toronto: PIMS, 1980), 180–1.

81 British Library MS Harley 45, fol. 119v, cited in Carole Rawcliffe, *Leprosy in Medieval England* (Woodbridge: Boydell, 2006), 82.

82 'þæt innan heora husum nan unhal cild sy geboren, ne crypol, ne dumb, ne deaf, ne blind, ne ungewittes'. Mary Clayton and Hugh Magennis (eds), *The Old English Lives of St Margaret* (Cambridge: Cambridge University Press, 1994), 168.

83 Avicenna, *A Treatise on the Canon of Medicine of Avicenna: Incorporating a Translation of the First Book*, 'General Discourse upon the Treatment of Disease', Book I, Part IV, section 21, 1032, in edition and translation by Oskar Cameron Gruner (London: Luzac, 1930), 509–10; also Richard C. Scheerenberger, *A History of Mental Retardation* (Baltimore and London: Brookes, 1983), 28.

84 Passage 807b28, also at 806b22, 807b19–28, 810b19, 811a8, 811a29, 811b30 and 812a5–7, in *Seeing the Face, Seeing the Soul: Polemon's Physiognomy from Classical Antiquity to Medieval Islam*, ed. Simon Swain, with contributions by George Boys-Stones … [et al.] (Oxford: Oxford University Press, 2007) [hereafter Polemon], 645. Generally on physiognomy: Voula Tsouna, 'Doubts about Other Minds and the Science of Physiognomics', *The Classical Quarterly (New Series)*, 48 (1998), 175–86.

85 Modern edition Dominic O. O'Meara, *Michaelis Pselli Philosophica Minora*, vol. 2 (Leipzig, 1989).

86 Christine Hummel, *Das Kind und seine Krankheiten in der griechischen Medizin. Von Aretaios bis Johannes Aktuarios (1. bis 14. Jahrhundert)* (Frankfurt-am-Main: Peter Lang, 1999), 84–5, 179; cf. Otto Auburger (ed. and trans.), 'Michael Psellos: Die Entstehung von Intelligenz und Schwachsinn (um 1059)' (diss., Technische Universität München, 1978); R. Volk, *Der medizinische Inhalt der Schriften des Michael Psellos* (Munich: Institut für Byzantinistik, 1990); a more recent study is Stratis Papaioannou, *Michael Psellos: Rhetoric and Authorship in Byzantium* (Cambridge: Cambridge University Press, 2013).

87 Kellenberger, *Schutz der Einfältigen*, 12n8.

88 Cited in Goodey, *History of Intelligence*, 225.

89 'Im Sinne der im *Buch der Natur* ausgebreiteten Logik gibt es eine kausale Beziehung zwischen dem Äußern und Inneren. Die andersartige Hirnstruktur ist daher auch an der Kopfform bei den natürlichen Narren ablesbar.' Ruth von Bernuth, *Wunder, Spott und Prophetie. Natürliche Narrheiten in den 'Historien von Claus Narren'* (Tübingen: Niemeyer, 2009), 39.

90 Modern edition by Robert Luff and Georg Steer, *Konrad von Megenberg: Buch der*

Natur. Texte und Textgeschichte (Berlin: De Gruyter, 2003), 77. The old edition by Franz Pfeiffer, *Konrad von Megenberg. Das Buch der Natur* (Stuttgart, 1861), 43–8, gives the round face as a 'sinwel antlütz (fecies vehementer rotunda)'.

91 'wie dez menschen gestalt vnd seiner glider schickung vns bezaichent sein natuerleich siten, vnd die ler wil ich setzen als sie Rasis hat gesetzt in seinr artztey', cited von Bernuth, *Wunder, Spott und Prophetie*, 39.

92 'Daz prueft man dar an, daz si vngeschicktev haubt habent, aintweder ze groz oder ze clain.', Book VIII, 2, cited von Bernuth, *Wunder, Spott und Prophetie*, 39.

93 'wurkent nicht nach den werchen menschleicher sel vnd habent doch menschen sel sam di chint', Book VIII, 2, cited von Bernuth, *Wunder, Spott und Prophetie*, 39.

94 'Die mentale Differenz der natürlichen Narren erklärt sich lediglich aus einer seit Geburt bestehenden andersartigen Hirnstruktur, die nicht als Krankheit zu verstehen ist. Ihre Devianz ist vielmehr ale eine einzigartige außergewöhnliche Erscheinung zu sehen und rechtfertigt damit ihre Aufnahme in den Abschnitt über die *wunder menschen.*' Von Bernuth, *Wunder, Spott und Prophetie*, 40.

95 David M. Turner, *Disability in Eighteenth-century England: Imagining Physical Impairment* (New York and Abingdon: Routledge, 2012), 4; cf. Jonathan Andrews, 'Begging the Question of Idiocy: The Definition and Socio-cultural Meaning of Idiocy in Early Modern Britain: Part 2', *History of Psychiatry*, 9 (1998), 179–200, at 183.

96 Angelika Groß, *'La Folie'. Wahnsinn und Narrheit im spätmittelalterlichen Text und Bild* (Heidelberg: Carl Winter Universitätsverlag, 1990), 86; cf. Franz Pfeiffer (ed.), *Konrad von Megenberg. Das Buch der Natur* (Stuttgart, 1861), 486.

97 Groß, *'La Folie'*, 86; cf. Pfeiffer (ed.), *Konrad von Megenberg*, 488.

98 Hugo Schulz (ed.), *Das Buch der Natur von Conrad von Megenberg* (Greifswald: Julius Abel, 1897), 418.

99 Schulz (ed.), *Das Buch der Natur von Conrad von Megenberg*, 419–20.

100 Von Bernuth, *Wunder, Spott und Prophetie*, 33–4.

101 Folker Reichert, *Das Bild der Welt im Mittelalter* (Darmstadt: Primus Verlag, 2013), 43; cf. Michael Rothmann, '*Mirabilia vero dicimus, quae nostrae cognitioni non subiacent, etiam cum sint naturalia.* "Wundergeschichten" zwischen Wissen und Unterhaltung: der "Liber de mirabilibus mundi" ("Otia imperialia") des Gervasius von Tilbury', in Martin Heinzelmann, Klaus Herbers and Dieter R. Bauer (eds), *Mirakel im Mittelalter. Konzeptionen, Erscheinungsformen, Deutungen* (Stuttgart, 2002), 399–432.

102 *Confessions*, 10.35 and 5.3 on curiosity as pride.

103 Reichert, *Bild der Welt im Mittelalter*, 44.

104 Reichert, *Bild der Welt im Mittelalter*, 28, 46.

105 S. E. Banks and J. W. Binns (eds), *Gervase of Tilbury: Otia imperialia. Recreation for an Emperor* (Oxford Medieval Texts) (Oxford: Clarendon Press, 2002), 558–9; this supercedes the older edition *Otia imperialia ad Ottonem IV imperatorem*, in Gottfried Wilhelm Leibniz (ed.), *Scriptores rerum Brunsvicensium* ... (Hanover: Nicolaus Foerster, 1707), 960, as was cited by Lorraine Daston and Katharine

Park, *Wonders and the Order of Nature, 1150–1750* (New York: Zone Books, 1998), 23.

106   Banks and Binns, *Gervase of Tilbury*, lvii n193.

107   On wonder: C. W. Bynum, 'Wonder', *American Historical Review*, 102 (1997), 1–26; J. Le Goff, *The Medieval Imagination*, trans. A. Goldhammer (Chicago and London: University of Chicago Press, 1988), 27–44.

108   Daston and Park, *Wonders and the Order of Nature*, 109.

109   Daston and Park, *Wonders and the Order of Nature*, 110.

110   Daston and Park, *Wonders and the Order of Nature*, 394n18.

111   Von Bernuth, *Wunder, Spott und Prophetie*, 36.

112   Groß, *'La Folie'*, 86.

113   Nicole Oresme, 'De causis mirabilium', in Bert Hansen ed. and trans., *Nicole Oresme and the Marvels of Nature* (Toronto: PIMS, 1985), 234, cited by Sylvia Huot, *Madness in Medieval French Literature: Identities Found and Lost* (Oxford: Oxford University Press, 2003), 87.

114   Huot, *Madness in Medieval French Literature*, 87.

115   John Metham, *The Works of John Metham, including the Romance of Amoryus and Cleopes*, ed. Hardin Craig, Early English Text Society, os 132 (London, 1916), xi. He was not, as Goodey erroneously claimed, a physician.

116   C. F. Goodey, 'Mental Retardation', in G. Gerrios and R. Porter (eds), *A History of Clinical Psychiatry: The Origins and History of Psychiatric Disorders* (London: Athlone, 1995), 239–50, at 248–9. Note that the excerpts cited are in fact from the *Physiognomy*, not the *Days of the Moon* as Goodey believed.

117   Metham, *Works of John Metham*, 122 short and great head, 123 uneven head, 132 ears, 133 round ears, 135 nostrils and neck, 139 flat feet.

118   G. Sarton, *The Appreciation of Ancient and Medieval Science During the Renaissance 1540–1600* (Pennsylvania, 1955), 46.

119   Beek, *Waanzin in de Middeleeuwen*, 113–14, citing Pieter Van Foreest, *Observationum et curationum medicinalium ac chirurgicarum libri XXVIII*, in *Opera omnia X*, obs. 31: De stultitia (Frankfurt, 1609), fol. 354.

120   Neaman, *Suggestion of the Devil*, 161.

121   Hans Bertram, 'Die Entwicklung der Psychiatrie im Altertum und Mittelalter', *Janus*, 44 (1940), 81–122, at 110.

122   Scheerenberger, *A History of Mental Retardation*, 33.

123   Bertram, 'Die Entwicklung der Psychiatrie', 111.

124   Bertram, 'Die Entwicklung der Psychiatrie', 111. Full text of the *Stadtbuch* accounts 1465x78 given in Johann Mach, *Von Aussätzigen und Heiligen. Die Medizin in der mittelalterlichen Kunst Norddeutschlands* (Rostock, 1995), 106–7: 'Witlik zy alse denne beth herreto de armen dullen unde asynnigen lude, in de kisten vor dem borchdore unde molendore sittende, nicht so wol mit alle erer nottraft besorgt sind geworden, alse en nach erer legenheid wol van noden wäre, also nemliken in etende, drinkende in leger unde in kledinge na vorlope derer tyd des iares.' (It may be known that until now the stupid and those who lost their minds,

who sit in the mad-chests in front of the Castle Gate and the Mill Gate, are not provided for according to their necessities, that concerns food and drink, bedding and clothing, requisite for the seasons of the year.)

125 Bertram, 'Die Entwicklung der Psychiatrie', 116.

126 Jonathan Andrews, Asa Briggs, Roy Porter, Penny Tucker and Keir Waddington, *The History of Bethlem* (London and New York: Routledge, 1997), 94.

127 Timothy Stainton, 'Medieval Charitable Institutions and Intellectual Impairment c.1066–1600', *Journal on Developmental Disabilities/Le journal sur les handicaps du développement*, 8:2 (2001), 19–29, at 24, citing David Knowles and R. N. Hadcock, *Medieval Religious Houses: England and Wales* (London: Longman, 1971), 351.

128 R. Stewart-Brown, 'The Hospital of St John at Chester', *Transactions of the Historical Society of Lancashire and Cheshire*, 77 (1926), 66–106, is the only study of this hospital, with no mention of 'silly persons', 'idiots', 'innocents' or 'naturals' as having been present there.

129 Clarke, *Mental Disorder in Earlier Britain*, 81, citing as source J. M. Hobson, *Some Early and Late Houses of Piety* (London, 1926), 161 n.

130 Stainton, 'Medieval Charitable Institutions', 24.

131 A. Quiney, *Town Houses of Medieval Britain* (New Haven and London, 2003), 223; cf. G. Cowie, *The History of Wyggeston's Hospital, the Hospital Schools and the Old Free Grammar School, Leicester, AD 1511–1893* (London, 1893), 13–14.

132 Emilio J. Dominguez, 'The Hospital of Innocents: Humane Treatment of the Mentally Ill in Spain, 1409–1512', *Bulletin of the Menninger Clinic*, 31 (1967), 285–97, at 288; cf. Domingo Simo and Calatayud Baya, *El Primer Hospital Psiquiatrico del Mundo* (Valencia: Diputacion Provincial de Valencia, 1959); P. Bassoe, 'Spain as the Cradle of Psychiatry', *American Journal of Psychiatry*, 101 (1945), 731–8; R. D. Rumbaut, 'The First Psychiatric Hospital of the Western World,' *American Journal of Psychiatry*, 128:10 (1972), 1305–9.

133 Dominguez, 'The Hospital of Innocents', 289; cf. Fernando Domingo Simo, 'Historia de la Fundación del Hospital dels Ignoscents, Folls e Orats de Valencia', *Archivos de Neurobiologia*, 21 (1958), 84–96.

134 Antje Sander-Berke, '"Dulle und Unsinnige". Irrenfürsorge in norddeutschen Städten des Spätmittelalters und der frühen Neuzeit', in Peter Johanek (ed.), *Städtisches Gesundheits- und Fürsorgewesen vor 1800* (Städteforschung A Band 50) (Cologne/Weimar/Vienna: Böhlau, 2000), 111–24.

135 Christian Laes, 'Learning from Silence: Disabled Children in Roman Antiquity', *Arctos*, 42 (2008), 85–122; Augustine, *Contra Iulian. op. imperf.* 3, 161, *PL*, vol. 45, col. 1314–15.

136 Nigel Walker, *Crime and Insanity in England: Vol. 1. The Historical Perspective* (Edinburgh: Edinburgh University Press, 1968), 31.

137 T. O. Cockayne, *Leechdoms, Wortcunning and Starcraft of Early England*, Rolls Series 35 (London, 1864–66), part 2, 137–9. See Stefan Jurasinski, 'Madness and Responsibility in Anglo-Saxon England', in Tom Lambert and David

Rollason (eds), *Peace and Protection in the Medieval West* (Toronto: PIMS, 2009), 99–120.

138 Cockayne, *Leechdoms, Wortcunning and Starcraft*, part 2, 143, Leechbook I, chapter lxvi.

139 J. R. Clark Hall, *A Concise Anglo-Saxon Dictionary* (Toronto: University of Toronto Press, 4th edn, 1960), s.v. *ungemynde, dysgung*.

140 Harvey, *The Inward Wits*, 8.

141 Clarke, *Mental Disorder in Earlier Britain*, 111.

142 Stanley W. Jackson, 'Unusual Mental States in Medieval Europe. I. Medical Syndromes of Mental Disorder: 400–1100 A.D.', *Journal of the History of Medicine*, 27 (1972), 262–97, at 287.

143 Jackson, 'Unusual Mental States in Medieval Europe', 289.

144 Harvey, *The Inward Wits*, 2.

145 Harvey, *The Inward Wits*, 28. See also Vincent of Beauvais, *Speculum naturale* (Douai, 1623), Liber XXIII, ca. xliv, who defined spiritus as in between the terms body and soul, citing Ibn Gabirol, *Fons vitae*: 'spiritus, qui est medius inter animam et corpus.'

146 Albertus Magnus, *Quaestiones super de animalibus*, III, q. 4, in *Opera Omnia*, ed. B. Geyer, xii, 126, line 6; and Thomas Aquinas, *ST*, I, question 76, article 7, ad 2.

147 Thomas Aquinas, *ST*, I, question 75, article 4.

148 Harvey, *The Inward Wits*, 54.

149 Harvey, *The Inward Wits*, 3.

150 Harvey, *The Inward Wits*, 3.

4

THE INFANTILE AND THE IRRATIONAL: MIND, SOUL AND INTELLECTUAL DISABILITY

Consider the case of two persons of whom one has a more penetrating grasp of a thing by his intellect than does the other. He who has the superior intellect understands many things that the other cannot grasp at all. Such is the case with a very simple person who cannot at all grasp the subtle speculations of philosophy. But the intellect of an angel surpasses the human intellect much more than the intellect of the greatest philosopher surpasses the intellect of the most uncultivated simple person.[1]

The boundaries between theology, philosophy and psychology as they are today were non-existent in the Middle Ages. Soul (*anima*) and mind (*animus*) are linked for the Christian philosopher; the human soul therefore is a thinking soul as well as being an animating force. Philosophically, and subsequently judicially, medieval ID was considered the absence of reason, the irrational, which contrasted the intellectually disabled with the bowdlerised Aristotelian concept of man as the rational animal. The 'rational animal' was a concept that came to be ubiquitously cited in natural philosophy and theology of the Middle Ages, although Aristotle himself did not leave such a foundational sentence on human psychology to posterity. The absence of reason could, in rare instances, be valued positively, as in the 'innocence' of childlike folly and the occasional 'holy fool' who finds his way towards God along an alternative path of seeking knowledge and truth, as was posited in relation to a number of Byzantine saints, notably Basil and Andrew.

The eleventh century saw the rise of the arrogance of the literati, who expressed in their writings 'bottomless contempt for those who did not share their [clerkly] skills', formulated in the 'hostility of the *clericus* towards the *illiteratus, idiota, rusticus*'.[2] Coupled with this was an academic interest in topics like the soul, intellect and rationality, which the growth of the universities and the rediscovery of the Aristotelian corpus influenced in the themes in philosophy that were being treated in the twelfth and thirteenth centuries: the scholastic 'influx of information which stimulated the intellect could not fail to stimulate the examination of the phenomenon of intellect'.[3] According to Goodey, from only around 1200 onwards 'a body of intellectuals', meaning theologians, natural philosophers and medical authors, 'armed with learned texts on abstraction and logical reasoning began to speak a shared language with social administrators',[4] meaning legal professionals. This is too simplistic a picture. Late antique and early medieval authorities already debated the importance of intellectual abilities, especially logical reasoning and abstraction, for example Nemesius in his tractate on the soul. This chapter will enhance and rectify our current understanding of how late antique through to medieval notions of reason, intellect and the definition of being human had informed a discourse of ID.

The importance of medieval psychological concepts is that they describe, obviously according to the understanding of the times, the process of cognition, based both on sensory perception and abstraction. 'From as early as Augustine, "rationality" referred to the characteristic of being created both as human and in the image of God.'[5] This set the scene, and throughout the period the workings of rationality were being considered. One of the most succinct yet comprehensive descriptions of rationality and abstract reasoning may be found in the words of Ibn Khaldûn, a fourteenth-century Islamic scholar, statesman, jurist, historian and intellectual, tutored by some of the best-known Arabic scholars of his day, who in his later life applied himself to the study of Arabic Aristotelianism. His great historical work forms the earliest attempt by a scholar to discover patterns in the changes that occur in political and social organisation, rather than being restrained by traditional historiography (annals, chronicles, great events). Therefore he presented a kind of theory of history, in support of which he included discussions of the physical environment and its influence on human civilisation, as well as discussions of the nature of humanity, psychology and cognitive science – to put it in modern language.[6]

In the introduction to his work on history, completed in 1377, the *Muqaddimah*, Chapter 6 (various kinds of sciences and man's cognitive ability), prefatory discussion, section 1 (man's ability to think), Ibn Khaldûn explained how brain and intellect, mind and matter, work together.

> Man has this advantage over other beings: he can perceive things outside his essence through his ability to think, which is something beyond his senses. It is the result of (special) powers placed in the cavities of his brain. With the help of these powers, man takes the pictures of the *sensibilia*, applies his mind to them, and thus abstracts from them other pictures. The ability to think is the

occupation with pictures that are beyond sense perception, and the application of the mind to them for analysis and synthesis. The ability to think has several degrees. The first degree is man's intellectual understanding of the things that exist in the outside world in a natural or arbitrary order, so that he may try to arrange them with the help of his own power. This kind of thinking mostly consists of perceptions. ... The second degree is the ability to think which provides man with the ideas and behaviour needed in dealing with his fellow men and in leading them. It mostly conveys apperceptions, which are obtained one by one through experience, until they have become really useful. ... The third degree is the ability to think which provides the knowledge, or hypothetical knowledge, of an object beyond sense perception without any practical activity (going with it). This is the speculative intellect. It consists of both perceptions and apperceptions. ... By thinking about these things, man achieves perfection in his reality and becomes pure intellect and perceptive soul. This is the meaning of human reality.[7]

The construction of a link between psychological and social inferiority may be traced back to ancient Greece, and what with medieval writers' frequent reference to 'authorities' such as Plato and Aristotle, the book must also investigate some antique aspects of ID underpinning and influencing medieval notions. The reception of antique ideas found its way into those very medieval sources that will be cited below.

Rationality and antiquity

'A core paradigm in the negative construction of intellectual disability in Western society is that human value is directly associated with human reason.'[8] Plato, according to Stainton, is a paternalist, who on the one hand denied virtue and agency to those with insufficient intelligence, but on the other hand advocated lenient legal and moral treatment. Stainton then in the very next sentence bluntly sweeps across 2500 years of history by stating: 'This position is almost identical to that followed in the West from this time forward, now more commonly referred to as "mental capacity determination," which dictates the scope of one's moral and legal agency.'[9] With regard to classical authors on ID, Plato, the arch-philosopher, allegedly considered mental disabilities to be inconsequential and unproblematic.[10] His pupil Aristotle suggested that people with ID are like children, who in turn are like dwarfs.

Those whose upper parts are abnormally large, as is the case with dwarfs, have abnormally weak memory, as compared with their opposites, because of the great weight which they have resting upon the organ of perception, and because their mnemonic movements are, from the very first, not able to keep true to a

course, but are dispersed, and because, in the effort at recollection, these movements do not easily find a direct onward path. Infants and very old persons have
bad memories, owing to the amount of movement going on within them; for the
latter are in process of rapid decay, the former in process of vigorous growth; and
we may add that children, until considerably advanced in years, are dwarf-like
[nanôdês, i.e. in their bodily structure].[11]

But the defects of dwarfs and animals go beyond memory. In *Parts of Animals*
Aristotle had classified all animals, with the exception of humans, as 'dwarfish'
(*nanôdês*), by which he meant not deformed, but the natural arrangement
of disproportionate weight and stature in the upper trunk, and inadequate
parts below, i.e. the lower limbs, so that upright posture is simply biologically
not possible for animals, whereas four-footedness was intended by nature.
However, because of their dwarfish structure, for Aristotle animals are less
intelligent than humans.

> This [dwarfish construction] is why all the animals are also more stupid than
> human beings. For even in humans – for instance children as compared with
> men and those who are natural dwarfs among the adult population, even if they
> have some other strength to an unusual degree, yet as regards possession of intel-
> lect they are lacking. The explanation, as was said before, is that the source of the
> soul is excessively hard to move and encumbered with body.[12]

Discussing this passage, Osborne helpfully points out: 'It is simply a physical disability, like disabilities in dwarfs: animal souls would be as intelligent
as ours if they were put in suitably slender, upright bodies that would permit
them to operate their higher faculties.'[13] Quadruped animals and human
dwarfs (as well as children) therefore share a common 'defect', in that, for
perfectly 'natural' reasons of course, they are unable to attain the same levels
of intelligence as adult human males. These kinds of sentiments, irrespective
of the 'scientific' language they are couched in, set the future course for treating dwarfs as pet-like entertainment and curiosity (see Chapter 6 below). The
patronisation of certain human members of a household, such as children,
women, servants and entertainers – and thus dwarfs and fools – has been compared to the abuse of power that is also exercised over non-human creatures,
commonly referred to as pets; all of these could simultaneously be highly
valued and severely controlled, trained to be obedient, entertaining playthings
while also held in some affection.

The passages in Aristotle, *De anima*, Book III.iv (429a10, 21–2; 429b),
contain probably 'the most intensely studied sentences in the history of
philosophy',[14] where it is attempted to describe the transition of the human
intellect from its original unthinking state to a subsequent thinking state.

According to Aristotle, the human intellect was at the beginning, i.e. at birth, 'potentially [everything] thinkable but actually nothing at all', compared famously to a *tabula rasa*, a blank tablet which is ready to be written on but 'on which nothing is so far actually written'.[15] People with ID were alleged not to have voluntary control over emotional reactions. Aristotle described a false *apatheia*, whereby emotional reactions, such as fear, pity or anger, are stunted and apparently not fully developed, so that emotional non-reaction is a kind of deficiency. In the *Nicomachean Ethics* Aristotle said: 'The deficiency, whether it is called unanger or whatever, incurs blame; for people who do not get angry over what they should seem silly [*êlithioi*]... They seem not to notice those things nor to be distressed by them.'[16] The Greek term *êlithios* meant 'stupid, foolish, simple-minded', also 'in vain'. There was also a social element to intellectual weakness. On discussing why contemplation sometimes gets drawn down to earthly things, that is, the image of the Platonic Reality, Plotinus (c. 204–70) used this example: 'Children of dull intelligence [*ohi nôthesteroi tôn paidôn*] bear witness to this, in that, incapable of intellectual and theoretical study, they descend to the crafts and manual labour.'[17]

The main criteria for evaluating intellect and reasoning were, however, animality and language. In late antique philosophy humans are rational, mortal animals; they share with animals (and plants) the qualities of being alive, i.e. 'animated' by a soul which enables sensation, movement, nutrition and growth. Humans also possess a rational soul, the most characteristic sign of which is the ability to express thoughts in language – language which is inevitably oral. Reason is absent in non-human animals, and as yet undeveloped in human children. This means they cannot be aware of their surroundings, to the extent that they cannot act according to decisions made by them – they lack the rational capacity for decision making and judgement. They are thus not moral agents.[18] Graeco-Roman philosophy held two standard assumptions, going back at least to Plato: firstly, that humans are rational animals, and secondly, that 'it is right for reason to rule over unreason. "Reason" means not just intellectual capacity, but the aspect of human beings which is closest to God, so it is both an intellectual and a spiritual force.'[19]

Language and intellectual abilities

The art of rhetoric by Quintilian (c. 35–c. 100) was not just an instruction for public speaking, but above and beyond such simple aims concerned itself with educational theories in general and also, like no comparable antique text, provides an insight into the entire Graeco-Roman educational system. His influence during the Middle Ages and the Renaissance was immense. In his *Institutio oratoria* he said:

> Reason then was the greatest gift of the Almighty, who willed that we should share its possession with the immortal gods. But reason by itself would help us but little and would be far less evident in us, had we not the power to express our thought in speech; for it is the lack of this power rather than thought and understanding, which they do to a certain extent possess, that is the great defect in other living things.
>
> (Rationem igitur nobis praecipuam dedit eiusque nos socios esse cum dis immortalibus voluit. Sed ipsa ratio neque tam nos iuvaret neque tam esset in nobis manifesta, nisi, quae concepissemus mente, promere etiam loquendo possemus, quod magis deesse ceteris animalibus quam intellectum et cogitationem quandam videmus.)[20]

Thus what differentiates the human from all other living creatures is the ability to speak. Humans were given reason as the most excellent gift of the highest god, as a way of almost making humanity the equal of the gods; but even reason could not help us all too much and would not be so effective in us if we could not also express our thoughts by speech, something which apparently the other creatures are lacking more than they lack reason or a certain ability to think. Quintilian leaves open the possibility that other creatures might possess reason and thinking powers, these rational capabilities not being unique to humans, but speech is. Quintilian makes an analogy to people born speechless, saying that they are also without reason: 'Finally, how little the heavenly boon of reason avails those who are born dumb (*Denique homines, quibus negata vox est, quantulum adiuvat animus ille caelestis*).'[21] Thus congenital sensory impairment also impairs reasoning abilities. Language is one of several uniquely human skills, alongside reason, bipedalism, facial expressions, humour, scientific abilities, future planning, formulation of generalising concepts and morality that 'were claimed as human prerogatives' by classical antiquity.[22] Human infants are referred to literally as 'non-speakers' in the famous term *alogon*. Galen provided some interesting thoughts on animals: 'Whether the so-called unreasonable animals are not at all partaking in reason (*logos*) remains obscure. Although they have no expression through voice, which one can define as communication, perhaps they all have a reasonable soul which we define as innate (*endiathetos*, literally deep-seated), some more, some less ... But only man can acquire knowledge at will.'[23] The Greek words are difficult to translate, since voice, speech, reason and intellect were expressed by the same word *logos*.

With regard to language, one late antique philosopher, Porphyry (born Malkos of Tyre around 233, teaching philosophy at Rome from the 240s until 268), argued for the possibility that non-vocal, non-oral forms of expression, such as that made by animals, can be true language, and thus human speech alone is not the defining characteristic of *logos*. In his treatise *On abstinence from killing animals*,[24] Porphyry presented the novel notion that animals as well as humans possess language and therefore also *logos*, that is, the capacity for rational thought.

> Now since that which is voiced by the tongue is *logos* [discourse] however it is voiced, whether in barbarian or Greek, dog or cattle fashion, animals which have a voice share in *logos*, humans speaking in accordance with human customs and animals according to the customs each has acquired from the gods and nature. [...] For we are aware only of noise and sound, because we do not understand (say) Scythian speech, and they seem to us to be making noises and articulating nothing: they just make a sound which sometimes lasts a longer time and sometimes a shorter time, but the modification to convey meaning does not strike us at all. Yet to them their speech is easy to understand and very distinct, just as our accustomed speech is to us; and similarly in the case of animals, understanding comes to them in a way which is peculiar to each species, but we can hear only noise deficient in meaning, because no one who had learned our language has taught us to translate into it what is said by animals.[25]

This is essentially a relativistic argument, whereby all utterances are accorded the status of *logos*, and difficulty in understanding resides in the ignorance of the listener, not in the lack of *logos* in the speaker. But Porphyry goes still further than this, and even presents an argument that *logos* need not be voiced.

> How can it not be ignorant to call only human speech *logos*, because we understand it, and dismiss the speech of other animals? It is as if ravens claimed that theirs was the only language, and we lack *logos*, because we say things which are not meaningful to them. [...] But surely it is absurd to judge rationality or irrationality by whether speech is or is not easy to understand, or by silence or voice.[26]

By extrapolation, what Porphyry stated about animals and 'barbarian' non-Greeks, must also hold for speech-impaired humans, and ultimately for people with such ID that their language ability is reduced.

Augustine followed the distinction between humans and animals, creatures with reason and those without (in Greek *aloga zôa* 'living beings without language').[27] In his tractate on the soul, Nemesius asserted that God 'linked articulate speech to thought and reasoning, making it a messenger of the movements of the intellect'.[28] And Isidore in the *Etymologies* defined the infant as the non-speaker. 'A human being of the first age is called an infant (*infans*); it is called an infant, because it does not yet know how to speak (*in-*, 'not'; *fari*, present participle *fans*, 'speaking'), that is, it cannot talk.'[29]

By the thirteenth century Albertus Magnus, in *Liber de Animalibus*, treated pygmies as below human but above monkeys in the chain of being, due to their lack of abstraction, for although pygmies can speak, 'they do not argue or speak about the universals of things ... Reason has two principles. One comes from sense and memory, where the perception of experience lies; the other is that which it possesses when elevated to a unitary intellect, i.e. that which is capable of eliciting universals ... The pygmy, however, has only the first of these.' But there are also humans who cannot abstract, whom Albertus calls *moriones*, following Augustine. They are fully human but are 'foolish [*stulti*] by nature because they are incapable of apprehending reason, and their speech utterances resemble the pygmy's. But the pygmy lacks reason by nature, whereas *moriones* do not lack possession of reason but rather the use of it, as a result of melancholy or some other accident.'[30] This is a highly interesting point, because according to Albert's classification people with ID never lose their status as fully human, their inherent rationality is not in doubt, only damageable by accident.

Intellect and dominance

Giles of Rome (c. 1243–1316) regarded as 'natural' the domination over those who were physically strong but intellectually weak: 'He is naturally a slave who, being strong in his physical powers is deficient in intellect; thus, he naturally dominates [who is] strong by the industry of his mind and ruling prudence.'[31] In *Summa against the Gentiles*, Aquinas had also stated intellectual ability was justification for rule over others, having picked up such ideas from Aristotle: 'those men who excel in intellect naturally dominate; those who are deficient in intellect, but with strong bodies, seem made by nature for serving, just as Aristotle says in his *Politics*'.[32] Then, in *Summa theologiae* Aquinas argued that even in a state of grace and without sin, as in the prelapsarian state, those people who excelled in knowledge and virtue would have governed over the rest (like a Platonic philosopher-ruler), not punishing, since there would have been no need to punish, but guiding by instruction, on the basis of moral authority of a paternalistic kind.[33] 'In other words, Aquinas's view of government was based upon an assumption of an intellectual inequality among men, an inequality that meant that those in power rightly exercised control over the lives of the innocent.'[34] But there was also the notion of the equality of all in a sinless state. Augustine had already framed the argument that inequality (of wealth, power, stature or for that matter abilities) in human societies is the result of sin. In heaven there would be no need for social strictures like government, but on earth people were differentiated by their wealth, poverty, strength, weakness or size,[35] which however did not preclude a commonality of rationality for all. Peter the Chanter (d. 1197) had held an absolute egalitarian view of humanity, in that he was committed to the view that all men were equally rational, and thence, in an ideal state of grace without having done anything wrong, the morally good needed no government (of any kind, whether political in the larger community or 'state', or paternalistic in the sense of people being educated). But by the time of Thomas Aquinas certain developments in the way the new intelligentsia were seen meant that this absolute egalitarianism was being modified. According to studies by Buc and Moore, from the twelfth century onwards the term *clerici* came to mean not just men in priestly orders, but the subgroup among them of *literati*, those who had pursued the new courses of higher education emerging from the schools (and that would by the thirteenth century form the universities).[36] Both *clerici* and their subgroup *literati* 'had an exclusive claim to the title of *rationales*, giving them authority over all *laici*, whom these clerics also called *illiterati* and *simplices*'.[37] Rationality thus became associated with being learned or educated, which in turn contested the earlier notion of the equality of all in terms of rationality as a human condition, and further led to arguments for the purpose of knowledge as a tool with which to dominate others – after all, knowledge is deemed to be power. Such domination was grounded in that (in)famous concept 'the greater good', so that it was no longer just sinners that were to be correctly guided, but also those who simply had less understanding. The *literati* defined what 'greater good' actually meant, with the result that their power over the unlearned rested on the intellectual foundations of an arbitrary socio-cultural construct. Buc claimed that the emergence of the vocabulary of *rationales* and *simplices* was an attempt on the part of the doctors of the Church – the *clerici* – to claim the same total authority over their fellow men that men claimed to exercise over animals.[38] But the theses of Buc and Moore omit to mention that the predominance of the rational over the irrational goes back at least to antiquity – these are not new ideas, all that is new is that a newish class of people, the clergy or intelligentsia, are trying to jostle for power with an older class of people, the landholders, the nobility and the established secular rulers. Greek intelligentsia and slaveholding landholders had been one and the same class. This was no longer so by the early Middle Ages, where the worldly powerful were often illiterate in the modern sense of the word, but the holders of knowledge, of book learning, were the comparatively powerless monks, later the secular clergy.

What this meant in practical and less purely philosophical terms was that 'idiocy' could be associated with specific groups of people. The influential *De proprietatibus rerum* by Bartholomaeus Anglicus included a section on

servants, childishness and mental capacity. There is a similarity in the disenfranchised legal capacities of children, of people with ID and of certain types
of servant (what Bartholomaeus calls bonded servants, commonly referred
to as serfs or villeins). He describes bonded servants thus: 'for þey mowe not
selle noþir 3eue awey here owne good and catelle, noþir make contractes,
noþir fonge office of dignite, noþir bere witnes wiþoute leue of here lordes.
And þei3 [though] þey be not in childehode þey ben ofte ipunyschid wiþ
peynes of childehode.'[39] When noting the character traits of the 'bad' servant
(*serui mali*), Bartholomaeus lists a number of biblical passages that refer to
servants as 'slow' and idle, so that an unconscious association is formed with
the – deliberate – slowness of the 'evil' servant and the involuntary, 'natural'
slowness of the person with ID.[40] And in a miracle play of the late fourteenth
century, *Un parroissian esconmenié*, where a prince poses as a fool for peni-
tentiary reasons in similar fashion to the more common holy fool, the figure
of the assumed fool is described as impervious to the physical and mental
abuse the people of the town impose on him, hence like an animal in the lack
of understanding as to what is going on and being done to him: 'He has no
more memory nor sense than a dumb animal: he enjoys the pain inflicted on
him, and to him it seems pleasurable.'[41] Canon law also voiced opinion on the
assumed insensitivity of the mad and the young, and by implication the natural
fools, similar to that idea found in the fourteenth-century miracle play, that
the mad can feel no pain. The *Corpus iuris canonici* held that the insane and
the very young were incapable of suffering pain, arguing that those who were
used to ill-treatment, as presumably madmen and children were by physical
chastisement – beatings if not worse abuse – did not suffer. Habituation supposedly engenders endurance. 'In this way, canon law legitimizes our eternal
desire to believe that the mad cannot feel or that they do not know what others
do to them.'[42] Canon law betrays a stereotypical attitude especially found
towards people with ID, reflected in calling them dull, insensitive and thereby
insinuating that such people are less likely to feel emotions or physical pain. It
is the arrogance of the intellectually and socially superior to insist that lesser
folk, be they slaves, peasants, idiots or animals, because of their unrefined,
brutish nature, are insensitive to all kinds of hardships (cold temperatures,
starvation, hard physical labour) that the delicate upper classes can perceive.
The fairytale of the princess and the pea is just at one extreme end of the
spectrum that expresses such attitudes.

Augustine on intellect

Augustine could consider that while people with ID 'may not be particularly valued in this world, they are at least part of the divine plan and as such
human'.[43] God's grace is accessible to anyone, regardless of their ability to
reason and to think rationally, so that 'grace and faith act as a buffer, accommodating those excluded by a purely reason-based assessment of value' as
both classical antiquity did and modern society still does.[44] In fact, as later
critics of the church and of religion were only too keen to point out, the
church, especially the 'medieval' church in the full pejorative usage of the
word, was deemed anti-rational and therefore anti-science.[45] But Augustine, in
De peccatorum meritis, praises the man with ID who believes in Christ far more
strongly than the majority of the population, and who vehemently defends
Christian beliefs when a 'normal' person made derogatory remarks about Jesus
Christ.

> Chapter 32. – The Case of Certain Idiots and Simpletons. [...]
> If we follow those persons who suppose that souls are oppressed with earthly
> bodies in a greater or a less degree of grossness, ... who would not affirm that
> those had sinned previous to this life with an especial amount of enormity, who
> deserve so to lose all mental light, that they are born with faculties akin to brute
> animals, – who are (I will not say most slow in intellect, for this is very com-
> monly said of others also, but) so silly as to make a show of their fatuity for the
> amusement of clever people, even with idiotic gestures,[46] and whom the vulgar
> call, by a name, derived from the Greek [*môros*], Moriones? And yet there was
> once a certain person of this class, who was so Christian, that although he was
> patient to the degree of strange folly with any amount of injury to himself, he
> was yet so impatient of any insult to the name of Christ, or, in his own person,
> to the religion with which he was imbued, that he could never refrain, whenever
> his gay and clever audience proceeded to blaspheme the sacred name, as they
> sometimes would in order to provoke his patience, from pelting them with
> stones; and on these occasions he would show no favour even to persons of rank.
> Well, now, such persons are predestinated and brought into being, as I suppose,
> in order that those who are able should understand that God's grace and the
> Spirit ... does not pass over any kind of capacity in the sons of mercy ... They,
> however, who affirm that souls severally receive different earthly bodies, more or
> less gross according to the merits of their former life, and that their abilities as
> men vary according to the self-same merits, so that some minds are sharper and
> others more obtuse, and that the grace of God is also dispensed for the liberation
> of men from their sins according to the deserts of their former existence: – what
> will they have to say about this man? How will they be able to attribute to him
> a previous life of so disgraceful a character that he deserved to be born an idiot,

and at the same time of so highly meritorious a character as to entitle him to a preference in the award of the grace of Christ over many men of the acutest intellect?[47]

The narrative is mainly concerned with arguing against the theory of transmigration of souls, but sheds incidental light on Augustine's notion of 'idiocy'. Further on in the same text Augustine criticises the fact that apparently sensible people should find amusement in the infirmities of others. Augustine had argued for a comparison between children and so-called *moriones* – a late antique term perhaps best equated with the medieval 'fool' – relating the anecdote of a father who on the one hand may be amused by such silliness, while on the other hand dreading the prospect of his own son turning out to be such a 'fool'. Chapter 66 relates to the behaviour of infants, who are foolish and ignorant, but through no fault of their own.

> these small freaks [i.e. the infants] are not only borne in very young children, but are actually loved, – and this with what affection except that of the flesh, by which we are delighted by a laugh or a joke, seasoned with fun and nonsense by clever persons, although, if it were understood literally, as it is spoken, they would not be laughed with as facetious, but at as simpletons? We see, also, how those simpletons whom the common people call *Moriones* are used for the amusement of the sane; and that they fetch higher prices than the sane when appraised for the slave market. So great, then, is the influence of mere natural feeling, even over those who are by no means simpletons, in producing amusement at another's misfortune. Now, although a man may be amused by another man's silliness, he would still dislike to be a simpleton himself; and if the father, who gladly enough looks out for, and even provokes, such things from his own prattling boy, were to foreknow that he would, when grown up, turn out a fool, he would without doubt think him more to be grieved for than if he were dead.[48]

On the question of the soul, Augustine struggled with the problem of a 'defective' soul that was nevertheless of divine creation, asking for advice in a letter to Jerome.

> What shall I say [regarding] the diversity of talent in different souls, and especially the absolute privation of reason in some? This is, indeed, not apparent in the first stages of infancy, but being developed continuously from the beginning of life, it becomes manifest in children, of whom some are so slow and defective in memory that they cannot learn even the letters of the alphabet, and some (commonly called idiots) so imbecile that they differ very little from the beasts of the field. Perhaps I am told, in answer to this, that the bodies are the cause of these imperfections. But surely the opinion which we wish to see vindicated from objection does not require us to affirm that the soul chose for itself the body which so impairs it, and, being deceived in the choice, committed a blunder; or

that the soul, when it was compelled, as a necessary consequence of being born, to enter into some body, was hindered from finding another by crowds of souls occupying the other bodies before it came, so that, like a man who takes whatever seat may remain vacant for him in a theatre, the soul was guided in taking possession of the imperfect body not by its choice, but by its circumstances. We, of course, cannot say and ought not to believe such things. Tell us, therefore, what we ought to believe and to say in order to vindicate from this difficulty the theory that for each individual body a new soul is specially created.[49]

On the basis of these textual excerpts, one may summarise Augustine's position as strongly ambivalent, torn between negative and positive evaluations of ID. Primarily, Augustine regarded ID as a 'defect' of small children who have not yet knowingly sinned. He cites the fool in Ecclesiasticus 22:12–13, corresponding to the person with innate mental deficiencies and as part and parcel of the imperfections of children. Elsewhere Augustine enumerates the defects that children may be born with: physically impaired children, as well as impulsive, angry, frightened, forgetful, ponderously thinking children, those without sense, and so foolish that one would rather cohabit with animals than with them.[50] Augustine pondered the question regarding the conception of intellectually disabled children, specifically the issue of how and when the soul enters the body. He came up with four contradictory answers.

1   Each individual soul exists perpetually, eternally and timelessly in spiritual form in God; as punishment for some misdemeanour a soul enters a corporal being. More and more, Augustine came to reject this thesis, which is derived from Plato and Pythagoras, because it is a kind of transmigration of souls.[51]
2   The soul is a part of God, a kind of emanation – a thesis Augustine rejects once he turns away from the Manichaeans, who supported a dualistic view of the universe (soul is divine, matter is devilish).
3   At the moment of parental conception a soul is implanted in the foetus. This is rejected by Augustine as too materialist – although Tertullian (c. 160–c. 225) supported the idea.
4   Every soul is individually created by God at the moment of conception. This came to be Augustine's favoured position.[52]

An assessment of the different positions was also made by Augustine's contemporary Nemesius, who accepted the position of Origen (d. 253/4) that souls existed before bodies did, which is similar to Augustine's first proposition; the third proposition, that souls are in effect inherited from their parents, was held by Apollinaris (d. 390); while the fourth proposition, that souls are created by God at the same time as bodies, was also subscribed to by Eunomius (d. 393).[53] But this is exactly where ID poses problems for Augustinian thinking, for if God creates each soul individually (proposition 4), then that entails that the soul of a person with ID is also created directly by God, and God would then be creating something imperfect and deficient. Augustine did not want to end up having to argue that the creator creates imperfect and defective beings, therefore he would perforce have to turn to his third answer, that it is the parents who create the soul of their child at the moment of conception – thereby blaming generations of parents for the next 1500 years for the birth of mentally disabled children. But essentially, Augustine, even after turning to his older colleague Jerome for advice, could never solve this philosophical and psychological problem.

The Augustinian problem of how such a perfect entity as a soul can neverthe-less appear to be defective, how exactly the soul enters the body and how that can affect the mentally defective state of a child was never satisfactorily solved. 'It was never settled, by Augustine or his successors, whether each soul was freshly created when a child was conceived, or whether the soul was somehow generated with the body.'[54] Bede (d. 735), in *De Natura Rerum*, revisited this problem; in the Carolingian period a number of commentators were aware that neither Augustine nor Jerome could solve that issue; Cassiodorus (d. 585), in *De anima*, said that Augustine stated the impossibility of clarifying whether the soul was created (by God for each new body) or generated (by the process of physical conception); Alcuin (d. 804) avoided the issue completely by saying it is best left a mystery known only to God, since both Christian and pagan thinkers were stumped by this problem, and even Augustine and Jerome had failed to provide guidance for future theologians; and Rhabanus Maurus (d. 856) backed up Augustine's uncertainty in this case.[55]

De anima: treatises on the soul

There were numerous tractates called *De anima*, in a multitude of different versions, with amendments, new additions or condensations, throughout the Middle Ages, starting with Nemesius around the year 400, which all have something to say (even if not much individually) on mental (in)capacity. In his tract on the soul, Nemesius described autonomy as a result of our rational nature and described the faculties of the soul.

> Of the rational element [of the soul] one aspect is theoretical, another practical; that which comprehends the nature of what there is is theoretical, the delibera-tive element that determines the right rule for practical matters is practical. They also call the theoretical element intellect, the practical one reason [...] there is

every necessity that he who is able to deliberate should also be in control of his actions; for if action were not in his power his capacity to deliberate would be superfluous. If that is the case autonomy necessarily exists alongside the rational element: for either the rational element will not exist, or if the rational element exists it will be in control of actions. But if it is in control of actions it must certainly be autonomous.[56]

What Nemesius called 'superfluidity' is used as an argument to prove the point that nothing is created by god in a superfluous manner, everything has a purpose. But by linking rationality and agency, this leaves the position of people with ID in limbo: if they cannot deliberate because they do not possess reason, does that make them autonomous? According to Nemesius' argument the answer must be 'no'. 'The will was acknowledged by all Christian medieval scholars to be that part of the rational soul, or mind, that was responsible for choice and initiation of behavior.'[57] The implication is that someone whose rational faculty is damaged or congenitally absent, as in persons with ID, will also have no will, hence no capacity for choice or control over behaviour, which of course are the deciding criteria for legal evaluation of intellect. The will forms part of the mind, and is found in humans but not in animals.[58] Nevertheless, will is not deemed essential to life. Similar arguments were propounded by Isidore of Seville in the early seventh century. In the *Etymologies*, on human beings and their physical constitution on the relationship between soul and will, Isidore says they are the same, but soul is characteristic of life and mind of intention.

> Whence the philosophers say that life can continue to exist even without the will, and that the soul can endure without the mind (*mens*) – which is why we use the term 'the mindless' (*amens*). ... Because of this, 'mind' is not the word we use for the soul, but for that part which is the superior part in the soul, as if the mind were its head or its eye. ... 13. Indeed, memory is mind, whence forgetful people are called mindless. Therefore it is soul when it enlivens the body, will when it wills, mind when it knows, memory (*memoria*) when it recollects, reason (*ratio*) when it judges correctly, spirit when it breathes forth, sense (*sensus*) when it senses something.
> (Unde dicunt philosophi etiam sine animo vitam manere, et sine mente animam durare: unde et amentes. ... Quapropter non anima, sed quod excellit in anima mens vocatur, tamquam caput eius vel oculus. ... 13 Nam et memoria mens est, unde et inmemores amentes. Dum ergo vivificat corpus, anima est: dum vult, animus est: dum scit, mens est: dum recolit, memoria est: dum rectum iudicat, ratio est: dum spirat, spiritus est: dum aliquid sentit, sensus est.)[59]

Medieval philosophy recognised so-called powers of the soul. These could vary in number and type, depending on the text. For example, while Aristotle had spoken of five powers – in *De anima* they are the vegetative [*threptikon*], sensory [*aisthetikon*], intellectual [*dianoêtikon*], appetitive [*orektikon*] and locomotive [*kinêtikon*] – Hugh of St Victor (*Didascalion*) postulated three, namely a power of the soul which animated the body, another which enabled to evaluate sensory perception, and a third which possessed reason. Others came up with different schemata: Augustine (*De Trinitate*) divided the soul into only rational and irrational faculties, while Aquinas (*Summa theologiae*) added a further set of cognitive powers called 'interior senses' which extended beyond the senses.[60] As was discussed above in the previous chapter, sense (*sensus* or *sensualitas*), imagination (*imaginatio*), reason (*ratio*) and under-standing (*intelligentia* or *intellectus*) were regarded as faculties, hence material, physiological entities, of the rational soul which enabled the perception and organisation of ideas. To recapitulate, the outside world was observed through the senses. This information was then turned into an image in the brain, which although not existent in physical actuality mirrored the character or essence of something that could be sensorily perceived. The faculty of reason then applied analysis, ordering and conceptualising the sensorily observed things. Understanding likewise specialised in the analysis and ordering of things, but this time of immaterial things made by the imagination. 'The two higher faculties [of reason and understanding] thus abstract from the concrete.'[61] Aristotle's implied but not explicitly made differentiation between potential and active intellect sparked commentary, exegesis and speculation in antique and medieval philosophers, notably, for the purposes of this investigation of medieval notions of ID, by Alfarabi (d. 950), Avicenna (980–1037) and Averroes (1126–98), whose writings were in turn received and expanded upon by Western Christian theologians and natural philosophers. [62]

Alfarabi postulated three stages of human intellect. 'The initial stage is the "natural disposition" for thought, also called "rational faculty," "material intellect," and "passive intellect," with which all normal men are born.'[63] It follows that if a person was already born without this initial stage being intact or 'normal', then any chance of ever progressing to acquisition of the two fol-lowing, higher stages of intellect was null. For Avicenna, intellect resides in an incorporeal soul, which is completely empty at birth and only a potential-ity. As the child develops, so does the potentiality of the soul, in three stages. Using for intellectual development the analogy of learning the skill of writing, Avicenna describes the potentiality for writing/thought in an infant as being an 'unqualified disposition' or 'unqualified potentiality' (*potentia absoluta materialis*, where the potentiality for either exists only in so far as the infant has an in-built capability to learn writing or thinking); the second stage is said to have a 'possible potentiality' (where the child becomes familiar with the tools of writing/thought and acquires rudimentary skills), while the third stage culminates in 'perfect' potentiality for writing/thought (*intellectus in habitu*, meaning a scribe accomplished in his art and able, at will, to exercise this skill).[64] Children who are cognitively impaired will never, according to this proposition, progress from the empty potentiality, or at best only to the next stage, doomed as adults to remain for ever at the lowest level of human intellect. Avicenna also postulated a cogitative faculty which resided in the brain and was, unlike thought, an actual physical entity, which in turn meant that the cogitative faculty was prone to errors, or damages. In the process of thinking, the cogitative faculty was to provide an appropriate image, 'an image that will prepare the soul for conjunction with the active intellect. The soul is thereby able to receive the active intellect's emanation and think the given thought.'[65] By implication, persons with brain damage (sustained through trauma) or congenital abnormalities of the brain (as present in some ID), would have reduced cogitative input and hence reduced capacity for thought as well.

The Persian scholar Suhrawardi (1155–91) produced an allegorical tale, *Avaz-i Par-i Jibra'il* (The Sound of Gabriel's Wing), in which Avicenna's philosophy is laid out. In this fable, 'a young man, who obviously represents the human soul, leaves the women's quarters of his house; the women's quarters represent the domain of sense perception. On his way to the men's quarters, to the domain of intellect, the young man meets an elderly sage, who is clearly the active intellect, the cause of human intellectual development.'[66] What is interesting here is the hierarchical comparison of female with sensory, male with intellectual capacities – as for Costa ben Luca, women are believed never to attain the heady intellectual heights of men, while (male) children at least, if they are not 'defective', have the potential capacity to blossom into fully intellectually competent human beings.

Among medieval Jewish scholars, Judah Hallevi (c. 1085–c. 1140) and Maimonides (1135–1204) picked up on Avicenna's theories and introduced them to a wider audience, their original Arabic works being rapidly translated into Hebrew. Pertinent to consideration of the aetiologies of ID, Hallevi argued (in his *Sefer ha-Cuzari*, or dialogues before the king of the Turkish Chazars) that the human soul cannot be purely an intellectual substance, but must have a material basis and be individuated, otherwise men 'would not lose consciousness when they fall asleep, become intoxicated, have brain fever, suffer brain concussions, grow old and feeble'.[67] Such notions allow, at least theoretically, for a medical or anatomical explanation of cognitive impairment. Maimonides meanwhile, in his *Guide of the Perplexed* (Arabic: Dalalat al-Ha'irin; Hebrew: Moreh Nebukim), characterised the human rational faculty as a power in a body and as a disposition in the human organism, thus deviating from Avicenna by describing the human soul as a corporeal element. While Maimonides does not categorically assign stages to the human soul, nevertheless like the philosophers mentioned above he does distinguish between 'potential' or 'material intellect' on the lowest level, to be followed by 'actual intellect' and culminating with 'acquired intellect'.[68] Again, the implication is that if the potential or material intellect is somehow defective, a person can never develop intellectual capacities beyond those innate to the infant.

Averroes treated the subject of the human intellect in no less than seven of his compositions, especially with regard to the nature of the material intellect.[69] Since the material intellect, as we have seen, was regarded by most philosophers, including Averroes, as the lowest and most 'primitive' of the stages the human intellect was presumed to traverse, it is worthy of special consideration here. In the Epitome of the De anima, Averroes postulated that intelligible thoughts depend on the sensory input, so that a person who was congenitally sensorily impaired (such as blind or deaf from birth) would never be able to form the general concepts that non-impaired people with intact senses could form. Similarly, this line of thinking, although Averroes is not concerned enough with it to mention it in this text, allows the supposition that persons with impaired cognitive functions could also never form such intellectual concepts. Averroes does posit circumstances when the 'imaginative faculty is destroyed', and therefore 'comprehension is defective',[70] but this assumes acquired disability, rather than congenital ID.

In his Muqaddimah, Ibn Khaldûn put forward his theories on holy folly: it was seen not as an illness like 'regular' insanity, but such people lack the rational intellect ('aql) that would enable them to make a living and/or be culpable under the law, and they are 'stupid' from birth, whereas they should be differentiated from the insane who lost their minds during their lifetime due to natural physical accidents.[71]

Chapter 1 (on human civilisation in general), sixth prefatory discussion (on human types):

Among the adepts of mysticism are fools and imbeciles who are more like insane persons than like rational beings. ... they are not legally responsible. ... They are not bound by anything. They speak absolutely freely about it and tell remarkable things. When jurists say they are not legally responsible, they frequently deny that they have attained any mystical station, since sainthood can be obtained only through divine worship. This is an error. The attainment of sainthood is not restricted to the correct performance of divine worship, or anything else. When the human soul is firmly established as existent, God may single it out for whatever gifts of His He wants to give it. The rational souls of such people are not non-existent, nor are they corrupt, as is the case with the insane. They merely lack the intellect that is the basis of legal responsibility. That intellect is a special attribute of the soul. It means various kinds of knowledge that are necessary to man and that guide his speculative ability and teach him how to make a living and organize his home. ... Now, a person who lacks that special attribute of the soul called intellect still does not lack the soul itself, and has not forgotten his reality. He has reality, though he lacks the intellect entailing legal responsibility, that is, the knowledge of how to make a living. This is not absurd. God does not select His servants for gnosis only on the basis of the performance of some legal duty. If this is correct, it should be known that the state of these men is frequently confused with that of the insane, whose rational souls are corrupted and who belong to the category of animals. There are signs by which one can distinguish the two groups. One of them is that fools are found devoting themselves constantly to certain exercises and divine worship, though not in the way the religious law requires, since, as we have stated, they are not legally responsible. The insane, on the other hand, have no particular devotion whatever. Another sign is that fools were created stupid, and were stupid from their earliest days. The insane, on the other hand, lose their minds after some portion of their life has passed, as the result of natural bodily accidents. When this happens to them and their rational souls become corrupt, they are lost.[72]

One may compare Ibn Khaldûn, on the insane as alike to animals because they have lost their rational soul, to the following statement by Henry of Ghent (born around 1240, became master of theology at Paris in 1275, died 1293; the disputation that is labelled Quodlibet I was held 1276, so precedes Ibn Khaldûn by a century). Without previous knowledge of the intellect the will cannot act. 'As a result, in insane persons whose intellects are destroyed, there is no appetite of the will, but only the sensitive appetite of an animal. For, if the intellect is taken away, the human being remains only as an animal.'[73]

In western medieval Europe, the twelfth century brought a plethora of translations of Greek and Arabic philosophical works into Latin, so that the authors cited above became known, at least in parts of their work, to a Christian intelligentsia. The vocabulary of knowledge was still forming in the twelfth and thirteenth centuries, especially with regard to the technical terms used in philosophical texts; e.g. the opening lines of Aristotle's *Posterior Analytics*, which were translated in the twelfth century and set out his views that all learning and every intellectual discipline relies on pre-existent knowledge, were using different words for 'intellect'. Thus James of Venice had *intellectiva*, the Anonymous (Joannes) had *deliberativa*, Gerard of Cremona had *cogitativa* and William of Moerbeke had *ratiocinativa*.[74] One could equally point to the fluid vocabulary at that time concerning the opposite of intellect, 'idiocy', especially considering that the main way of defining 'idiocy' was in oppositional terms to intellect.

John Blund on soul and intellect

John Blund (d. 1248) had lectured on Aristotle at Oxford and Paris before being passed over in election to archbishop of Canterbury in 1232, after which he became chancellor of York. His main inspiration for the tractate on the soul was Avicenna's *De anima*, but also many works of Aristotle. As an avowed Aristotelian, Blund was among the first thinkers in Western Christendom to employ these new ideas, including Avicenna's, in a coherent way with regard to the soul, not just citing and regurgitating Aristotle and the Arabian philosophers, but trying to further develop their doctrines.[75] But very interestingly Blund states that in those cases where the soul is separated from the body, and therefore has lost the powers of sensation on which the incorporeal soul relies for information input, no soul is more wise than another.[76] Blund then poses the question of whether the soul of a philosopher, once separated from the body, is more wise than the soul of some *idiota* – leaving aside the question for the moment of who exactly is meant by *idiota* – whose soul has also been separated from his body; answering immediately that such a soul is not wiser, as may be seen by the preceding argument.[77] One may observe that Alexander of Aphrodisias, a contemporary of Galen and through his commentaries on Aristotle an influential source for Arabic and thence Western scholastic Aristotelian philosophy, distinguished between philosophers, on the one hand, and *idiotai*, on the other, by which he meant people lacking thinking abilities.[78] And Albertus Magnus, in *De anima*, described *idiotae* as people who 'do not discern the universal from the particulars', therefore those people who do not make abstractions.[79]

The reference to 'idiot' might at first be interpreted here in its meaning of the unlearned, the layperson, not the congenitally intellectually impaired, but nevertheless this is a highly equalising statement, and could theoretically be expanded upon to mean the souls of people with ID. Blund in a way resolves the problem Augustine had hinted at, as to how it could be feasible that a perfect, incorruptible soul of divine creation could exist in a debased, corruptible, imperfect form such as allegedly in people with ID (lacking various faculties, especially the powers of intellect and reason). If all souls in separation from the body are equal in essence, and none is wiser than the other, then it must follow that defects of intellect or reason are purely due to corporeal, physical defects and not due to corruption of the soul itself. Blund continues:

> We say that the soul separated from the body can make use of the intellect, and one soul understands more than another and is wiser than another; because inasmuch as a soul participates more in the enlightenment proceeding from

pure truth, which is supremely bright and immutable through this purification
it has a keener intellect, and greater wisdom than the soul which is oppressed
by the millstone of sins, and participates less in the nature of enlightenment.
For just as light makes for operation of the senses, so also enlightenment by
pure truth makes for operation of the intellect. Whence we are right to conclude that the soul of a certain *idiota*, when it is separated from the body, is
wiser than the soul of a philosopher, if that soul that belonged to an *idiota* participated more in pure truth and the light shining from it than the soul of a philosopher participated; for this reason it happens that a less wise soul receives
wisdom from the wiser one by looking at it and that which is in it. Nevertheless
it is likely that the soul of the philosopher may know more than the soul of the
idiota, even if the latter participates in pure truth, and it knows more about
the things that it receives by bodily teaching, which do not concern divine
contemplation.

(Dicimus quod anima separata a corpore intellectu uti potest, et una intelligit
plus alia et est sapientior alia; quia quanto anima magis particeps est illumina-
tionis procedentis a pura veritate, que summe lucida et incommutabilis est, illa
purificatione habet intellectum perspicaciorem, et maioris est sapientie quam
illa que mole peccatorum est oppressa, minus existens particeps nature illumina-
tionis. Sicut enim lux facit ad operationes sensus, ita et illuminatio pure veritatis
facit ad operationem intellectus. Unde bene concedimus quod anima cuiusdam
idiote, quando est separata a corpore, est sapientior quam anima philosophi,
si anima ille que fuerit idiote fit magis particeps pure veritatis et lucis ab ea
irradiantis quam anima philosophi sit particeps; et propter hoc contingit quod
anima minus sapiens scientiam recipit a sapientiori intuendo eam et quicquid
est in ea. Probabile tamen est quod anima philosophi plus sciat de quibusdam
quam anima idiote, licet ipsa sit particeps pure veritatis, et de illis plus scit
ipsa que recipit per receptionem discipline in corpore que non sunt de divina
contemplatione.)[80]

While in many texts the dualisms philosopher/unlearned (or *idiota*), or cleric/
layperson, refer to *idiota* purely as ignorant in a specific sense (no Latin, cannot
read or write), in this case there is some qualifying material embedded in the
text. The reader may care to remember that Blund followed up his description of the quality of the immortal, divine soul by contrast with the material
soul. It is here that Blund's allusion to the sensory input does not make sense
(pun unintended) unless read as an opposition between someone who has
functioning sensory input (in the case of the philosopher the best functioning,
due to training) and someone who has some damage to their sensory input
and the way this input is processed cognitively. The crucial passage declares:
'it knows more about the things that it receives by bodily teaching, which do
not concern divine contemplation (*de illis plus scit ipsa que recipit per receptionem discipline in corpore que non sunt de divina contemplatione*)'. If the text

is concerned just with opposing layman with philosopher, why should this sensory input matter?

Regarding the question of how the soul can know things without the aid of the senses, Evans commented on the passage regarding the idiot: 'Blund asked whether the soul of a philosopher is wiser when it is separated from the body than the soul of a fool when it is separated from its own, again puzzling over the degree to which the soul depends on the body to obtain knowledge or wisdom.'[81] Finally, Blund turns to a discussion of free will. He concludes, having argued that rationality consists of the power to arbitrate by rational thinking (or evaluating) if something is good or bad, true or false (*quoniam in eo est ratio quod est potestas arbitrandi per ratiocinationes quid sit bonum et quid malum, quid verum et quid falsum*), by stating that rationality is free will (*ratio est libertas arbitrii*).[82] This is similar to the argument put forward already by Nemesius, that human autonomy is due to rationality, which begs the question of how this applies to people with ID, who by definition lack rationality, therefore by implication must also lack autonomy.

Albertus Magnus and his pupil Thomas Aquinas on intellect

Albertus Magnus, in *Ethica*, considered the three things within the soul that guide action and truth, namely sensory perception, intellect and the appetitive urge (*sensus, intellectus et appetitus*). 'For it has been said that the action of a person as person resides in rationality. Therefore that is not an action of a person, which does not proceed from the person according to rational thought.'[83] According to this argumentation, people with ID are devoid of agency. Possessing sensory perception alone is not enough to constitute agency: 'For there is nothing in a person in which the entire principle of their action may reside, other than rationality and intellect.'[84] Albertus then continues with a most interesting comparison:

> But where sensory perception is separated from rationality, as it is in brute animals, there it reacts (literally: *agitur*, is acted upon) rather than that it acts. For such a soul is moved immediately by that which is seen, and it follows or avoids that seen without possessing anything inside it by which the impulse might be curbed or moderated. That is why we say they react and do not act, and such a reaction is immediately a state of being moved by that which is seen.'
>
> (Ubi autem sensus a ratione separatus est, sicut in brutis, ibi magis agitur quam agat. Talis enim anima statim visis movetur et visa prosequitur vel fugit, nihil in se habens quo talis impetus fraenetur vel moderetur. Propter quod aguntur et non agunt, et tale agi statim movere est a visis.)[85]

In this fashion, then, people with defective intellect are put on a par with animals in terms of reasoning powers, or lack thereof.

With Albertus' pupil Aquinas, in *Summa theologiae*, reason reached its medieval apogee – although it is worth recalling that in his lifetime Aquinas was not uncontroversial.

> Reason and intellect cannot be different powers in human beings. This is clearly seen if one considers the activities of both. Understanding is an immediate grasp of an intellectual truth. Reasoning is passing from the understanding of one thing to the understanding of another thing in order to reach knowledge of intellectual truth ... So reasoning is to understanding as motion is to rest, or getting to having.
>
> (Ratio et intellectus in homine non possunt esse diversae potentiae. Quod manifeste cognoscitur, si utriusque actus consideretur. Intelligere enim est simpliciter veritatem intelligibilem apprehendere. Ratiocinari autem est procedere de uno intellecto ad aliud, ad veritatem intelligibilem cognoscendam ... Patet ergo quod ratiocinari comparatur ad intelligere sicut moveri ad quiescere, vel acquirere ad habere.)[86]

In *Summa theologiae* Aquinas made arguments against the Platonic concept that the human intellect contained all possible intelligible ideas but was prevented by physical matter (i.e. the body) from knowing them and using them:

> the falsity of this theory appears obvious from the fact that when a certain sense is lacking, there is lacking also the scientific knowledge of things perceived by that sense. A blind man, for instance, cannot have any knowledge of colours. This would not be the case if the soul's intellect were naturally endowed with the concepts of all intelligible objects.
>
> (manifeste apparet huius positionis falsitas ex hoc quod, deficiente aliquo sensu, deficit scientia eorum quae apprehenduntur secundum illum sensum; sicut caecus natus nullam potest habere notitiam de coloribus. Quod non esset, si animae essent naturaliter inditae omnium intelligibilium rationes.)[87]

One can use this to explain Blund's passage on the soul of the philosopher versus the soul of the idiot as being unequal only in so far as knowledge gained by the senses is concerned.

Aquinas, in *Summa theologiae*, discussed *De stultitia*, here rendered as 'stupidity', in three articles, with the first article on whether stupidity is to be seen in opposition to wisdom (*utrum stultitia opponatur sapientiae*), the second on the question whether stupidity is a sin (*utrum stultitia sit peccatum*) and the third on whether stupidity is to be regarded as one of the daughters of luxury (*utrum stultitia sit filias luxuriae*). In the first article he touched on the difference between two types of 'stupidity, namely *stultitia* and *fatuitas*:

Stultitia [Folly] seems to take its name from 'stupor'; wherefore Isidore says: 'A fool [*stultus*] is one who through dullness [*stuporem*] remains unmoved.' And folly differs from fatuity, according to the same authority, in that folly implies apathy in the heart and dullness in the senses, while fatuity denotes entire privation of the spiritual sense. Therefore folly is fittingly opposed to wisdom. (Et differt stultitia a fatuitate, sicut ibidem dicitur, quia stultitia importat hebetudinem cordis et obtusionem sensuum; fatuitas autem importat totaliter spiritualis sensus privationem. Et ideo convenienter stultitia sapientiae opponitur.)[88]

Aquinas responds to the first article that stupidity (*stultitia*) is to be distinguished from idiocy (*fatuitas*), the latter being a total lack of spiritual sense and therefore a complete negation and, unlike stupidity, not an opposition to wisdom. For the idiot lacks discretion (*sensus judicandi*), while the stupid person still has that even if blunted (*stultus autem habet, sed hebetatum*). The criterion for distinguishing stupidity from idiocy is therefore the presence of the ability to form judgements.[89] Taking this further, considering the second question, whether stupidity is a sin, Thomas responds 'It would seem that folly is not a sin. For no sin arises in us from nature. But some are fools naturally. Therefore folly is not a sin. ... [dullness in judgment may come] from a natural indisposition, as in the case of idiots, and such like folly is no sin.'[90] Thus in the second article Aquinas distinguished holy folly (unconcern for worldly things) from simple stupidity: 'Sometimes however it is the result of a man's being simply stupid about everything, as may be seen in idiots, who do not discern what is injurious to them, and this belongs to folly simply.'[91] Stupidity is then a sin if someone deliberately and willingly loosens their sense from the spiritual and turns towards the worldly. It is a different case for artificial fools, since they deliberately act foolishly, hence, then, folly can be a sin. In yet another article Aquinas dealt with the question 'whether reviling or railing is a mortal sin'. Making mockery of the impairments and defects of other people is a sin, Aquinas stated, and a small or large sin depending on whether one makes fun of small or large defects; plus, mockery is a greater sin than simply making fun of, since mockery turns the defects of a person to something worse, as if they were a fool, by which he dishonours such a person more than someone just making fun.[92] Explaining the morality of making fun of people and their character traits, Aquinas argued that the 'object of derision is always some evil or defect' but the very fact that one person is making light of another's 'defect' and not taking it seriously as a great evil means that 'this defect may be considered as a slight evil in relation to the person, just as we are wont to think little of the defects of children and imbeciles [*puerorum et stultorum*]'.[93]

In *Summa theologiae* Aquinas also dealt with the question of whether madmen and imbeciles should receive baptism, first presenting the objections that such people should not be baptised because they lack the use of reason, that lack of reason renders madmen and imbeciles like animals who are also irrational, and that such people are like those asleep in terms of not having reason and we do not baptise sleeping people. Especially the second objection draws on the age-old link between children and people with ID: 'But madmen and imbeciles lack the use of reason, indeed in some cases we do not expect them ever to have it, as we do in the case of children.'[94] In reply, Aquinas posits that if infant baptism is perfectly acceptable, then so should be the baptism of other irrational persons. Furthermore, he points out: 'Madmen and imbeciles lack the use of reason accidentally, i.e. through some impediment in a bodily organ; but not like irrational animals through want of a rational soul. Consequently the comparison does not hold.'[95] Finally, Aquinas summarises the advice on baptism, categorising the mentally ill and the mentally disabled according to four types.

> In the matter of madmen and imbeciles a distinction is to be made. For some are so from birth, and have no lucid intervals, and show no signs of the use of reason. And with regard to these it seems that we should come to the same decision as with regard to children who are baptized in the Faith of the Church … But there are others who have fallen from a state of sanity into a state of insanity. And with regard to these we must be guided by their wishes as expressed by them when sane: so that, if then they manifested a desire to receive Baptism, it should be given to them when in a state of madness or imbecility, even though then they refuse. If, on the other hand, while sane they showed no desire to receive Baptism, they must not be baptized. Again, there are some who, though mad or imbecile from birth, have, nevertheless, lucid intervals, in which they can make right use of reason. Wherefore, if then they express a desire for Baptism, they can be baptized though they be actually in a state of madness. And in this case the sacrament should be bestowed on them if there be fear of danger otherwise it is better to wait until the time when they are sane, so that they may receive the sacrament more devoutly. But if during the interval of lucidity they manifest no desire to receive Baptism, they should not be baptized while in a state of insanity. Lastly there are others who, though not altogether sane, yet can use their reason so far as to think about their salvation, and understand the power of the sacrament. And these are to be treated the same as those who are sane, and who are baptized if they be willing, but not against their will.[96]

With regard to this passage, where Aquinas distinguishes four types of insanity, Pickett surmised the fourth one (those who are mentally deficient but can take thought for their salvation) to mean 'those who are not really insane but rather feeble-minded'.[97] Ultimately this is all irrelevant, because infant baptism is the rule from the time of the early church onwards, so that 'most of the insane with whom the Church would have to do, whether idiots, imbeciles or persons who had enjoyed the use of reason but had subsequently suffered the loss of it, would have been baptized before their mental handicap had any bearing on the matter'.[98]

Aquinas had similar concerns over who can or cannot receive the Eucharist, again based on the prerequisite of possessing reason. Children, who are only temporarily irrational and of course eventually 'grow out' of this state, are not given the Eucharist, therefore neither should those adults deprived of reason be given it. But in a compromise solution Aquinas allows some 'irrational' people to receive this sacrament, since, as for baptism, there are different degrees and varieties of unreason.

> Men are said to be devoid of reason in two ways. First, when they are feeble-minded [*habent debilem*], as a man who sees dimly is said not to see: and since such persons can conceive some devotion towards this sacrament, it is not to be denied them. In another way men are said not to possess fully the use of reason. Either, then, they never had the use of reason, and have remained so from birth; and in that case this sacrament is not to be given to them, because in no way has there been any preceding devotion towards the sacrament: or else, they were not always devoid of reason, and then, if when they formerly had their wits they showed devotion towards this sacrament, it ought to be given to them in the hour of death; unless danger be feared of vomiting or spitting it out.[99]

Thus there are those who are not totally irrational or congenitally insane, but only 'feeble-minded' – a category which notably might include people with ID – and therefore may receive the Eucharist. Second, there are those who are congenitally irrational who should not be given the Eucharist, but the third group, those with lucid moments, might. So, according to Aquinas the feeble-minded are deemed to possess a varying measure of reason, whereas the congenitally and permanently insane lack *all* reason. Furthermore, the sacrament of anointing of the sick should not be conferred on children, on the mad or on imbeciles, since, unlike baptism, which is chiefly a remedy for original sin, the sacrament of anointing requires a movement of the free will, which none of these groups is deemed to have.[100]

The *Decretals* of Gregory IX contain a passage which derived from a query (incidentally, on the occasion of Becket's murder) by the bishop of Exeter to Pope Alexander III (1159–81), where a distinction is made of kinds of knowledge according to 'whether the delinquent was sane, insane or mentally deficient (*An sit discretus, vel non sane mentis, vel minus discretus*)'.[101] In the mid-twentieth century interpretation of this passage by Pickett, those entirely without the use of reason include infants whose mental immaturity does not permit them to have intellectual cognition and perpetually insane persons; while those without sufficient use of reason include children past the age of seven who have not in fact reached the normal mental maturity expected at that age (i.e. developmentally disabled) and adult idiots, whose understanding and mental development remained immature, for a variety of reasons (which of course would be of no interest to the church, only psychiatrists and educators), and in many cases of indeterminable causes.[102]

Although more than half a century old, this summary still neatly describes how the terminology of medieval church law might be matched with (relatively) contemporary modern categories. With regard to the question of whether children can take vows of religion Aquinas was of the opinion:

> It would seem that children cannot bind themselves by vow to enter religion. Since a vow requires deliberation of the mind, it is fitting that those alone should vow who have the use of reason. But this is lacking in children just as in imbeciles and madmen [*amentibus vel furiosis*]. Therefore just as imbeciles and madmen [*amentes et furiosi*] cannot bind themselves to anything by vow, so neither, seemingly, can children bind themselves by vow to enter religion.[103]

Aquinas, like Augustine before him, struggled to explain how original sin could be transmitted across the generations from Adam onwards, and used the example of heredity of idiocy to highlight the problem: 'granted that some bodily defects are transmitted by way of origin from parent to child, and granted that even some defects of the soul are transmitted in consequence, on account of a defect in the bodily habit, as in the case of idiots begetting idiots [*ex fatuis fatui generantur*]'.[104]

ID as perpetual childishness?

Having touched on the theme of the 'childishness' of persons with ID, it is worth taking a closer look at the connection between children and the intellectually disabled, starting with antiquity. Properly controlled emotions are rational judgements which can in turn control the irrational forces, such as physical, involuntary movements and reactions ('instinct', 'automatic emotional system' or 'lower brain functions' in modern parlance), that the human person is subject to. According to ideas developed by the Presocratic philosophers, Plato and Aristotle, the emotions are themselves a cognitive process, a concept taken up and further developed by the Stoics, Neoplatonists and Christians.[105] Emotions allow for value judgements, permitting the distinction between good and bad.[106] The problem is that animals never develop beyond such 'basic instincts', while in the normal course of individual human development from infant to adult the instinctive reactions are gradually added to and augmented by higher cognitive functions. Thus by the age of 14, according to the Stoic Posidonius (c. 135–c. 51 BC), the rational side of cognitive processes should be developed enough to take control of the emotions and of physical movements: 'This [rational element] is small at first and weak, but finishes up large and strong around the fourteenth year, by when it is right for it, like a charioteer, to take control (*kratein*) and rule (*arkhein*) over the pair of horses naturally conjoined with it, appetite (*epithumia*) and anger (*thumos*).'[107] The education of children is hence an important aspect of gaining understanding of the nature of things that allows a person to develop rational thought. Posidonius, as related by Galen, allowed for the existence of emotions without judgement in animals and children, 'especially appetite for pleasure (*epithumia*) and anger (*thumos*).'[108] Both animals and children are naturally aggressive and have a wish for domination for its own sake, while being without reason: 'We see [children] being angry (*thumousthai*) and kicking and biting and wishing (*ethelein*) to win (*nikân*) and dominate (*kratein*) their own kind, like some of the animals, when no prize is offered besides winning itself.'[109] This kind of 'impulsive' behaviour is seen often enough in toddlers, but also in adults with ID. The key difference between antique and modern notions appears only to be that while antique philosophers saw such behaviour as 'bestial', and as evidence for the intellectual and cognitive similarity of children to animals, modern disciplines of psychology and sociology apply different labels, e.g. inappropriate behaviour, but describe the same phenomena. Antique commentators like Posidonius emphasised the uncontrollable urges of appetite and anger, stating that 'animals use the appetitive and irascible (*epithumêtikê, thumoeidês*) capacities, but that humans alone have the rational (*logistikê*) principle',[110] yet this rationality is subject to development and at birth is small and weak. Children are thus like animals and, like animals, possess the non-rational powers of the soul; but while animals 'are not capable of understanding (*epistêmê*), but only of a non-rational habituation (*ethismos alogos*), such as might be given to horses',[111] children possess a faculty for rational thought but cannot yet control it when this faculty appears. Hence children are the hardest to deal with by their master/educator, they must be trained (*paideia*), curbed and moderated, and in a way children must be treated like the slavish beings that animals are characterised as. This goes back to a famous passage in Plato, *Laws* VII 808de, where children are compared to sheep, slaves and wild animals, but of all of these the child is the most intractable since, if 'the fountainhead of all wisdom' (*pêgên tou phronein*) goes untrained, the child can turn into a 'treacherous, cunning and shameless thing'.

Physical movement, especially uncontrolled, involuntary movement, is obstructive to intelligence, as Plato says in the *Timaeus*, effected 'by shaking the circuits of the soul', previously in the bodies of humans when they were first created, but nowadays in newborn infants.[112] It is not too far fetched to see in this description, perhaps, the origins of the idea that the repetitive, 'excessive' or inappropriate physical movement of people with ID is characteristic of the wider phenomenon: one may think in modern times of the child diagnosed with Attention-Deficit Hyperactivity Disorder, or the rocking motion so typical of institutionalised 'patients'. Proper movement, correctly directed, could, however, be beneficial and contribute to the education of the child. 'The therapeutic value of nurses rocking babies and singing ... is based on the bodily movements calming the movements of the soul.'[113]

Such concepts travelled a long way down the centuries. *De proprietatibus rerum* by Bartholomaeus Anglicus included a section on children and child behaviour, if not to say child psychology. Book Vi.v on (male) children (*de puero*) between the ages of seven and fourteen, when they reach the age of discernment ('knoweþ good and euel') and begin formal education (are 'sette to lore vndir tutours'), described children thus:

> Þan soche children [ben] neisch of fleisch, lethy and pliant of body, abel and li3t to meuynge, witty to lerne caroles, and wiþoute busines, and þey lede here lif wiþoute care and busines, and tellen pris [courage] onliche of merþe and likynge, and dreden no perile more þan betinge wiþ a 3erde [rod]. And þey louen an appil more þan gold. ... When þey ben preised or schamed or blamed þay sette litil þerby. For mouynge of hete of fleisch and of humpours þey ben eþeliche [lightly] and sone wrooþ and sone iplesed and for3euen sone. And for tendirnes of body þey bene sone ihurt and igreued, and þey mowe not wel endure harde trauaile.[114]
>
> Seþ smale children often han iuel maneres and tacchis, and þinken onliche on þinges þat beþ and recchiþ nou3t of thingis þat schal be, hy loueþ playes and game and venytes and forsake most þingis worth, and a3enward, for most worth þey holde lest worth or nou3t worth. Þey desiren þat is to hem contrarye and greuous, and tellen more of þe ymage of a childe þan of þe ymage of a man, and maken sorowe and woo and wepiþ more for þe losse of an appil þanne for þe losse of þeire heritage. And goodnes þat men doþ for hem þey late it passe out of mynde. Þey desiren and coueiten all þinges þat þey see, and prayeþ and askeþ hem wiþ voys and wiþ honde. Þey loue talkynges and counsailes of suche children as þey bene and forsaken and voyden companye of olde men. They holde no counsaile but þey wreyen [?] and tellen alle þat þey see and here. Sodeynly þey lau3e and sodeynly þey wepe. Always þey crie and iangle and iape and make mowes; vnneþe þey ben stille while þey slepe. Whanne þey bene iwassche of filthe and hore anon þey defoulen hemself eft. Whanne þe modir wasschiþ and

kembiþ hem þey kyken [kick] and praunsen [sprawl] and putte with feet and hondis, and wiþstonde with al here my3t and strengþe.[115]

The immature 'childish' behaviour, not knowing about consequences or ignoring them, led by their passions, no control over emotive outbursts, no forward thinking, no concept of the worth of things as defined by adults, not knowing what is good for them, driven by desire and passions, bursting out with their feelings and physically restless – all these things could equally be said of the behaviour ascribed to persons with ID.

Unguided and uneducated, children, animals and hence, by inference, people with IDs, will have emotions that cannot develop into judgements. Sometimes the will, and reason, can be completely overcome by the sensory appetites and by passions. 'When people are overpowered by passion so as to deprive them of reason and will, they effectively become animals whose behavior is always determined by their appetites.'[116] One philosophical question posed is whether living minds have to be rational minds, which leads on to the question whether brute animals are incapable of knowing anything. Augustine had refuted this, by giving the example of Odysseus's dog, which recognised and therefore 'knew' his master after his return from an absence of twenty years.[117] But the dog cannot sin in the same way as a supposedly rational human can, and sin is the key to lack of knowledge in patristic and medieval thought. 'It may be that rational minds, when they belong to sinful creatures, are more likely to get things wrong than a dog, which, though limited, can at least see clearly that which he does know.'[118] This, interestingly, compares with Blund's statement on the soul of an idiot being more perfect than the soul of a philosopher.

Medieval scholastic texts concerned with what we now categorise as psychological topics went a long way, describing the human mind and human behaviours in many details, but failed 'to develop a systematic account of developmental psychology'.[119] This is even more so the case when one considers that numerous passages in medieval writing are concerned with children, and especially with the psychological difference between adults and infants/ young children. As we have seen, children before a certain age were not accorded the same degrees of rationality as adults. A few further examples demonstrate the pervasiveness of this concept. Isaac Israeli (c. 855–955) was a Jewish Neoplatonist philosopher and physician, whose *Book of Definitions* was translated from Arabic into Latin by Gerard of Cremona in the twelfth century as *Liber de Definicionibus*. This passage on the intellect concerns intellectual potential and the trajectory of knowledge: 'When it acquires knowledge, that which had been in potentiality passes into actuality – like the intellect of a child which is in him potentially until he grows up, studies, and acquires knowledge, so that what had been in him potentially passes into actuality and he becomes a possessor of knowledge.'[120] Albertus Magnus, in *Quaestiones super De Animalibus*, also regarded children as mentally deficient: they are intermediate between man and animals because 'like brutes they spend all day eating and drinking', a simile extended to adult inebriates, for 'drunks and the intemperate' in their 'defects are childlike'.[121] And in his *Summa contra Gentiles*, Aquinas had explained:

> Now, *understanding is a kind of undergoing*, as is stated in [Aristotle] *De anima* III [III, 4, (429a 13)]. Therefore, since the child is potentially understanding, even though he is not actually understanding, there must be in him a potentiality whereby he is able to understand. And this potentiality is the possible intellect. Hence, there must already be a union of the possible intellect to the child before he understands actually. Therefore, it is not through the actually understood form that the possible intellect is brought into connection with man; rather, the possible intellect itself is in man from the beginning as part of himself.[122]

The 'debility' of infants was often discussed by scholastic theologians, based on a passage in Augustine where he wondered how so perfect a being as Christ had begun so ignominiously in a baby, responded to by Hugh of St Victor and Peter Lombard in the mid-twelfth century, then by Albertus Magnus, Bonaventure and Aquinas in the thirteenth.[123] The terminology used by these latter is *pueri, filii, proles* (children or offspring), as well as *parvuli*, but the context makes it clear that they were referring to children in the first stage of infancy, when as yet they could not walk or speak. The inability to speak is the chief distinction of the first stage of childhood from the next (although of course in real life this inability does not extend for the seven-year span that the first stage represents).

Augustine (*City of God* 5.11) had already emphasised the differences between irrational and rational elements within the make-up of the human soul. When God created human beings certain faculties were given to the soul: 'To the irrational soul also He gave memory, sense, appetite, to the rational he gave in addition intellect, intelligence and will.'[124] If will is a characteristic of the rational soul, and if children, animals and by implication the intellectually disabled do not have a fully developed rational soul, then it follows that none of these three beings possess will either. The next step in this line of thinking is not far off: if certain beings have no rational soul, and no will, then it is only right that those beings (e.g. adult humans with full mental faculties) who have both rational capabilities and will are put in charge over those lacking these capacities. This troubled Cassiodorus as much as it had Augustine. 'If God creates perfect and rational souls, why are infants not thus and children too? Can their limited capacity for knowing be explained by their comparative bodily weakness? Is this something like what happens when a fire is confined in a narrow vessel and cannot burn freely?'[125] Evans posited that one way for the medieval philosopher to look at this problem is to surmise 'that faculties will reach as far as they can if nothing impedes them. So it might be that we could extend this account of the problem of immaturity by suggesting that a given soul has an *inepta habitatio* from its mother's womb, as in the case of the mentally handicapped and thus is impeded from the full use of its powers.'[126] Because of such impediments people with ID are seen as perennial children. Therefore, as Evans concludes, '[h]uman capacity for knowledge is also affected, as divine and angelic knowing is not, by the need for human beings to grow up from immaturity. Angels do not have to grow up. The weakness of young bodies means that their senses and members cannot yet fully discharge their functions. Immaturity is imperfection.'[127] This is the basis of the philosophical argument for the domination over animals, children and, due to the child-like state ascribed to them, also the mentally disabled (the same argument was furthermore used to justify slavery).

In his tractate on the soul, Nemesius also addressed the link between children, irrationality and animals.

> For even if, when children are extremely young, they exhibit only non-rational behaviour, we still say that they have a rational soul, since, as they grow, they exhibit rational activity. But a non-rational animal at no age exhibits rationality and would have a rational soul superfluously, since rational ability was going to be absolutely useless. For everyone is agreed with one voice that nothing was brought to be by God that was superfluous. If that is so, a rational soul that would never be able to exhibit its function would have been inserted into domestic and wild animals superfluously, and it would have been a reproach to him who provided an unsuitable soul for the body.[128]

This raises interesting questions for people with ID: do they have a rational soul? If so, is that an example of superfluity, since people with ID are not using, or cannot use, their rational soul? Since superfluity is an absurdity that is not possible in the ordered scheme of divine creation, does that mean people with ID do not have a rational soul? If so, are they then to be categorised with animals? Such philosophical conundrums followed the preoccupation with the cognitive development of children, from a state of cognitive impairment in neonates and infants to the gradual acquisition of reason as part of growing up.[129]

Augustine had complained that it was less physical infirmity but the 'appalling ignorance, an infirmity that is not of the flesh but of the mind'[130] which infants had that was worrying for the human condition overall, especially since such infirmity was the direct result of original sin. Augustine was bothered by the fact that even Christ started off in ignorance whilst a baby, and concluded that there should not have been babies at the beginning of the world (because they are imperfect and because they are the result of original sin). Augustine did not regard infants as particularly innocent, stating in his *Confessions*: 'It is the feebleness of infantile limbs that is innocent not the intent [*animus*] of infants', plus the greedy, spiteful acts of infants 'are blandly tolerated not because they are nothing or a small matter, but because they will pass away with age'.[131] In response to this, in the 1130s Hugh of St Victor had argued that child growth and gradual development was part of a natural process, and since what was 'natural' was part of a divine plan, hence even in a prelapsarian state any children born to Adam and Eve would have followed the same gradual development as infants do today.[132] Around the same time, Odo of Lucca also covered this theme. Peter Lombard's synthesis of earlier authors argued similarly for the natural condition being one of gradual development of cognitive and physical abilities. Reynolds summed up Peter Lombard's views: 'Those who object that ignorance is a penalty for sin fail to appreciate the distinction between ignorance and mere nescience, for ignorance is the lack of knowledge of what one *ought* to know.'[133] Then Albertus Magnus, in the 1240s, dealt with the impairments of infancy in his *Commentary on the Sentences*. In *Summa theologiae* Aquinas wrote on child development and the idea that very small children do not yet have the use of free will: 'As long as he does not have the use of reason, the child does not differ from an irrational animal.'[134] And a Franciscan writer on anthropology in the 1260s picked up the theme in the work *Summa fratres alexandri*, where he argued that the infirmity of modern infants (i.e. that they do not possess intelligence or rational faculties at birth) is due to original sin. In general, in the thirteenth century the scholastics agreed on the natural weakness of babies, which therefore would have been natural in paradise also. All scholastics, except for Albertus Magnus, said that the hypothetical paradisiac infants would have been quicker in developing than postlapsarian infants are; the explanation normally given is that excess moisture in the brain of infants is, especially according to Albertus Magnus, the cause for the low level of development in infants. These statements can be found in Albertus Magnus' texts on cognitive development. Furthermore, the thirteenth-century scholastics made a distinction, where Augustine had made none, between immaturity (which is natural) and corruption (which is due to original sin), hence the scholastics were more accepting of infants and their apparent imperfections than Augustine had been. But they did not

regard infancy as something positive or valuable in itself, merely as a necessary prelude to 'proper' humanity (i.e. the mature person – implying male
– of around thirty, at the height of their powers). Overall, therefore, infantile
development is 'natural', and infantile nescience equally so, because it takes
time to develop and acquire cognitive abilities, except that the fictitious infants
of Eden would have done so more quickly and easily, plus would have been
imbued with a kind of instinctive basic knowledge of practical and moral
matters.[135]

Medieval scholastic authorities, such as Aquinas and Albertus Magnus,
stated that children are, in fact, born with a rational soul, but opinions differed
as to the exact development of the soul. Aquinas believed that the foetus in
the womb went through a series of stages in which a succession of souls, first
vegetative, then sensitive and finally the rational soul inhabited the growing
body.[136] This view has interesting implications for the birth of pre-term babies,
for miscarriage or for abortion, in that the earlier a foetus exited the maternal
womb, the lower down the developmental scale its soul would be, and presumably, if the pre-term baby died or miscarried, would be stuck with an un(der)
developed, pre-rational soul, and hence the inability to access limbo, let alone
heaven. In contrast, Albertus Magnus presented a graded (and almost evolutionary) developmental theory, in which the soul gradually grew in capacity
and ability to acquire new faculties.[137] Some attempt was made by Aquinas to
explain why the neonate, although fully human in all other respects, was not
fully rational, arguing, in common with many other medieval authorities, that it
was the excessive moisture of the brain of neonates that prevented intellectual
thought, but also that newborn infants simply had not acquired enough knowledge yet to make use of reason.[138] In conclusion, it is important to remember
that the schoolmen regarded infants as incomplete human beings, not incomplete per se, but incomplete because they had not fulfilled their potential. From
the scholastic point of view, human perfection was reached in the 'youthful
age' (aetas iuvenilis), which was deemed to be around the age of thirty, a figure
chosen because Adam was created and Christ died at that age; in addition, it
was commonly believed that everyone, regardless of their actual age at death,
would be resurrected as a perfect thirty-year-old.[139] 'Hence Thomas Aquinas
assumes that the typical life span was a cycle proceeding from deficiency to perfection in humanness and then declining to deficiency again.'[140] And of course,
according to such arguments, people with ID never go through the cycle, never
reach perfection, are permanently stuck in defect. This was echoed in Arabic
Aristotelianism. In the Muqaddimah, Chapter 6, prefatory discussion, section
6 (man is essentially ignorant, and only acquires knowledge), Ibn Khaldûn
remarked on the trajectory of knowledge acquisition.

Man's ability to think comes to him only after the animality in him has reached perfection. It starts from discernment. Before man has discernment, he has no knowledge whatever, and is counted one of the animals. His origin, the way in which he was created from a drop of sperm, a clot of blood, and a lump of flesh, still determines his (mental make-up). Whatever he attains subsequently is the result of sensual perception and the ability to think God has given him.[141]

Arguably, therefore, following Ibn Khaldûn's exposition, neonates and people with severe ID are at the first stage of ignorant existence, the difference being that babies mature into infants, children and then adults, acquiring the various levels of discernment along the way, but people with ID remain forever below the discernment threshold.

Poor in spirit, not in mind

One final theological aspect of ID needs comment. The Sermon on the Mount (Matt. 5:3–10) opens with the famous beatitude 'Blessed are the poor in spirit: for theirs is the kingdom of heaven'. All too often the phrase regarding the poor in spirit seems to have been read as meaning those lacking in mind, that is, the mentally disabled. But on closer inspection there is no evidence for this interpretation.

> The word *poor* seems to represent an Aramaic *'ányâ* (Hebrew *'anî*), bent down, afflicted, miserable, poor; while *meek* is rather a synonym from the same root, *'ánwan* (Hebrew *'ánaw*), bending oneself down, humble, meek, gentle. ... The blessed ones are the poor 'in spirit', who by their free will are ready to bear for God's sake this painful and humble condition, even though at present they be actually rich and happy.[142]

Augustine wrote an early treatise around 394 entitled *On the Sermon on the Mount*, where the poverty of the spirit is referred to already as deliberate humility, and has nothing whatsoever to do with ID.[143] The idea that the phrase 'blessed are the poor in spirit' is meant to refer to people who are poor in intellectual capacities seems to have crept in via a German theologian named Karl Friedrich August Fritzsche, who published his influential *Lateinische Kommentare zu Matthäus* in 1826. Since then, this reading has held a firm and unshakeable place in German theology as well as in histories of disability. For example, in his social history of disability, Fandrey committed the typically German scholarly faux pas of assuming that the poor in spirit means the mentally disabled.[144] But Anglophone history need not rest on its laurels either, since influential medical historians have also made the same misinterpretation. In an overview of medical history, it has been claimed that 'blessed are the poor in heart' referred to the simple-minded, leading to the following rather fanciful historiographic depiction: 'Many authors exalted the village idiot, singing cheerfully, if tunelessly, to the glory of God; in fact, as well as in the word's etymology, the cretin thus represented the true Christian.'[145] This is a gross over-simplification on all counts, linguistic as much as analytical, and serves nothing else but to perpetuate one of the modern myths (outlined in the introduction), here the 'village idiot' myth of a rose-tinted, happily integrated, pre-modern past. As the next chapter shows, the legal situation of persons with ID during the Middle Ages was everything other than 'inclusive' in the modern sense.

Notes

1 Thomas Aquinas, *Summa contra Gentiles. Book One: God*, trans. and intro. Anton C. Pegis (Notre Dame, IN: University of Notre Dame Press, 1975), 64, Chapter 3.4.

2 R. I Moore, *The Formation of a Persecuting Society* (Oxford: Blackwell, 1987), 139.

3 Judith S. Neaman, *Suggestion of the Devil: Insanity in the Middle Ages and the Twentieth Century* (New York: Octagon Books, 1978), 142.

4 Christopher Goodey, *A History of Intelligence and 'Intellectual Disability': The Shaping of Psychology in Early Modern Europe* (Farnham: Ashgate, 2011), 282.

5 B. B. Price, *Medieval Thought: An Introduction* (Oxford: Blackwell, 1992), 169.

6 Ibn Khaldûn has been termed the true father of historiography and sociology, amongst others by none other than Arnold J. Toynbee, *A Study of History* (London: Oxford University Press, 2nd edn 1935), vol. 3, 322, who called the *Muqaddimah* 'undoubtedly the greatest work of its kind that has ever yet been created by any mind in any time or place'. As the author himself of a monumental world history, Toynbee spoke as one who should know. Monumental, universal histories may currently have fallen somewhat out of academic fashion, but that is no reason to belittle the achievements of the past.

7 Ibn Khaldûn, *The Muqaddimah: An Introduction to History*, translated by Franz Rosenthal, abridged and edited by N. J. Dawood (London: Routledge and Kegan Paul, 1967), 333–4.

8 Tim Stainton, 'Reason and Value: The Thought of Plato and Aristotle and the Construction of Intellectual Disability', *Mental Retardation*, 39 (2001), 452–60, at 452.

9 Stainton, 'Reason and Value', 456.

10 As argued by C. F. Goodey, 'Mental Disabilities and Human Values in Plato's Late Dialogues', *Archiv für Geschichte der Philosophie*, 74 (1992), 26–42.

11 Aristotle, *De memoria et reminiscentia*, 453a31–453b7; English in J. I. Beare (trans.), 'On Memory', in Jonathan Barnes (ed.), *The Complete Works of Aristotle:*

The Revised Oxford Translation (Princeton: Princeton University Press, 1984), 720.

12 Aristotle, *Parts of Animals*, 4.10, 686b23–9.

13 Catherine Osborne, *Dumb Beasts and Dead Philosophers: Humanity and the Humane in Ancient Philosophy and Literature* (Oxford: Clarendon Press, 2007), 115.

14 Herbert A. Davidson, *Alfarabi, Avicenna, and Averroes, on Intellect: Their Cosmologies, Theories of the Active Intellect, and Theories of Human Intellect* (New York and Oxford: Oxford University Press, 1992), 3.

15 'en grammateiôi ôhi mêthen enuparkhei entelekheia gegrammenon', Aristotle, *De anima*, Book III.iv (429b30–430a2); see Davidson, *Alfarabi, Avicenna, and Averroes*, 259.

16 Book 4, cap. 5, 1126a3, Aristotle, *Nicomachean Ethics: Books II–IV*, trans. C. C. W. Taylor (Oxford: Clarendon Press, 2006), 51.

17 *Enneads*, III 8.iv, cited in John Gregory, *The Neoplatonists: A Reader* (London and New York: Routledge, 1999), 58.

18 For the foregoing summary of late antique philosophy, see Gillian Clark, 'Preface', *Body and Gender, Soul and Reason in Late Antiquity* (Farnham: Ashgate, 2011), ix.

19 Gillian Clark, 'The Fathers and the Animals: The Rule of Reason?', in A. Linzey and D. Yamamoto (eds), *Animals on the Agenda* (London: SCM Press, 1998), 68.

20 Book II 16, 14–15, *The Institutio oratoria of Quintilian*, trans. H. E. Butler (Loeb Classical Library 124) (Cambridge, MA: Harvard University Press/London: Heinemann, 1980), vol. I, 322–4/323–5.

21 Book II 16, 17, *Institutio oratoria*, vol. I, 324/325.

22 Catherine Atherton, 'Children, Animals, Slaves and Grammar', in Yun Lee Too and Niall Livingstone (eds), *Pedagogy and Power: Rhetorics of Classical Learning* (Cambridge: Cambridge University Press, 1998), 214–44, at 214; see R. Sorabji, *Animal Minds and Human Morals* (London, 1993), 89–93 for a discussion of the sheer variety of characteristics allegedly unique to human beings.

23 Rudolph E. Siegel, *Galen on Psychology, Psychopathology and Function and Diseases of the Nervous System* (Basel: Karger, 1973), 140, citing Galen in condensed form via ed. D. C. G. Kuehn, *Galeni opera omnia*, 22 vols (Leipzig, 1821–33), vol. 1, 1–2;

24 Porphyry of Tyre, *On Abstinence from Killing Animals*, trans. Gillian Clark (London: Duckworth, 2000).

25 Porphyry of Tyre, *On abstinence* 3.3.3–5. Translation given in Gillian Clark, 'Translate into Greek: Porphyry of Tyre on the new barbarians', in *Constructing Identities in Late Antiquity*, ed. R. Miles (London: Routledge, 1999), 119–20.

26 Porphyry of Tyre, *On abstinence* 3.5.2–3. Translation given in Clark, 'Translate into Greek', 120–1.

27 Some of Augustine's philosophical thoughts on animals and un/reason may be found in his tract '83 Questions on Various Topics', *Corpus Christianorum*

Series Latina (Turnhout: Brepols, 1953–) [hereafter *CCSL*], vol. 44A, 20; see also R. Renehan, 'The Greek Anthropocentric View of Man', *Harvard Studies in Classical Philology*, 85 (1981), 239–59.

28 Section 1[4.20], *Nemesius: On the Nature of Man*, trans. with intro. and notes R. W. Sharples and P. J. van der Eijk (Liverpool: Liverpool University Press, 2008), 40.

29 'Infans dicitur homo primae aetatis; dictus autem infans quia adhuc fari nescit, id est loqui non potest.' Book XI.ii.11, *The Etymologies of Isidore of Seville*, trans. and intro. Stephen A. Barney, W. J. Lewis, J. A. Beach and Oliver Berghof (Cambridge: Cambridge University Press, 2010, 241; Latin from http://penelope.uchicago. edu/Thayer/E/Roman/texts/Isidore/home.html (accessed 21 January 2013).

30 Albertus Magnus, *Liber de Animalibus*, 21.1.1, ed. R. Stadler (Munich, 1916), cited by Goodey, *A History of Intelligence*, 303.

31 'Sicut est naturaliter servus qui pollens viribus deficit intellectu: sic vigens mentis industria et regitiva prudentia, naturaliter dominatur.' *De regimine principum*, bk. 3, prologue, cited and English trans. by Robert W. Carlyle and Alexander J. Carlyle, *A History of Mediaeval Political Theory in the West*, vol. 5: *Political Theory from the Tenth Century to the Thirteenth* (Edinburgh: Blackwood, 1903), 24.

32 'Nam illi qui intellectu praeeminent, naturaliter dominantur; illi vero qui sunt intellectu deficientes, corpore vero robusti, a natura videntur instituti ad serviendum; sicut Aristoteles dicit in sua politica.' Aquinas, *Summa contra gentiles*, ed. P. Marc, C. Pera et al., 3 vols (Turin: Marietti, 1961–67), vol. 3, 116, Book III, chapter 81; cf. Aristotle, *Politics*, I, 5.

33 *ST*, Ia, question 96, article 4.

34 Katherine Chambers, '"When We Do Nothing Wrong, We Are Peers": Peter the Chanter and Twelfth-Century Political Thought', *Speculum*, 88:2 (2013), 405–26, at 420.

35 Augustine, *De Quantitate Animi*, ix.15, ed. in *CSEL* vol. 89.

36 Philippe Buc, *L'ambiguïté du livre: Prince, pouvoir, et peuple dans les commentaires de la Bible au moyen âge* (Paris: Beauchesne, 1994), 75–96; Moore, *Formation of a Persecuting Society*, 151.

37 Chambers, 'When We Do Nothing Wrong', 425.

38 'La capacité du prélat de se refaire à l'image de Dieu par la contemplation et la vertu justifie sa domination sur "l'homme animal"; ce gouvernement est assimilé à celui exercé par la raison sur la chair et ses passions'. Buc, *L'ambiguïté du livre*, 82.

39 Book Vi.xv, *On the Properties of Things: John Trevisa's Translation of* Bartholomæus Anglicus De proprietatibus Rerum. *A Critical Text*, Vol. I, eds M. C. Seymour and Colleagues (Oxford: Clarendon Press, 1975), 312.

40 Book Vi.xvi, *On the Properties of Things*, 312. Bartholomaeus cites 'slow' in *Prouerbium* 30 (probably Ecclesiasticus 19:1), 'slow3' in *Mathei* 18 (Matthew 18:23–4), and 'slowe' in *Luk* 19 (Luke 19:20).

41 'Il n'a ne memoire n'assens/ Plus qu'aroit une mue beste:/ Des maulx c'on li

fait a grant feste,/ Et grant solaz estre li semble.' *Miracles de Nostre Dame par personnages*, eds Gaston Paris and Ulysse Robert, 8 vols, Société des Anciens Textes Français (Paris, 1876–93), verses 874–7, cited by Sylvia Huot, *Madness in Medieval French Literature: Identities Found and Lost* (Oxford: Oxford University Press, 2003), 66. But elsewhere in same text treatment of the 'fool' is put in perspective: 'This wretched fool here suffers so many blows and so much filth that I don't know how he stands it.' 'Cilz meschans soz yci presens/ Reçoit tant de corps et d'ordure/ Que je ne scé conment il dure.' *Miracles de Nostre Dame par personnages*, eds Gaston Paris and Ulysse Robert, vv. 460–2, cited Huot, *Madness in Medieval French Literature*, 73.

42 Neaman, *Suggestion of the Devil*, 101; cf. *Corpus iuris canonici*, ed. Aemilius Richter and Friedberg, 2 vols (Graz: Akademische Druck und Verlagsanstalt, rpt 1959), C.2, C.XV, q.1.

43 Tim Stainton, 'Reason, Grace and Charity: Augustine and the Impact of Church Doctrine on the Construction of Intellectual Disability', *Disability & Society*, 23:5 (2008), 485–96, at 491.

44 Stainton, 'Reason, Grace and Charity', 492.

45 See James Latham, *God's Philosophers: How the Medieval World Laid the Foundations of Modern Science* (London: Icon, 2010) for a counter view on this stereotype.

46 Schaff translation notes: 'We here follow the reading *cerriti*; other readings are, – *curati* (with studied folly), *cirrati* (with effeminate foppery), and *citrati* (decking themselves with *citrus* leaves).' Edgar Kellenberger, *Der Schutz der Einfältigen. Menschen mit einer geistigen Behinderung in der Bibel und in weiteren Quellen* (Zurich: Theologischer Verlag Zürich, 2011), 100–1, 146 follows the reading *cirrati* and translates as the curly-haired, linking in with his findings that often in the ancient world the mentally afflicted (whether psychologically or intellectually disabled, mad or foolish) are portrayed as having dishevelled hair.

47 Augustine, *De peccatorum meritis et remissione et de baptismo parvulorum ad Marcellinum*, I.32, CSEL, vol. 60 (1913); English trans. by Philip Schaff, *Nicene and Post-Nicene Fathers*, Series I, vol. 5, 151, full text via www.ccel.org/ccel/schaff/npnf105.pdf (accessed 28 January 2013).

48 Augustine, *De peccatorum meritis* I.66, trans. Schaff, Series I, vol. 5, 153. See also Kellenberger, *Schutz der Einfältigen*, 100, and 135n237, mentioning further writings of Augustine on fools, simpletons, *moriones*: *Letters* 143.3; 166.17; *Contra Julian* III.10; the phrase 'born a *fatuus*' appears in *Enchiridion* 103; *Letters* 187.25; *Contra Julian* IV.16; V.18; VI.1–2; *Opus imperfectum* I 54; III 155, 160–1 and 191; IV 8, 75, 114–15, 123, 125 and 134; V 22; VI 9, 14, 16 and 27; other terms for fools used in *Opus imperfectum* III 198; V 1 and 11; cf. E. Kellenberger, 'Augustin und die Menschen mit einer geistigen Behinderung. Der Theologe als Beobachter und Herausgeforderter', *Theologische Zeitschrift*, 67 (2011), 25–36.

49 Letter 166 from Augustine to Jerome, chapter 6 para. 17, at www.newadvent.org/fathers (accessed 5 December 2012).

50 Augustine, *Opus imperfectum* VI 16.
51 Origen controversially thought that souls enter into bodies as a kind of punishment; *Nemesius*, 6.
52 See Kellenberger, *Schutz der Einfältigen*, 100, 137.
53 *Nemesius*, 6.
54 G. R. Evans, *Philosophy and Theology in the Middle Ages* (London and New York: Routledge, 1993), 93.
55 Bede [Ps.-Byrhtferth on Bede], *De Natura Rerum*, PL, vol. 90, cols 190–1; Cassiodorus, *De anima*, VII, PL, vol. 70, col. 1292; Alcuin, PL, vol. 101, col. 645; Rhabanus Maurus, PL, vol. 110, col. 1112.
56 Section 41 [117.20–5], *Nemesius*, 201.
57 Simon Kemp, *Medieval Psychology* (New York: Greenwood Press, 1990), 82.
58 Kemp, *Medieval Psychology*, 83; cf. Aquinas, *ST*, I, question 2, article 40, 3.
59 Book XI.i.11–13, *Etymologies*, 231–2; Latin from http://penelope.uchicago.edu/Thayer/E/Roman/texts/Isidore/home.html (accessed 21 January 2013).
60 G. R. Evans, *Getting It Wrong: The Medieval Epistemology of Error* (Leiden: Brill, 1998), 32–3. Aristotle, *De anima*, Book II.iii (414a29–32); Hugh of St Victor, *Didascalion*, I.iii; Augustine, *De Trinitate*, I.400, ed. in *CCSL* vol 50; Aquinas, *ST* I, question 78, article 4.
61 Evans, *Getting It Wrong*, 34.
62 A number of post-Aristotelian Greek texts and later Arabic texts influenced Alfarabi, Avicenna and Averroes; some of the pertinent examples include Alexander of Aphrodisias (*De anima*), Plotinus (*Enneads*), Themestius (paraphrases of Aristotle's *De anima* and *Metaphysics*), a number of commentaries attributed to John Philoponus, a paraphrase of the Aristotelian *De anima* attributed to Ishaq ibn Hunain (d. 876) and the ninth-century writings of Al-Kindi; see Davidson, *Alfarabi, Avicenna, and Averroes*, 7–9 for summary.
63 Davidson, *Alfarabi, Avicenna, and Averroes*, 49. The second stage is actual intellect and the third, culminating stage, is acquired intellect.
64 Davidson, *Alfarabi, Avicenna, and Averroes*, 83–4. Also explained in E. Ruth Harvey, *The Inward Wits: Psychological Theory in the Middle Ages and the Renaissance* (London: Warburg Institute, University of London, 1975), 48.
65 Davidson, *Alfarabi, Avicenna, and Averroes*, 98.
66 As summarised by Davidson, *Alfarabi, Avicenna, and Averroes*, 162.
67 Davidson, *Alfarabi, Avicenna, and Averroes*, 189.
68 Davidson, *Alfarabi, Avicenna, and Averroes*, 200–1.
69 They are, respectively, Averroes' Epitome of the Aristotelian *De anima*, the Middle Commentary on the *De anima*, the Long Commentary, the *Epistle on the Possibility of Conjunction*, two short pieces on conjunction with the active intellect, and a commentary on sections of Alexander of Aphrodisias' *De intellectu*; see Davidson, *Alfarabi, Avicenna, and Averroes*, 262–4, for description of surviving manuscripts in Arabic, Hebrew and Latin.
70 Davidson, *Alfarabi, Avicenna, and Averroes*, 267.

71 Michael W. Dols (ed. Diana E. Immisch), *Majnûn: The Madman in Medieval Islamic Society* (Oxford: Clarendon Press, 1992), 421.

72 Ibn Khaldûn, *Muqaddimah*, 86–7.

73 Henry of Ghent, *Quodlibetal Questions on Free Will*, trans. and intro. Roland J. Teske (Milwaukee, WI: Marquette University Press, 1993), 31, Quodlibet I, Question 15.

74 Evans, *Getting It Wrong*, xi.

75 See D. A. Callus, 'The Introduction of Aristotelian Learning to Oxford', *Proceedings of the British Academy*, 29 (1943), 229–81.

76 'Ergo nulla anima alia est sapientior.' XXV.iii.369, Iohannes Blund, *Tractatus de anima*, eds D. A. Callus and R. W. Hunt (London: British Academy/Oxford University Press, 1970), 101.

77 'Item. Potest similiter hic queri, utrum anima philosophi cuiusdam sit sapientior separata a corpore quam anima alicuius idiote post separationem ipsius a corpore. Quod non sit sapientior videtur per proximam rationem precedentem.' XXV.iii.370, Blund, *Tractatus de anima*, 102.

78 R. W. Sharples, 'Alexander and pseudo-Alexander of Aphrodisias, *Scripta Minima*. Questions and Problems, Makeweights and Prospects', in W. Kullmann, J. Althoff and M. Asper (eds), *Gattungen wissenschaftlicher Literatur in der Antike* (Tübingen: Günter Narr Verlag, 1998), 383–403, 171.28; 172.5; 189.12; and *Alexander of Aphrodisias On Fate*, ed. and trans. R. W. Sharples (London: Duckworth, 1983), 131.

79 'Sunt autem quidam homines idiotae non discernentes universale a particulari.' Albertus Magnus, *De anima*, Liber I, tractatus I, cap. 6, in B. Geyer (ed.), *Opera Omnia*, vol. VII, pars I (Münster: Aschendorf, 1968), 12.

80 XXV.iii.372, Blund, *Tractatus de anima*, 102.

81 Evans, *Getting It Wrong*, 27.

82 XXVI.i.385, Blund, *Tractatus de anima*, 107.

83 'Dictum est enim quod actus hominis ut homo est ratio est. Propter quod actio hominis non erit quod secundum rationem ab homine non procedit.' Albertus Magnus, *Ethica*, liber VI, tr. I, cap. 4, in Albertus-Magnus-Institut (ed.), *Albertus Magnus und sein System der Wissenschaften. Schlüsseltexte in Übersetzung Lateinisch-Deutsch* (Münster: Aschendorff, 2011), 342–3.

84 'Nihil enim in homine est in quo sit totum principium sui actus, nisi ratio vel intellectus.' Albertus-Magnus-Institut (ed.), *Albertus Magnus und sein System der Wissenschaften*, 342–3.

85 Albertus-Magnus-Institut (ed.), *Albertus Magnus und sein System der Wissenschaften*, 344–5.

86 *ST*, I, question 79, article 8, 3 and *ad* 3, in Anthony Kenny, *Aquinas on Mind* (London and New York: Routledge, 1993), 55, 164n14.

87 *ST*, I, question 84, article 3, in Kenny, *Aquinas on Mind*, 91, 168n2.

88 *ST*, II-II, question 46, article 1, contra.

89 See Angelika Groß, *'La Folie'. Wahnsinn und Narrheit im spätmittelalterlichen Text*

und Bild (Heidelberg: Carl Winter Universitätsverlag, 1990), 56–7; Annie Kraus, *Der Begriff der Dummheit bei Thomas von Aquin und seine Spiegelung in Sprache und Kultur* (Münster: Aschendorff, 1971), 138–43.

90   *ST*, II-II, question 46, article 1, obj. 1.

91   *ST*, II-II, question 46, article 1, resp. to obj. 4; 'Quandoque autem contingit ex hoc quod homo est simpliciter circa omnia stupidus, ut patet in amentibus, qui non discernunt quid sit iniuria. Et hoc pertinet ad stultitiam simpliciter.'

92   *ST*, II-II, question 72, article 2.

93   *ST*, II-II, question 75, article 2.

94   *ST*, III, question 68, article 12, obj. 2.

95   *ST*, III, question 68, article 12, resp. ad obj. 2.

96   *ST*, III, question 68, article 12, resp.

97   R. Colin Pickett, *Mental Affliction and Church Law: An Historical Synopsis of Roman and Ecclesiastical Law and a Canonical Commentary* (Ottawa, Ontario: The University of Ottawa Press, 1952), 51

98   Pickett, *Mental Affliction and Church Law*, 32.

99   *ST*, III, question 80, article 9, resp.

100 *ST*, Supplement to III, question 32, article 3; on the effects of grace and possession of free will see also II pars I, Question 113, article 3, reply to objection 1 concerning the insane [*furiosis et amentibus*] who have never had free will.

101 C. 6, X, *de homicidio, etc,* IV, 12, Pickett, *Mental Affliction and Church Law*, 65.

102 Pickett, *Mental Affliction and Church Law*, 103–4.

103 *ST*, II-II, question 88, article 9, a. 1.

104 *ST*, II-I, question 81, article 1, resp.

105 Richard Sorabji, *Emotion and Peace of Mind: From Stoic Agitation to Christian Temptation* (Oxford: Oxford University Press, 2000), 17, 19–28.

106 Sorabji, *Emotion and Peace of Mind*, 29–33.

107 Posidonius, lost compostion *On Emotions*, but preserved in Galen, *De placitis Hippocratis et Platonis*, 5.5.34, ed. and trans. P. de Lacy, Corpus Medicorum Graecorum (Berlin: Akademie Verlag, 1978–84), 324, cited in Sorabji, *Emotion and Peace of Mind*, 96; the metaphor of the charioteer stems from Plato, *Phaedrus* 246 A-257 B; this psychodynamic tug between reason and two irrational forces had even influenced Sigmund Freud, 'The Ego and the Id', Standard Edition, vol. 19, 25.

108 Sorabji, *Emotion and Peace of Mind*, 125.

109 Posidonius, *On Emotions*, in Galen, *De placitis Hippocratis et Platonis*, 5.5.4–5, ed. de Lacy, 316, 318, cited in Sorabji, *Emotion and Peace of Mind*, 129.

110 Sorabji, *Emotion and Peace of Mind*, 125; see Posidonius, *On Emotions*, in Galen, *De placitis Hippocratis et Platonis*, 5.6.38, 5.5.34, ed. de Lacy, 334, 324; Galen actually denies any reason at all to children (*De placitis* 5.5.2, at 316).

111 Sorabji, *Emotion and Peace of Mind*, 128; see Posidonius, *On Emotions*, in Galen, *De placitis Hippocratis et Platonis*, 5.5.35, ed. de Lacy, 324.

112 Sorabji, *Emotion and Peace of Mind*, 117; Plato, *Timaeus* 43 A-44 B.

113   Sorabji, *Emotion and Peace of Mind*, 117; see Plato, *Laws* 790 D-791 B.

114   Book Vi.v, *On the Properties of Things*, 300.

115   Book Vi.v, *On the Properties of Things*, 301.

116   Kemp, *Medieval Psychology*, 84; cf. Aquinas, *ST*, I, question 2, article 10, 3.

117   Augustine, *De Quantitate Animi*, xxvi.50.

118   Evans, *Getting It Wrong*, 209.

119   Kemp, *Medieval Psychology*, 160.

120   *Book of Definitions*, cap. 4, Isaac Israeli: *A Neoplatonic Philosopher of the Early Tenth Century*, trans. Alexander Altmann and Samuel M. Stern, foreword Alfred L. Ivry (Chicago: University of Chicago Press, 1958, new edition 2009), 36.

121   Albertus Magnus, *Quaestiones super De Animalibus*, in *Opera Omnia*, ed. B. Geyer (Münster, 1955), vol. xii, 171.

122   Chapter 60, 6, Aquinas, *Summa contra Gentiles. Book Two: Creation*, trans. and intro. James F. Anderson (Notre Dame, IN: University of Notre Dame Press, 1975), 185.

123   Philip L. Reynolds, 'The Infants of Eden: Scholastic Theologians on Early Childhood and Cognitive Development', *Mediaeval Studies*, 68 (2006), 89–132; see also Philip L. Reynolds, 'Thomas Aquinas and the Paradigms of Childhood', in *The Vocation of the Child*, ed. Patrick McKinley Brennan (Grand Rapids, MI: Eerdmans, 2008), 154–88. Augustine, *De peccatorum meritis et remissione et de baptismo parvulorum ad Marcellinum libri tres* 1.37.68, ed. C. F. Urba and J. Zycha, *CSEL*, vol. 60 (Vienna, 1913), 68–9; Hugh of St Victor, *De sacramentis christianae fidei*, writtten 1130/31–37; Peter Lombard, *Sentences*, Book 2, distinction 20, written 1154–57; Albertus Magnus, *In II Sent.* 20.7, completed 1249; Bonaventure, *In II Sent.* 23.2.1, probably 1254–56; Thomas Aquinas, *Scriptum super libros Sententiarum* 20.2.1 and *ST* I, question 101.

124   Cited in Sorabji, *Emotion and Peace of Mind*, 335.

125   Evans, *Getting It Wrong*, 159, paraphrasing Cassiodorus, *De anima*, VII.549, ed. in *CCSL*, vol. 96: 'Si divinitas perfectas et rationabilies animas cret, cur aut posito sensu vivunt infantes aut iuvenes inveniuntur excordes? Se quis non intendat animas parvulorum imbecillitate corporis nec officia sensuum nec ministeria posse explicare membrorum? Ut si ignem anbusto vase concludas, [?]ltum, ut illis moris est, nequit appetere, quia eum artissimum obstaculum constat operire.'

126   Evans, *Getting It Wrong*, 160, refering to Cassiodorus, *De anima*, cap. VII, ed. J. W. Halporn, *CCSL*, vol. 96, 549–50: 'Sic stultis iuuenibus obuiat quod aut imparilitate partium aut crassitudine humorum materni utero uitio suscepto, anima inepta nimis habitatione deprimitur et uim suam exercere non praeualet, inconuenientis domicilii sede praepedita; quod stultis accidere hodieque conspicimus quos Graeci *niniones* uocant. Nam ut de usuali quoque dicamus euentu, quam multi morbis accidentibus aut onerato cerebro aut praecordiorum stupore confusi acumen solitae sapientiae perdiderunt.'

127   Evans, *Getting It Wrong*, 207.

128   Section 2 [35.15–36.1], *Nemesius*, 74.

129 Reynolds, 'The Infants of Eden', 117–26.
130 'propter horrendam ignorantiam atque infirmitatem non carnis, sed mentis', *De peccatorum meritis* 1.37.68, cited Reynolds, 'The Infants of Eden', 69.
131 'Ita imbecillitas membrorum infantilium innocens est, non animus infantium ... Sed blande tolerantur haec, non quia nulla uel parva, sed quia aetatis accessu peritura sunt', 1.7.11, *Confessionum libri XIII*, ed. L. Verheijen, CCSL, 27 (Turnhout, 1981), 6.
132 Reynolds, 'The Infants of Eden', 94–6.
133 Reynolds, 'The Infants of Eden', 98.
134 *St Thomas Aquinas on Politics and Ethics*, trans. and ed. Paul E. Sigmund (New York and London: Norton, 1988), 63; *ST* II-II, question 10, article 12.
135 Reynolds, 'The Infants of Eden', 117–26.
136 Kemp, *Medieval Psychology*, 161; cf. Aquinas, *ST*, I, question 76, article 3 and I, question 118, article 2.
137 Kemp, *Medieval Psychology*, 161; cf. Katherine Park, 'Albert's Influence on Late Medieval Psychology', in James Weisheipl (ed.), *Albertus Magnus and the Sciences: Commemorative Essays* (Toronto: PIMS, 1980), 501–35.
138 Aquinas, *ST*, I, question 101, articles 1–2.
139 Irina Metzler, *Disability in Medieval Europe: Thinking about Physical Impairment during the High Middle Ages, c.1100–1400* (New York and London: Routledge, 2006), 56–7.
140 Reynolds, 'The Infants of Eden', 130; cf. Thomas Aquinas, *In II Sent.* 20.2.1 resp.: 'in hominis vita est quaedam circulatio, eo quod a defectu incipit, in statum debitae perfectionis deveniens, ex quo iterum in defectum terminatur.'
141 Ibn Khaldûn, *Muqaddimah*, 339.
142 Catholic Encyclopedia, at www.newadvent.org/cathen/02371a.htm (accessed 4 October 2012); Vulgate: 'beati pauperes spiritu quoniam ipsorum est regnum caelorum'.
143 *De sermone Domini in monte libros duos*, ed. A. Mutzenbecher, CCSL 35 (Turnhout: Brepols, 1967), 3–4, 7–8, 11; *Commentary on the Lord's Sermon on the Mount*, trans. D. J. Kavanagh, The Fathers of the Church 11 (Washington, DC: Catholic University of America Press, 1951).
144 Walter Fandrey, *Krüppel, Idioten, Irre. Zur Sozialgeschichte behinderter Menschen in Deutschland* (Stuttgart: Silberburg-Verlag, 1990), 22.
145 Lawrence I. Conrad, Michael Neve, Vivian Nutton, Roy Porter and Andrew Wear, *The Western Medical Tradition 800 BC to AD 1800* (Cambridge: Cambridge University Press, 1995), 185.

5

NON-CONSENTING ADULTS: LAWS AND INTELLECTUAL DISABILITY

Although early English law had little to say on the subject of the vulnerability of the insane, the danger that the inheritances and possessions of idiots and madmen would be exploited by those who were supposed to be looking after them was certainly recognized. Indeed, the risk to the mentally impaired was even greater than that posed to another especially vulnerable group, fatherless children, because fatherless children, if they do not die, eventually reach adulthood and can then fight back. Idiots, however, never emerge from mental and legal childhood; the same is true of some lunatics.[1]

Ever since laws have become transmissible across the bounds of history, by virtue of being encoded in writing, it seems that infants and the insane, among whom the intellectually disabled have all too frequently been included, have been placed in the category of those who had diminished or no responsibility. But lack of responsibility also more often than not meant lack of rights. Thus, while medieval 'idiots' were pardoned for many infringements of the law, they were also excluded from many property rights, mainly relating to inheritance. For instance, in his will, in the fifteenth-century, John Baret of Bury St Edmund wrote a clause to ensure that mentally incompetent heirs were excluded and 'jumped over' in the family succession: 'But I wil that in no wyse noon ydiot nor fool occupye the seid goods, but refuse hym and take anothir that is next.'[2] Certain conditions, such as dementia, learning disabilities, brain injury and neuro-disability, as they are labelled in modern medical parlance, affect a person's mental capacity, especially the ability to make decisions for themselves. In many modern societies, various legal systems set out what should happen if someone is unable to make a particular decision for themselves, in other words if they are deemed to lack mental capacity. Part of the assessment process includes evaluating if and how a person lacks mental capacity, a process in modern times involving health and social care professionals, as well as family members. As legal records demonstrate, forms of assessments and evaluations did take place in the high and later Middle Ages regarding a person's mental capacity, permitting comparison of the modern assessment processes with their medieval counterparts.

Pre-modern laws mainly concentrated on the dis/ability of ID for agency and contractual powers, inheritance, also culpability and guardianship. Thus there is a long history of law codes that assign guardians to minors and to those deemed mentally incapable, already dealt with by Roman law (i.e. inheritance and legal controls over the mentally disturbed), which influenced canon law and the secular laws of France, England and Germany (via customary law). Civil law, being concerned with a person's ability to account for their actions – the question of culpability – in criminal cases, and equally concerned with the ability of an individual to administer property – testate, inherit – allows the modern researcher to gain a quantitatively valuable picture of medieval ID. Differentiation appears to be the key concept throughout medieval legal texts. All of these sources refer to a range of mental conditions and afflictions, in particular the distinction between intellectually disabled from birth and becoming cognitively impaired later in life. This range of medieval terminological richness sits uneasily with previous authors' fusing together of such terms under the heading 'madness' or 'mental disability'.

Antecedents and comparisons: Judaic and Islamic law

For the social position of the mentally incapacitated in Judaic society, one may turn to the Mishnah, the collection of oral law developed over some seven hundred years on the basis of the Old Testament: the most disabling conditions in rabbinic culture 'were those which prevented a person from participating in that culture and from being able to recognize its orally transmitted rules and norms: that is, deaf-muteness, mental illness (insanity), and mental disability (retardation)'.[3] Furthermore, in the culture that the Mishnah idealises, 'those who lack cognitive, cultural, moral, auditory, or oral skills will be deemed nonparticipants in that culture insofar as their impairments reduce their *da'at*'.[4] A *midrash* (commentary) on Leviticus 21:16–24, *Sifra Emor*, added the invisible 'blemishes' of speech and hearing disabilities, mental disabilities (strictly speaking, here meaning mental illness) and intoxication to the visible defects (lame, hunchback, dwarf) that disqualified someone from the priesthood. Speech and hearing disabilities, mental disorders and drunkenness all share the same functional deficit, in that people affected by these conditions were deemed unsuitable to perform ordered actions, communicate reliably and hence be in a state of ritual purity. The child or minor was also excluded in *Sifra Emor*, even if none of the categories of 'blemishes' applies. Although the *Sifra* did not state so explicitly, the lumping together of the deaf or dumb, insane, intoxicated and children as unsuitable prefigures the wider cross-cultural practice – later Roman or medieval laws – of excluding such persons deemed insufficiently mature or mentally adept enough to perform tasks related to legal or religious offices. According to the *Babylonian Talmud*, a person who was, in modern parlance, either mentally ill or intellectually disabled was considered a person without reason and, by extension, mentally and legally incompetent, which is why under-age children and severely hearing- and speech-impaired persons were also included in this category, and all of them could be appointed with guardians – none of these persons was accorded legal responsibility or culpability.[5]

Comparing the biblical texts with the Qumran literature, one may note that the Qumran texts went much farther than the biblical ones in designating people with mental disability among the classes of those persons (deaf, lame and blind) who were to be excluded from the assembly of the community; moreover, the Qumran texts employed terms cognate with 'madness', 'simple-mindedness' and 'foolishness' to designate specific groups. One such text, the *Damascus Rule* 15, excluded several kinds of disabilities from communal worship: 'No madman, or lunatic, or simpleton, or fool, no blind man, or maimed, or lame, or deaf man, and no minor, shall enter into the Community, for the Angels of Holiness are with [the congregation].'[6] Another such text, the *Messianic Rule*, curtailed the responsibilities of the 'simple' person, so that they were barred from holding judicial office or joining the army. Interestingly, the notion of mental capability appears here, in that the simple person should do only such work as they are capable of.[7] 'No simpleton shall be chosen to hold office in the congregation of Israel with regard to lawsuits or judgment, nor carry any responsibility in the congregation. Nor shall he hold any office in the war destined to vanquish the nations; his family shall merely inscribe him in the army register and he shall do his service in task-work in proportion to his capacity.'[8] Such differences between the attitudes to ID in the biblical and the Qumran texts might stem from the fact that, as a kind of sect within Judaism, the Qumran community, in common with many other minorities, had to be 'purer' than the surrounding groups, to give it the raison d'être for being a splinter group in the first place. Perhaps there is also a Hellenistic or Roman cultural influence, in that the curtailment of responsibilities echoes the Roman civil law as it later came to be collated in the Justinian legal corpus.

A brief overview of Islamic legal traditions shows that in legal matters, too, besides the philosophical notions discussed in the previous chapter, there were many similarities with the Western Christian situation during the Middle

Ages. The mentally ill and disabled possessed no legal rights, but equally did not have any obligations; they were seen as children who were not legal actors, but nevertheless protected by the law, and Islamic laws, like Christian medieval laws, emphasised the family unit as the prime provider of care – as well as of control – while property rights were mainly concerned with preservation. Terminology was just as varied as in the Western counterpart. The Hanafis, Islamic law schools dating from the eighth century, distinguished 'atâha, 'idiocy', from run-of-the-mill insanity. But this neat categorisation of mental incapacity was complicated by the fact that some Hanafis equated the idiot with the madman in legal terms, while others considered idiots to be only semi- or partially insane. Where an idiot was deemed legally the same as a madman, the congenital idiot (ma'tûh) was remarkable only by the less-violent behaviour, so that the term junûn referred to violent insanity, while 'atâha related to harmless idiocy. One Hanafi jurist opined: 'We can say that the ma'tûh is stupefied but not mad ... it is a question of an individual who understands with difficulty, who expresses himself in a confused manner, and whose behaviour is defective. Also he does not strike or insult [other people] like a real madman.'[9] Where an idiot was considered only semi-insane, the comparison was made to a legal minor who possessed discernment, so that such a person was permitted to enter into legal transactions – provided they were not detrimental – and was allowed to accept gifts and donations. 'Partial incapacity is also assigned by most of the schools to the foolish or prodigal (safîh) and the imbecile of simpleton (dhû l-ghafla), whose ability to conclude legal acts is limited.'[10] It seems that foolishness was regarded as a moral defect, and imbecility or simple-mindedness as a mental deficiency. Both were treated like children who had reached some level of discernment. They could perform only those legal acts that were to their advantage, and even if their guardian approved other acts, if these were potentially damaging, the fool or imbecile was not allowed to accept them. Marriage and divorce were considered valid legal acts, but some law schools disagreed with each other when it came to legal acts that might incur a risk to the fool or simpleton.

Roman law

In Roman law, Justinian's Institutiones 1.23 extended the principle of guardianship to imbeciles (mente capti) as well, not just, as earlier, only for the furiosi.[11] Rosen noted that the older Roman law, starting with the Twelve Tables, dating from about the fifth century BC, dealt mainly with furiosi, that is, the violently insane who posed a threat to public order and safety, and who were to be placed under guardianship, but in late antiquity 'the cura furiosi was extended to mental defectives (*mente capti, fatui*), the deaf, the dumb and to those subject to an incurable malady (*cura debilium*)'.[12] Whether impaired or insane, people with mental aberrations are described as perennial children because they cannot 'rule themselves', as so many legal texts put it. This is the precedent set by Roman law, best expressed in the *Institutes* of Justinian. As *Institutiones* 3.19.10 stated: 'A baby and a child barely past infancy hardly differ from the insane, in that they are too young to understand anything' (*nam infans et qui infanti proximus est non multum a furioso distant, quia huius aetatis pupilli nullum intellectum habent*).[13]

Old Irish laws on intellectual functions

Some of the most detailed legal sources pertaining to ID are the Old Irish law-texts, originating mostly in the seventh and eighth centuries, but often surviving only in manuscripts of fourteenth- to sixteenth-century date, which furthermore may be incomplete and/or corrupt.[14] A kind of entertainer referred to as *drúth* features prominently. Kelly notes: 'The word *drúth* can refer both to the congenital idiot and the professional entertainer who earns a living by imitating him. It is clear from literary references that the *drúth* might also provide entertainment by telling stories or composing satirical verse.'[15] In other words, with *drúth* we have the same problem as with the medieval 'fool': a figure who encompasses what today are considered two different categories of behaviour, but which in the (earlier) Middle Ages appear to have been undifferentiated.

In Old Irish laws there are categories of persons deemed 'legally incompetent, senseless' (*báeth, éconn*), including women, children and the insane (a category subsuming the mentally disabled), who all require guardians for any legal actions. In this the Irish laws are quite unexceptional, following the same pattern as both the earlier Roman laws and the later medieval civil laws. Sometimes the legal status is subject to change in the course of a person's life events, children growing up to be adults being the obvious example. But sickness and disability, too, can affect legal status and capacity. For instance, the rearing of children is usually considered the responsibility of both father and mother. However, 'a child is not reared by a mother who is insane, blind, deaf, maimed in one hand, leprous, or who suffers from a wasting sickness'.[16] There is wide-ranging terminology for persons with mental disorders, which makes it difficult to equate Old Irish with modern terms. However,

> the meaning of the three most frequent terms (*mer, drúth*, and *dásachtach*) seems clear. The *dásachtach* is the person with manic symptoms who is liable to behave in a violent and destructive manner. The *mer* (lit. 'one who is confused,

deranged') poses less of a threat to other people, and is normally permitted into the ale-house. The *drúth* appears to be a person who is mentally retarded. (The term *drúth* is also used of the professional clown or buffoon whose act would include imitations of the insane).[17]

A distinction was made in Irish laws between male and female fools, with female fools accorded a greater level of maintenance enforcement, since they could not find 'alternative employment' as entertainers like the male fools could.

The exceptional behaviour and hence legal consequences for such persons is what unites a disparate group. Responsibility for offences devolved onto the guardian (*conn*), who would ideally be a relative. While the laws try to protect society from the more dangerous and violent insane behaviour of the mentally ill, there is a sense of their inculpability; for instance, if a known *drúth* threw something and hit another person, this does not qualify for compensation, since the onus lies on the other person to keep out of the way in the first place.[18] Similarly, it is primarily a family responsibility to look after members regarded as being a *drúth* or *mer*, with one text stating that a defendant is excused delays if looking after a *drúth* or *mer*.[19] A fragmentary text, *Do brethaib gaire* 'on judgements of maintenance', deals with the family obligation to care for incapacitated members, with the first section concerning the physical disabilities of the aged, blind and deaf, while the second part, entitled *De druthbrethaib* 'on judgements relating to idiots', concerns the mentally incapacitated.[20] The legal curtailments were partly intended for protection. 'A contract with a person of unsound mind is invalid, and anyone who incites a *drúth* to commit a crime must himself pay the fine. A man who impregnates a *mer* is solely responsible for rearing the offspring, and a sane woman who bears a child to a *drúth* is similarly obliged to rear it unaided.'[21] Inheritance rights of land were dealt with in a late Old Irish tract (entitled *Do Drúthaib 7 Meraib 7 Dásachtaib* in the manuscript, meaning 'on idiots, insane persons and lunatics'), whereby under three conditions land could be inherited during the current owner's lifetime, these being if the owner was a *drúth*, or had 'parted from his sense' (i.e. was insane), or required support due to age.[22] In other words, people who are incapacitated in law are not entitled to possession of their inheritance (or ownership in the case of the old man), even if they may draw use from it which is, however, administered on their behalf by someone else, the next heir. Interestingly, this Old Irish law clearly distinguished between idiocy and two types of mental illness.

The practice of sick-maintenance, whereby the culprit who has injured another is responsible for the medical care of the injured party, provides details with regard to the perception of mental disability and insanity. The *Bloodlyings* tract made provision for care and custody of the person identified as mentally aberrant in the home by the family or wider kin group. Section 12 included classes of people who are to be kept at home but qualify for compensation because of high rank or want of reason. These are in Binchy's translations an idiot (*mer*), a fool (*drúth*), a lunatic (*dasachtagh*) and an unreasoning person (*econn*). Section 61 repeated some of these classes: fools (*drúth*), lunatics (*dasachtaig*), senseless people (*ecuind*) and half-wits (*docuinn*), but stated that they were not allowed to enter the house where someone else was being cared for. The word *drúth* was here a collective term for fools, madmen, male and female persons deemed irrational, while the word *mer* seems to have been a specifically female term for fool and mentally disordered female persons. Finally, section 32 mentioned various classes of women who were excluded from certain legal rights. These included the female versions of the male idiot and lunatic of section 12, plus, in the annotations by the Irish commentators, the so-called vagrant 'half-witted (*buicnech*) woman [who] goes with the fairies'.[23] The word *rath* (probably derived from *ratis*, a reconstructed Proto-Indo-European word for reason, via Latin *ratio*) is the Old Irish term for 'grace, virtue, gift, good fortune', and by implication also 'reason'. A *co rath* was someone with *rath*, a person with talent, hence a person who can work, while a *cen rath* was without talent, hence cannot work. Discussing the *Bloodlyings*, Clarke noted that the text made some distinction between ID and mental illness. 'The word *econn* is translated "unreasoning person" and *ecuind* annotated as "the young 'senseless' one, or an idiot without grace"; *docuinn* (translated "half-wits") seems not far removed, with the annotation "or bad is his sense, the idiot without grace, or the little child". The word *buicnech*, translated as "half-witted", is applied to them to imply derangement.'[24] The word *mer* also means blackbird in Old Irish, associated with the idea that the blackbird goes alone, i.e. presumably relating to the non-flocking behaviour of this species (compare Latin *merulus*, and modern scientific name *turdus merula*).

Not just medical care, but also appropriate accommodation must be provided by the guilty party for the injured person and their retinue. Paragraph 61 of *Bretha Crólige* describes the standard of care and environment accorded to the victim and entourage:

> There are not admitted to him into the house fools or lunatics or senseless people or half-wits or enemies. No games are played in the house. No tidings are announced. No children are chastised. Neither women nor men exchange blows … No dogs are set fighting in his presence or in his neighbourhood outside. No shout is raised. No pigs squeal. No brawls are made. No cry of victory is raised nor shout in playing games. No yell or scream is raised.[25]

The 'quiet zone' imposed on the house for the injured party thus proscribes all sorts of noisy nuisances, and in this context the fools and other mentally unsound people are mentioned first. That could be because their uncontrolled vocalisations were regarded as particularly disturbing, or equally it could be because it may have been common practice to permit fools and others into one's house. The latter makes more sense in the context of this legal text, since the injured person is in a house provided by the aggressor, and the mention of 'enemies', who are likely to be the friends of the aggressor (hence enemies to the injured party), in the same line as fools, lunatics or half-wits, appears to group these categories of persons together.

Berkson mentioned an early Irish text called the *Law of Aicill*, which was probably proclaimed by King Cormac Mac Art at the end of the third century, but edited, supplemented and commented on up to the end of the eighth or the ninth century, which states: 'It shall be determined at the age of seven years whether a person is mentally deficient or has come to the use of reason, and at the age of fourteen years it shall be determined whether any person is permanently weak-minded or possesses ordinary intelligence.'[26] Concerning the milestones of achievement at ages seven and fourteen, one may note the Ages of Man theme here; such philosophical concepts may have entered the legal texts via Irish monasticism, especially if the laws were being re-edited in the eighth/ninth century. The *Law of Aicill* continued by setting out things that are familiar from the 'barbarian' codes and from Roman law, i.e. that the weak-minded are not liable for their crimes, that they cannot control any lands but they can inherit, that their families are liable for compensation for them, and that if a sensible person incites a weak-minded one to a criminal act, then the sensible person is the culpable one and is liable.

Another Old Irish law code, the laws of the *Senchus Mor* collection, discussed insanity in all its variations much along the same lines as Roman law. Thus 'no contracts are made binding on fugitives from a tribe who are proclaimed ... adulteresses, idiots, dotards, fools, persons without sense, madmen'. The concept of guardianship meant that fools, madmen, idiots and dumb people were exempt, but their guardians were the ones held responsible and distrained.[27] With regard to the *Cáin Lánama*, a text of the *Senchas Már*, related to the *Bloodlyings* tract, again some distinction seems to have been made between people classed as mentally deficient and mentally ill. In section 36.ix concerning the validity of marriage of such persons, any children issuing from the marriage were to be in the custody of those who had allowed the marriage in the first place. Presumably the grandparents had guardianship over both their own mentally incompetent children and any grandchildren. In the *Cáin Lánama, mer* is used for the male and *drúth* for the female, but *dasachtach* is used collectively for both. Modern editors have translated *mer* as 'fool', *drúth* as 'female fool' and *dasachtach* as 'madman', so that *mer* and *drúth* appear to signify ID, while *dasachtach* indicates mental illness. In the Irish law tracts '[m]ental defect and derangement can be thought to be distinguished by the descriptive adjectives employed, but the terminology seems to shift (like modern terminology), and one cannot be sure how far this sort of law-code discrimination of conditions – which was not necessarily the same as any medical or magical-cult one – was extended'.[28]

The Welsh 'Laws of Hywel Dda', dating from the tenth century, in section on the 'Nine accessories of homicide', mentioned that the 'relatives of an idiot (like those of a cleric, a leper, a dumb man) were excluded from *galanas* [life compensation] payment or active revenge'.[29] And the Laws of *Aethelred* VI, 52, treated unintentional crime (*unwilles oþþe ungewealdes*) – compare *unge-wollt* in modern German – as different from someone who offends by his own free will. But in early English laws the main evidence is on madness, that is, sudden and/or temporary states of mind, e.g. one of the Old English *Canons of Theodore* mentions that a 'man falls from his thoughts or from his mind' (*on his geðohtum oððe of his gewitte feole*); also that homicide occurs in a state of *ungewitte*, with the ambiguity of this term as either 'insanity' or 'idiocy, simple-mindedness'.[30] Therefore *ungewitte* seems to be similar to Latin *amens*, in the ambiguity of both meanings.

Medieval English law

In medieval laws in general, insanity (postnatally acquired and often tempo-rary) was differentiated from idiocy (congenital and insuperable), so that by the thirteenth century this distinction had become commonplace. The legal distinction became important primarily because it affected property owner-ship, as will be seen below with regard to the *Prerogativa Regis*. In general, it is worth noting that 'English law was therefore mainly concerned with estab-lishing idiocy; medical and literary authors, meanwhile, displayed far more interest in madness.'[31] The permanency of idiocy made it simpler to deal with than lunacy, since, once established, the idiot remains in that legal position for life. A 'reading' or lecture at the Inns of Court by Thomas Frowyk in 1495 noted that even 'if afterwards the idiot is restored to his memory by a miracle, the king will retain the land during his life, because the idiocy was once tried in chancery'.[32] Thus it seems that, although a number of fourteenth- and fifteenth-century English cases refer to people lapsing in and out of what they termed 'idiocy', by the late fifteenth century English legal experts were treating idiocy as a permanent condition that needed miraculous means to be cured.

England saw the development, dating from 1255x90, of some legal provision for both the 'idiot' and the non-congenital lunatic, associated with two clauses (11 and 12) in a summary of royal prerogative (privileged) rights known as *Prerogativa Regis*. Clause 11 stated:

> The king shall have the custody of the lands of natural fools taking the profits of them without waste or destruction and shall find them their necessaries ... And after the death of such idiots he shall render it to the right heirs, so that such idiots shall not alien nor their heirs ... be disinherited.[33]

This entailed lifelong guardianship for 'idiots' who held so-called 'feudal lands' (i.e. held by military service), according to the king's judgement. It seems that by the reign of Edward I this was established as a principle, even if it may have originated under Henry III. The king was able to control the funds released by the idiot's inheritance, while in return having to guarantee only the basic necessities. Clause 12 dealt with the mad person who 'happened to fail of his wit', in other words the person who had been deemed sane and mentally competent prior to some life event or episode, in which case the king had less exploitative financial control, since the lunatic and their family had to be supported competently and profits from the estate had to be put aside in case the mad person should recover.[34]

Neugebauer was the first modern commentator to take a serious look at the medieval evidence, in particular the *Prerogativa Regis*.[35] He provided still-useful observations on the differences between fools and idiots (phrase *fatui naturales*, to mean mental defectives), on the one hand, and persons termed *non compos mentis* and later called lunatics, on the other hand. Fools were developmentally affected persons whose intellectual capacities remained at the level of child, i.e. of a minor. The more precise term 'natural fool', or even in later English legal texts 'idiot', had the specific meaning of someone born with reduced intellect[36] and permanently remaining in that condition, a notion echoed in section 11 of the *Prerogativa Regis*. The medieval meaning of 'natural' was from birth, and is not to be mistaken with a view of 'natural' as postnatal, accidentally acquired disabilities, due to illness, age or even strong emotional reaction, such as grief. The meaning and synonymity of 'idiot' and 'natural fool' were summed up in an anonymous sixteenth-century legal dictionary:

> Idiot is he that is a fool natural from his birth and knows not how to account or number 20 pence, nor cannot name his father or mother, nor of what age himself is, or such like easy and common matters; so that it appears he has no manner of understanding or reason, nor government of himself, what is for his profit or disprofit.[37]

However, the phrase, still in use today in legal language, 'non compos mentis' carried a far more general meaning in medieval royal writs, so that in section 12 of the *Prerogativa Regis* it appears to include all mental afflictions, what we now call mental illness, but not those already observable at birth. People termed 'non compos mentis' could experience any number of lucid intervals or even recover entirely. Therefore all one can say with absolute certainty is that clauses 11 and 12 of *Prerogativa Regis* distinguished between congenital and acquired mental defects. 'For reasons that are not altogether clear, by the 15th century the term *lunatic* had replaced the phrase *non compos mentis* in legal discussions and in the administrative implementation of section 12. At the same time, too, *idiot*, rather than *natural fool*, became the preferred term for congenital subnormals.'[38] Perhaps, in answer to Neugebauer's rhetorical question, the reason why 'idiot' was preferred to 'fool' was that by the fifteenth century the keeping of fools as courtly entertainers was becoming more popular, and the legal language of the day needed accurate and precise terms to make it easier to differentiate between what elsewhere was termed an artificial fool, i.e. the entertainer, and a natural one, i.e. an idiot. One may add to the discussion of the evidence that Neugebauer had assembled the following criticism: he used 'disability/disabled' as having a faculty or capacity that may be switched off, disabled like a machine or device gets disabled, certainly not in the sense of Disability Theory; this means that, although citing various sources as to why and in what way lunatic and idiot were distinguished, Neugebauer could write about both lunatics and idiots as being disabled, which is confusing by modern standards. Instead, the distinction between idiots and lunatics made by medieval jurisprudence 'shows that professionals of the time already knew about the difference between the mentally ill and the "mentally retarded," thereby demonstrating signs of modern psychological expertise.'[39] This is too pointedly put. In defence of Neugebauer, one must also highlight that while, on the one hand, the legal 'professionals' of the time were making that distinction between mental illness and mental retardation, they were, on the other hand, not concerned with aetiologies, medical amnesis or treatment, hence the comparison to modern psychological expertise is completely misleading and beside the point. Nevertheless, Goodey's observation that 'it was the sudden public currency of the legal terminology that fed (along with other things) into modern psychological conceptualizations of intellectual disability',[40] rather than the other way around (psychological notions informing legal practice) is a valid one.

Not all people were subject to English 'feudal law', the prime exceptions being the citizens of boroughs, namely towns that had been granted a special status incorporating certain rights and privileges, including the right to hold jurisdiction over civil – but not criminal – cases. The magistrates of borough towns had some legal responsibility towards vulnerable groups like widows and orphans, a responsibility which in a handful of boroughs was extended to the mentally incapacitated. But from the comprehensive survey made by Bateson of medieval and early modern custumals, that is, collections of the customary law practices specific to a chartered borough, only two examples emerge (Bristol, dated to 1344, and Hereford, 1486) which are concerned with insanity in general, and then only one mentions idiocy in particular. In the Hereford example, idiots, as well as people who generally are not of sound mind, who inherit property are to be treated like children who are at risk of being defrauded, unless they have living relatives as guardians. This concerns 'any testator or other person alienating tenements [who] is in any way not of sound mind or an idiot (*vel sint non compos mentis vel ydiota*), in such case and the like, our chief bailiff ... shall examine them ... and if he be not of sound mind, it shall be done ... as is afore said of children who may be defrauded. And of idiots in the same way ...'.[41] Thus there is a functional amalgamation in this medieval administrative record of mental illness and ID, as we would call these conditions, by placing them into the same legal category.

English laws had different results for persons with ID, depending on whether they were subject to the *Prerogativa Regis* or to borough custom. Under the former, guardianship of the idiot may have been primarily intended to protect the next heir in line, but at least their legal affairs were supervised and regulated. But under borough custom, exploitation of the idiot by family and authorities alike was a distinct possibility. Then there was the problem of turning legal theory into practice, in that medieval concepts of ID and/or mental illness could sometimes get confused. Despite the best of theoretical intentions, writs, inquisitions and returns muddled up idiots and lunatics, referring to people as 'idiots from birth', but then reporting that such people are said to be worse at lunations and to rave with madness. *Prerogativa Regis* may have been one interpretation of the king's rights, but on the ground medieval officials and minor administrators did not always draw the same educated distinctions between types of mental incapacity. One may also note especially that what seems to have been of concern to the *Prerogativa Regis* was not whether someone was an idiot or insane, but whether the mental affliction was likely to be permanent.[42] In other words, with regard to *Prerogativa Regis* we need to remember that we are dealing with a document of law, an instrument of government, and not with a philosophical or medical text. We should be aware that it is not in the intentions of such a document to lay out clear, precise, 'scientific' definitions of ID, but only to arrive at practical solutions that offer some protection for the mentally disabled, and more importantly allow the king to farm out the possessions of his royal wards to the highest bidder. Scheerenberger had already noted that 'since the Crown took all the profits of an idiot's estate, relatives usually sought to have them classified as lunatics in order to retain control over their assets. Thus, the King's act probably was rarely used with mentally retarded persons.'[43] This may be hypothetical, and as a glance through the *Calendar of the Patent Rolls* volumes shows, the act *was* used to classify quite a number of people as 'idiots', but it does highlight the fact that the impact of the *Prerogativa Regis* needs to be carefully contextualised, with family interests and property concerns being the most obvious factors.

The pitfalls and fallacies of taking the *Prerogativa Regis*, and those investigations into the mental state of late-medieval English feudal tenants based on it, as record of a psychiatric assessment, as a modern expert witness would provide in court, can be seen in the following case. An aristocratic woman named Joan Fauconberg was served a writ by royal officials in 1463, insinuating that she had been an idiot from birth, and if she was proven an idiot, her property would, according to the oft-mentioned *Prerogativa Regis*, have fallen to the king. However, at this time Joan was aged nearly sixty and a widow (her second husband had just died, her first, incidentally, was William Neville, active in the Wars of the Roses). This confluence of events begs the question whether it was the fact that Joan was now a woman holding property in her own right, as a widow, which made it financially attractive to arraign her as a congenital idiot, and connected with this, whether her marriages 'protected' her from the attention of the escheators, since, while she was married, her property nominally fell under the control of her husbands. The fact that the 'congenital idiocy of Joan Fauconberg seems to have gone unremarked'[44] until 1463 could indicate several courses of events: the above scenario of 'idiocy' being hidden by marriage, or a simple failure of the legal officers to identify her as an 'idiot', or, more, cynically the accusation of an in fact non-idiotic Joan purely for reasons of fiscal greed. Joan's alleged idiocy is unconvincing. Perhaps the royal officials had less interest in pursuing cases of possible mental illness and/or disability, instead focusing their attentions on the wardship of under-age heirs, who were investigated with vigour, irrespective of familial connections. If royal officials did not 'go idiot hunting', then neither did administrators in the boroughs, it seems. Overall, neither customary nor royal law paid much attention to idiots or lunatics. One fifteenth-century civic London record incidentally mentions a woman who 'was in maner an idote and had nor knew no worldly reason', although she was married and, as far as one can tell, 'lived out her days without any external intervention'.[45]

Bracton on idiocy

By the end of the thirteenth century, four English jurists and their legal texts – Bracton, *Fleta*, the *Mirror of Justices* and *Britton* – had assimilated notions derived from those in the *Prerogativa Regis*, combined with older legal traditions regarding the position of intellectually disabled persons. In *De Legibus et Consuetudinibus Angliae* by Henry de Bracton, we find a more or less complete reception of the legal restrictions placed on idiots, the insane and deaf and mute people that the Justinian code had contained. With regard to inheritance, Bracton inquired who should do so, listing those to whom the right descended, including 'to idiots [*idiotis*] as well as those who have discretion, to lunatics [*mente captis*] as those of sound mind, which could be said of the insane, whether they enjoy lucid intervals or not'. While permanently insane persons could not acquire seisin (freehold possession of land or goods), 'stupid and weakminded persons [*stulti et idiotae*] may, because they are able to consent and dissent, which is not true of those mentioned above'.[46] As in so many legal codes, insanity and idiocy are distinguished. With regard to a specific legal question, the rights of tenant parceners (a kind of legal partner) in an essoin of bed-sickness (excuse for not attending court on grounds of illness), Bracton again advised separate treatment of idiots and the insane. 'If one is insane [*furiosus*] and enjoys no lucid intervals, the plea will remain until his death, because since he once began to possess *animo et corpore*, he may never cease to possess *animo*, once madness comes upon him. But if he enjoys lucid intervals, such time will be awaited. It is otherwise in the case of the fool and the idiot [*de fatuo et de stulto*], as will be explained more fully below in the tractate on exceptions.'[47] The passage on exceptions is as follows:

> It is clear that one who is dumb [*mutus*] can neither stipulate nor promise, since he cannot speak or utter the words appropriate to a stipulation. The same is true of a deaf mute [*surdus*], for it is essential that the stipulator hear the words of the promisor and the promisor those of the stipulator, unless one says that they may enter into a stipulation by a nod or a writing. What we have said applies not to one who is hard of hearing [*tardius audit*] but to him who is stone-deaf [*omnino non exaudit*]. That a stipulation and obligation may be created by a writing is obvious, because if it is written in an instrument that a person has promised, it is treated exactly as if an answer had been made to some preceding question. A lunatic [*furiosus*] cannot stipulate or conduct any transaction because he does not understand what he is doing. Nor can an infant or one just out of infancy (who does not greatly differ from a lunatic) unless what is done is to his advantage and done with the authority of his tutor.[48]

This passage is an amalgamation and reworking of several passages from the Justinian code, e.g. *Institutes* 3.19.7, 3.19.17, 3.19.8–10. Interestingly, the reasons why lunatics and children cannot stipulate are separated out from those why the deaf-mute cannot do so – for once there is a clear separation between deaf/mutes on the one hand and lunatics/infants on the other. However, in another passage Bracton does lump idiots, those born deaf and dumb, women and minors into the same bracket, as persons lacking reason. Persons may be excused for not putting in a claim if they were under-age or

> was then a madman [*furiosus*] or *non compos mentis* and of unsound mind, because in many ways a minor and a madman are considered equals or not very different, because they lack reason, which could be said of others, as idiots [*de idiotis*] and those born deaf and dumb [*naturaliter surdis et mutis*] and the like. But we must see whether they are excused forever or only for a time, that is, until the minor has reached full age or the madman has become sane.[49]

If we take this particular passage in isolation the impression emerges that, according to Bracton, the mental abilities of 'idiots' as well as of deaf-mutes are permanently fixed below the required level of rationality. A distinction is given by Bracton of legal ownership – *proprietas* and possession – which may reflect the treatment of property and ownership in the *Prerogativa Regis*. The right to property is available to all, but possession does not automatically follow. 'Sometimes the proprietary right is separated from possession, because the *proprietas* descends to … a madman [*furioso*] or one *non compos mentis*, an idiot or a fool [*stulto et fatuo*], or one born deaf and dumb [*surdo et muto naturaliter*], but possession is not at once acquired by such persons.'[50] Similar distinctions had already been made by the late Old Irish law discussed above, *Do Drúthaib 7 Meraib 7 Dásachtaib*, which had denied possession to the mentally incapacitated but had permitted use. Continuing with Bracton:

> A peremptory exception arising from the person of the demandant also lies for the tenant if the demandant is insane or of unsound mind [*furiosus fuerit vel non sanæ mentis*], so that he knows not how to understand or has no understanding at all [*quod discernere nesciat, vel quod omnino nullam habeat discretionem*], for such men are not far removed from brute beasts which lack reason [*brutis quæ ratione carent*] … But what is to be said of a fool [*fatuo*]? A fool [*fatuus*] may acquire, provided he has understanding in some matters. To such a curator is also given … But if he is a fool who cannot distinguish [*discernere*] between tenements or between rights, he does not acquire because he does not consent. But the decision on an exception of this kind is left to the discretion of the judge.[51]

Among the more usual terms for madness in all its forms (e.g. *furiosus, mente captus*) Bracton also uses the phrase *ratione carens*, that is, lacking responsible reason. The term could signify either understanding of the nature of one's actions or knowledge of one's wrongness (sin in the theological sense), and the insane might lack either. Bracton pondered what to say about the lunatic bereft of reason. 'And of the deranged, the delirious and the mentally retarded? ... *Quare* whether such a one commits a felony *de se* [if he commits suicide]. It is submitted that he does not, nor do such persons forfeit their inheritance or their chattels, since they are without sense and reason and can no more commit ... a felony than a brute animal.'[52] Bracton was not arguing that the mentally disabled or mentally ill were to be equated to wild beasts, but that if in mental disorder 'some physical defect prevents the mind from exerting its usual control' the 'resulting psychological state, and consequent behavior, then resembles that of an animal'.[53]

Fleta on idiocy

The legal tract *Fleta* mentions idiots a few times. *Fleta* (the author says he wrote it by the river Fleet or in Fleet Street, London) was completed around 1290–92, after Bracton (since *Fleta* cites Bracton) but before Britton (since Britton cites *Fleta*) and survives in a single manuscript (British Library, Cotton Junius B. viii). Book I, chapter 11, paragraph 8 'Of guardians of idiots' provides interesting context:

It is the custom to appoint guardians for the lands and persons of idiots and fools for the whole of their lives, and this has been lawful and permissable because of their inability to rule themselves, being adjudged ever to be, as it were, below full age. But because they were suffering many disherisons by reason of such wardships, it was provided and generally agreed that the king should have the perpetual wardship of the persons and inheritance of such idiots and fools from whatsoever lord they held their lands, provided that they were idiots and fools from birth – though not if they became so later – and that the king should marry them and preserve them from any disherison, with this proviso, however, that the lords of the fees and others interested should lose none of their rights.

(Solent enim tutores terras ydiotarum et stultorum cum corporibus eorum custodire suo perpetuo, quod licitum fuit et permissum eo quod se ipsos regere non nouerunt, nam semper indicabantur infra etatem vel quasi. Verum, quia plures per huiusmodi custodiam exheredaciones conpaciebantur, prouisum fuit et comuniter concessum quod rex corporum et hereditatum huiusmodi ydiotarum et stultorum sub perpetuis custodiam optineret, dum tamen a natiuitate fuerint ydiote et stulti, secus autem si tarde, a quocumque domino tenuerunt, et ipsos maritaret et ex omni exheredacione saluaret, hoc tamen adiecto quod dominis feodorum et aliis quorum interfuerit.)[54]

Therefore *Fleta* follows the *Prerogativa Regis* in principle, distinguishes congenital idiocy from acquired (as senility would be) and permits that idiots
could marry. Book VI, chapter 40, 'Of a plaintiff who is a fool, deaf, leprous
or insane' reiterated the comparison to wild beasts already found in Bracton:

> An exception ... arising out of the person of the demandant if he is insane or
> mentally disturbed so that he does not know how to discriminate or has no
> nous at all (*si fuerit furiosus vel non sane mentis ita quod discernere nesciat vel quod
> omnino nullam habeat discrecionem*). For such men are not far removed from
> brute beasts which lack feeling and reason, and dealings with such men during
> their madness ought not to be valid. (*Tales enim non multum distant a brutis qui
> sensu carent et racione, nec valere debet quod cum talibus agatur durante furore.*)[55]

In the following sections, *Fleta* stated that a different case is made for those
who enjoy lucid intervals (*dilucidis gaudere intervallis*), since legal actions
by them are approved, but in contrast those who are insane all the time (*qui
furorem habuerint perpetuum*) can make only invalid actions. 'Therefore, to
such men must needs be given curators and tutors by the lords of fees with
the consent of parents and friends' (*Talibus igitur de necessitate dandi sunt
curatores et tutores per dominos feodorum ex consensu parentum et amicorum*).
Exceptions are also made for the deaf or the dumb from birth because these
cannot give consent, while those who become so later on – acquired deafness –
can 'acquire property by procurators but not lawfully alien it' (*per procuratores
adquirere poterunt, set non legitime alienare*). Hence, although the text mentions
'fool' (*fatuo*) in the chapter title, it does not actually mention fools specifically,
and speaks only of permanent insanity – perhaps the writer was not particularly interested in the finer points of difference between mental disability and
mental illness, especially if the legal outcome is the same in both instances. The
material in *Fleta* on the deaf/dumb is taken from Bracton, and therefore incidentally an example of the inner-textual evidence that allows dating of *Fleta*.

The *Mirror of Justices* on idiocy

The *Mirror of Justices* (*Speculum Justiciariorum*) was written in Anglo-Norman
French, possibly between 1285 and 1290 according to Maitland's introduction to Whittaker's edition; the text survives today in just one fourteenth-
century manuscript (Cambridge, Corpus Christi College MS 258), but there
are several early printed editions.[56] The *Mirror* stipulates that those kinds of
people cannot be judges who are 'under the age of twenty-one, open lepers,
idiots, attorneys, lunatics, deaf mutes, the parties to the plea, those excommunicated by a bishop, nor criminal persons' (*ne nul demeins de age de xxj*

anz, ne meseals apertz, ne fous nastres, ne atturnez, continuelement arragez, ne sourz e muz, ne parties es plez, ne escomengez de evesqe ne homme criminal).[57] Furthermore, the law forbids to be an essoiner 'to women, infants, serfs and all who are within ward, to madmen, to excommunicates, to natural fools' (*a femmes, a enfanz, a serfs e a touz ceuz qi sunt engarde, as arrages, as escomengez, as foxnastres*).[58] An essoin is the excuse for a default due to some hindrance in the way to court. The following cannot be plaintiffs, that is, they cannot bring accusations and plaints in their own right: 'lepers, idiots without guardians, children under age without guardians, criminals, outlaws, exiles, banished men, women who are waived, serfs without their owners, married women without their husbands, men of religion without their guardians, excommunicated persons, deaf mutes without their guardians ...' (*meseals, ne fous nastres sanz gardeins, nenfanz dedenz age sanz gardeins, ne homme criminal, ne utlaguie, exille, bani, ou femme weive, ne serf sanz soun possessour, ne femme marie sanz soun mari, ne gent de religioun sanz lur gardeins, ne escomengez, ne sourz ne mutz sanz lur gardeins ...*).[59] Thus, here one finds the full catalogue of those persons disenfranchised by the laws of the time.

From the early twelfth century onwards one finds the categorisation of homicides as either culpable, excusable or justifiable, with legal actions respectively entailing capital punishment pardoning, or acquittal. 'Pardonable homicides were those committed by the insane, unintentional homicides and homicides committed in self-defence.'[60] By the late thirteenth century such pardons for homicide due to insanity, accident or self-defence were issued as a matter of course. The mentally disabled, falling under the category of the insane, will therefore invariably have been pardoned in cases of homicide. 'As early as the reign of Henry III, the patent rolls of England recorded any number of acquittals on the grounds of *furiosus* [sic] or *amentia* or *fatuitas*.'[61] The *Mirror*, too, postulated that homicide can be lawfully done (i.e. the death penalty on the order of judges after a trial), or unlawfully by 'those who have the will to kill but do not kill, e.g. those who abandon infants, old or sick folk in places where they intend them to die for want of help' (*ceux qi sont en voluntie doccire e point noccient, sicom est de ceus qi gettent enfanz, veillz e malades en tieux lus ou il entendent qil moergent pur defaute de eide*)[62] and by suicides. Then follows a list of all those who do not fit into the above three categories, i.e. 'physicians, leeches, justices, witnesses, those who strike but do not slay, fools, madmen, fugitives' (*de fisiciens, mirs, justices, testmoins, de ceus qi ferent e neqedent mie occire, de fous darragez* [MS has *de fous de fous darragez*, hence the editor translated as the two separate categories of 'fools, madmen'] *e de futifs*).[63] With regard to fools the *Mirror* makes further comment on their lack of culpability and lack of reason:

Then as to fools let us distinguish, for all fools can be adjudged homicides except natural fools and children within the age of seven years; for there can be no crime or sin without a corrupt will, and there can be no corruption of will where there is no discretion and an innocent conscience, save in the case of raging fools (?). And therefore Robert Walerand[64] ordained that heirs who were born fools should be in ward to the king, to be married along with their inheritances, of whosesoever fees those inheritances might be held.

(Des fous ausi distinctez, car touz fous sunt contables pur homicides quant al jugement forpris les foux nastres e enfanz de meinis de vij ans de eage, car crim ne se poet fere ne pecche si noun parmi voluntie corumpue, e corrupcion de volunte ne poet issi si de discrecion noun e innocente de conscins sauve fous ragie. E pur ceo ordena Robert Walraund qe fous nastres heirs soient en la garde le Roi pur marier ovesqe lur heritages de qi fieus qil tiegnent.)[65]

It seems that the *Mirror* has two categories of 'natural' fool, since it distinguishes between 'natural' from birth, i.e. congenital, and 'natural' arising postnatally, i.e. impairments developing with age or due to accidents, with 'accidents' meaning accidental happenings not willed by the person experiencing them. Finally, it is forbidden by law to make a contract with 'those who are in ward unless it be for their advantage, or with the deaf or the dumb, or with born fools, or with lunatics' (*ne a nul qest en garde si noun al profit de ceux en garde, ne as sourz ne a muz, ne as foux nastres, ne arragez*).[66]

Britton on idiocy

Britton, an Anglo-Norman law book of the late thirteenth century, was probably written during the reign of Edward I and appears to rely heavily on the earlier Bracton and *Fleta* for passages relating to idiocy and insanity. Concerning burglars, *Britton* opined: 'Infants under age, and poor people, who through hunger enter the house of another for victuals under the value of twelve pence, are excepted; as are also idiots and madmen, and others, who are incapable of felony' (*forpris enfauntz de eynz age, et povers qi par famine entrent pur aukun vitayle de meyndre value de xii. deners, et forpris fous nastres et arragez et autres, qi ne sevent nule felonie fere*).[67] Outlawry is invalid 'if the outlaw at the time of pronouncing the outlawry, was under the age of fourteen years, or out of his right mind, or deaf [or dumb], or an idiot' (*de utlagerie pronouncié fust de eynz age de xiiii. aunz, ou hors de sen, ou surd, ou muwet, ou folnastre*).[68] People who cannot appeal are 'an infant under the age of fourteen years, nor a madman, nor an idiot, nor one deaf, or dumb, nor a leper expelled from common society, nor a person in holy orders' (*ne enfaunt de eynz age de xiiii. aunz, ne homme aragé, ne fol nastre, ne muet, ne surd, ne mesel ostee de commune des gentz, ne homme ordeyné de eynz saintz odres).*[69] And these people cannot make gifts: 'Nor may infants within age, nor natural fools, nor madmen, nor deaf persons, nor dumb, nor lepers' (*Ne enfauntz de eynz age, ne fols nastres, ne gentz arragez, ne sourdz, ne mutz, ne mesels*). Also, infants cannot purchase anything without their guardian's consent, and neither can 'madmen, nor idiots, nor such as are incapable of consenting to a purchase, acquire anything without guardians' (*ne arragez, ne fous, ne ceux qi ne sevent assenter al purchaz, ne porount rien purchacer sauntz gardeyns*).[70] Wardship was discussed at length:

> And whereas it sometimes happens that the heir is an idiot from his birth, whereby he is incapable of taking care of his inheritance, we will that such heirs, of whomsoever they hold, and whether they be male or female, remain in our custody ... and that they so remain in our wardship as long as they continue in their idiotcy. But this rule shall not hold with regard to those who become insane by any sickness.
>
> (*Et pur ceo qe acune foiz avent qe acun heir est sot nastre, par quei il ne est mie able a heritage garder, voloms nous qe teus heirs, de qi qe il unques tienent, madles ou femeles, demurgent en nostre garde ... et issi remaignent en nostre garde, taunt cum il durent en lour sotie. Et ceo ne voloms nous mie de ceux qi deveignent fous par acune maladie.*[71]

This must be a reference to the *Prerogativa Regis*; note the 'get-out clause' allowing for the theoretical if unlikely possibility that idiots may recover their wits, in which case they would be released from wardship, this legal clause reflecting wishful thinking on behalf of property-conscious families, rather than erroneous medieval medical notions about the curability of permanent disabilities. On exceptions to the assise *Britton* stated: 'If the tenant is deaf and dumb naturally, and the same is not lately come upon him through sickness, or if he is a mere madman or an idiot from his birth, so as to be incapable of discretion, the assise shall stand over until he is in a better state' (*Et si le tenaunt soit sourd et muet naturelment, et nient de survenue par maladie, ou si il soit purement arragé, ou fol nastre ou de nativité, issint qe il ne sache point de descrescioun, en tel cas remeyndra la assise jekes au meillour estat*).[72] Nichols, the nineteenth-century editor/translator, noted that this is 'one of those instances in which Bracton or Fleta has been carelessly paraphrased. The direction to put off the assise refers to the case where the incapacity arises from sickness. ... In the other case, according to Bracton, *cadit assisa.*'[73] Britton got confused and seemingly only half-copied what Bracton had written earlier, garbling the words so that the sense of permanence of conditions from birth has got 'lost in translation'. People who cannot be summoned are defined: 'For an infant under age is not capable of receiving any summons except through his guardian ... nor a madman, nor one otherwise deprived of sense, as an idiot; nor deaf and dumb persons' (*Car enfaunt de einz age ne seet a receivere nule somounse, for qe par mi soen gardein, … ne ausi homme arragé ne autrement sauntz sen, sicum sount fols nastres; ne ausi sourdz ne mutz*).[74] In a final mention idiots and insane persons are referred to in the section on attorneys, where the following people are forbidden from making appearance by attorney: 'no child under-age, no-one deaf, mute, nor natural fool, no purely demented man, nor anyone else without discretion [i.e. rational sense], nor anyone accused of a felony … nor lepers ousted from the community of men' (*Chescun ne put mie fere attourné. Car enfaunt de eynz age, ne sourd, ne muet, ne fol nastre, ne homme purement aragé, ne autrement sauntz descrescioun, ne homme acusé de felonie, ne nul de qi nous le defendoms, ne mesel ousté de commune de gent, ne put mie fere attourné*).[75] This is similar to the earlier list in the *Mirror of Justices* which had forbidden certain people from becoming judges.

Medieval German examples

A German legal text, *Freisinger Rechtsbuch* of 1328, also mentions that people excluded from testifying as witnesses are simpletons and idiots, whose relatives have taken over their guardianship and custody of their property and they have caused this because of their idiocy.[76] The well-known German *Sachsenspiegel*, compiled by Eike von Repgow around 1230, had sections dealing with the legal exclusion of physically (and mentally) impaired persons. Most of these related to the rights to inherit property or make property transactions, similar to the stipulations already found in Roman law. Certain categories of impaired persons may not inherit: 'Neither tenancy nor hereditary property can devolve upon the feebleminded, dwarfs, or cripples. The actual heirs and their next of kin are, however, responsible for their care' (*Uf altvile unde uf getwerge erstirbit weder len noch erbe, noch uf kropels kint. Wer denne ir nehisten magen und erben sint, die enphan ir erbe und sollen si halden in ire phlage*).[77] In the *Sachsenspiegel* there is some evidence for a kind of 'protection' of the impaired and other people requiring special treatment in the law. So, for example, a woman with child 'may not be given a sentence more severe than flogging and the cutting of her hair. Neither shall fools nor the feebleminded be sentenced to punishment. If they cause harm to someone, their guardian shall pay compensation (*Man en sal obir kein wip richten, de lebende kint treit, hochir den zu hut unde zu hare. Ubir rechte thoren unde sinnelosen man en sal man ouch nicht richten. Wenne se abir schaden thon, ir vormunde sal ez gelden*).'[78] In this sense the *Sachsenspiegel* echoed earlier Roman law (appointment of guardians) and early medieval codes (in Anglo-Saxon law the congenitally deaf-mute are exempt from punishment). In all probability the dividing line between people with a sensory physical impairment such as speech or hearing difficulties, and people with a mental disability (the 'feebleminded') was not very clearly drawn.

Medieval French cases

Legal texts from France covered idiocy in similar vein. In the *Coutumes de Beauvaisis* by Philippe de Beaumanoir, composed around 1283 and heavily influenced by Roman law, reference is made to idiots, as people considered demented (compare modern senile dementia), or mad from birth and/or due to natural causes: 'the idiot, of whom it appears that he does not have good memory either because of age, or through natural madness, or through another illness, by which he is out of his previous memory' (*li ediote a qui il apert qu'il n'ëussent pas de bone memore ou pregnent viellece, ou par sotie naturele, ou par autre maladie, par quoi il sunt hors de lor ancienne memore*).[79] Furthermore, Philippe de Beaumanoir stated that 'one cannot sue on agreement made by ... an insane person, nor a natural mad person [i.e. a fool or person with ID] ... for ... neither an insane person nor a natural mad person [can make an agreement], because they do not know what they are doing' (*L'en ne puet suir de convenance ... forsené, ne fol naturel ... car ... ne li forsenés, ne li fous natureus pour ce qu'il ne sevent qu'il font*).[80] Beaumanoir also discussed the inheritance rights and ability to marry of mentally incapacitated people, which included the mentally disabled:

> Those who are natural mad people, so mad that they have no discretion through which they can understand how to maintain themselves, should not hold property if they have brothers or sisters, even though they are the oldest. Therefore if the oldest is naturally mad, the right of firstborn should pass to the oldest after him, because it would be a bad thing to leave any important thing in the hands of such a man; but always he should be honestly supported out of what would have been his if he had been a person who could hold land. But we understand this to apply to those who are so insane that they would not know how to maintain themselves if they were married or not; for if a person knew enough, and not any more, to be married so that he could have heirs, he and his property should be under guardianship until the time of his heirs.
> (Cil qui sont fol de nature, si fol qu'il n'ont en eus nule discrecion par quoi il se puissent ne ne sachent maintenir, ne doivent pas tenir terre puis qu'il aient freres ne sereurs, tout soit ce qu'il fussent ainsné. Donques se li ainsnés est fous natureus, l'ainsneece doit venir a l'ainsné après lui, car male chose seroit que l'en lessast grant chose en la main de tel homme; mes toutes voies il doit estre gardés honestement de ce qui fust sien s'il fust hons qui deust terre tenir. Mes se entendons nous de ceus qui par sont si fol qu'il ne se savroient maintenir ne en mariage ne hors mariage; car s'il se connoissoit en riens en tant sans plus qu'il

seust estre en mariage par quoi de lui peussent venir oir, il et li siens devroit estre
gardés dusques au tans de ses oirs.)[81]

In legal terms, then, a person who was deemed unsuitable (or incapable) of
marriage was also deemed incapable of inheritance with proper legal title,
although emphatically the due care and attention to care and guardianship
of the 'natural mad' person was proposed by Philippe de Beaumanoir. This is
similar to what was happening at the same time in the English legal system,
with guardians appointed in cases of 'madness', whether congenital or cyclical.
However, a key difference between French and English laws of the thirteenth
century was that 'in the French system, the ideal way of caring for the mad
was to keep them under the control of their families or neighbors', while the
English system often advocated royal guardianship.[82]

Legal texts often made comparison of mental states with that of idiots. In
such cases the word 'idiot' may be used as a marker to indicate that someone
is (behaving) *like* an idiot, not that they *are* an idiot. Examples can also be
found in French cases, where the ambiguity of the word 'idiot' points to
wide semantic meaning and variable usage of the term. In 1350 a swineherd
by name of Haninus Walet was accused of sodomising a fellow swineherd,
Thominus, who was then eight years old. Haninus was described as a *fatuus*
and as suffering from an evil illness called the illness of St John (*fatuus et malo
morbo qui dicitur morbus sancti Iohannis percussus*). Haninus was caught, but
on account of his illness was not punished but only sent away. But later, in
Lille, he was caught again in another sodomitic act with a boy, and this time
was tried and burned (*pro suis dementis* [sic] *tamquam sodomita combustus*).
Thominus too got drawn into this second affair, which is how the letter asking
for pardon came to be written that relates his and Haninus' story. The pardon
for Thominus was granted on account of his youth.[83] Beek cited the example of
Marion, a poor woman from the series of French remission letters, dating from
1394, who was described as not sensible and like an idiot (*qui est non sensible
et comme idiote*), in addition to which she is suggestive of manipulation by
others (*comme toute folastre tant par ce comme par temptacion de l'ennemi et que
jehan, son cousin lui demandoit à emprunter argent*).[84] Another case emerged in
1414 with Jehan Perrot, a poor, feeble-minded young man (*povre jeune homme
ydiot*). Jehan had a vision of a woman instructing him at night to get up and
follow him, telling him how to make a lot of money. Once he realised this was a
vision, he had masses read for the dead, the money for which he borrowed. He
started trading in wine, but an uncle told Jehan's customers that he was mentally ill (*Ne bailliez riens a mon nepveu, car il n'est que un fol*). Then one day he
committed theft, due to enchantment by the fiend, or because he was such an

idiot (*par temptacion d'Ennemy ou autrement par ce qu'il est si ydiot*). His elders threatened that he would be hanged, but he asked for a pardon, arguing that he was and still is an idiot who does not know what he does (*comme il fust et soit ainsi fol et ydiot par lunoisons telement qu'il ne scet qu'il fait*).[85] A further case from the French remission letters used by Beek concerned Jacques Mignon, a wheelwright and odd-job man, who by 1459 had been married to Mathurine Paynelle for six years; she was a fool with a very simple and hardly varied style of life (*estoit toute sote, de simple et tres petit gouvernement*). She could do no more than a small child (*en telle maniere qu'elle ne se savoit gouverner, non plus que ung petit enfant*). She could not run her household nor feed her children nor educate them, unless with the help and instruction of others (*ne savoit faire son mesnaige, gouverner ne nourrir ses enfants ne faire autre chose sans la conduicte et remonstrance d'aucune autre personne*). One day while out walking to visit Mathurine's parents, having left their five children at home in bed, Jacques pushed his wife into a river, where she drowned. Jacques pleaded that he was confused and impaired in his understanding (*perturbé et alteré de son entendement*).[86] Apparently we are confronted with the case of an 'idiot' murdered by her insane husband.

ID or mental illness?

In medieval English legal history, the judicial inquiry into the state of mind of Emma de Beston, who was certified an idiot in July 1383, is probably the best-known case.

> The said Emma, being caused to appear before them, was asked whence she came and said that she did not know. Being asked in what town she was, she said that she was at Ely. Being asked how many days there were in a week, she said seven but could not name them. Being asked how many husbands she had had in her time she said three, giving the name of one only and not knowing the names of the others. Being asked whether she had ever had issue by them, she said that she had had a husband with a son, but did not know his name. Being asked how many shillings there were in forty pence, she said she did not know. Being asked whether she would rather have twenty silver groats than forty pence, she said they were of the same value. They examined her in all other ways which they thought best and found that she was not of sound mind, having neither sense nor memory nor sufficient intelligence to manage herself, her lands or her goods. As appeared by inspection she had the face and countenance of an idiot.[87]

This is actually a rather misleading example, since it does not illustrate ID very well. For instance, the case of Emma omits to mention (or ask) about the length of time she has had her mental incapacity, so that it is not clear whether she had acquired her idiocy or had been an idiot since birth. Since Emma has had three husbands, even if her husbands all died within a short time of marriage to her, one may assume in the absence of any information given about her age that she is not the youngest any more, and that therefore her mental state may be due to senile dementia rather than congenital ID. It is worth observing the phrase used by the medieval source, 'she had the face and countenance of an idiot', implying that she looked like what the officials associated with an idiot, not that she was an idiot. Emma's case does not make for a completely convincing example of a woman with ID, rather for a woman whose stage of her life cycle or life experience (accident? head injury? psychological trauma?) led the jury to compare her to an idiot. In his pioneering study, Neugebauer cited this record, pointing out that at 'Emma de Beston's idiocy inquisition her 14th-century examiners concluded that her impairment resulted from "the snares of evil spirits"'.[88] Her case, then, was not in fact about congenital idiocy.

The problem of terminology is particularly well exemplified in the following example. John atte Berton was deemed not an idiot from birth, hence:

> the king commanded the said escheator to examine his state ..., and further to find by inquisition whether he were of sound mind or an idiot, and, if so, whether he was so from his nativity or from some other time and had any lucid intervals, and on its being found by the personal examination as well as by the inquisition that the said John from his infancy until his completion of the age of twenty-one years and more was of sound mind, having no kind of idiotcy, but, because of a great fright and excessive grief because of his father's death, he afterwards sustained almost total loss of memory and remained in that state for three years, although with occasional lucid intervals, after which he recovered and his memory was restored and remained so for more than five years before the date of the said inquisition.[89]

Hence, in fourteenth- and fifteenth-century English legal thinking 'idiocy' was something that was not permanent, and therefore conceptually treated more like an illness than a disability. Idiots can come and go, according to this thinking, and fall into idiocy as well as recover their senses again. Perhaps therefore, as in Emma's case, it is better to translate the medieval English legal term 'idiot' as meaning someone who acts *like* an idiot, rather than someone who *is* an idiot. The variance in how idiot is used indicates that idiot does not refer to a specific nosology in medical terms, nor even to a more general legal concept of incompetence. It seems that idiot is used as a benchmark signifier to describe the behaviour of certain people who act like an idiot. Legal writers had a concept of what kind of behaviour an idiot, as in a genuine idiot in the modern sense, e.g. the person with ID, demonstrates, and when talking about people with erratic behaviour or mental disorders used this known signifier to provide detail on such people. In judicial terms it hardly mattered, other than for the *Prerogativa Regis* cases, whether someone was a true idiot (person with ID) or behaved like an idiot (had some acquired mental disorder later in life), since in either situation the affected person was declared legally incompetent. The word idiot, then, just adds information about the aberrant behaviour, i.e. such people were more likely to act foolishly, irrationally and damage their own interests than to act violently against others (as *furiosi* might). The oft-cited Emma de Beston case is a prime example, in that Emma was obviously not born with ID, but in middle years started displaying behaviour deemed erratic and was described as being like an idiot. Harper also discussed her case, concluding that 'Emma's mental condition was ascertained principally by an analysis of the thought-processes rather than her appearance or behaviour'; Harper contrasted this with insanity, which he described as something that 'usually gave itself away'.[90] In other words, the madman was deemed to be highly visible, with very noticeable erratic and different behaviour, and different appearance to the norm, especially in the literary descriptions of madness which were, after all, the focus of Harper's study. A more straightforward case appears to concern John, the son and heir to John Brewes, who was labelled an *idiota*, but even here there may be some uncertainties, since John was in and out of wardship for twenty years (1348–68) even though he was consistently labelled an *idiota* during various examinations.[91]

Turner's study of several hundred later medieval English legal records indicates that with regard to mentally incapacitated landholders (i.e. the kind of people who also turned up in the *CPR* records discussed below) the term '*idiota* came into regular use sometime in the 1270s, and it quickly became used by clerks over forty percent of the time in reference to mentally incompetent landholders. This usage leveled off at approximately fifty percent of the total usage throughout the fourteenth and fifteenth centuries.'[92] But, as we have seen, *idiota* need not imply ID as per modern definition, since many of the individuals Turner has located in the records are described as having fallen into idiocy, or as enjoying lucid intervals.[93] We have better evidence denoting mental incompetence when qualifiers such as 'natural' or 'from birth' are added to the word *idiota, fatuus* or *stultus*. Turner cites John Thymolby, who would have held a manor but, because he was *fatuus naturalis*, became a ward of the crown in 1427;[94] Bartholomew Sakevill, who was certified '*fatuus* and an idiot ... from the time of his birth (*fatuus et idiota ... a tempore nativitatis sue*)' in an inquisition post mortem;[95] John Bertelot, who was described as *fatuus et idiota* and 'has existed as such since birth';[96] and John Cofe, who in 1360 was described as a natural fool without mental ability, 'Coof [Cofe] est fatuus natural et non compos mentis sue'.[97]

Congenital idiocy and English law: the case of the patent rolls

In the patent rolls, mentions of idiots in general, (natural) fools, or idiots since birth, occur in around 160 cases between 1216 and 1452, from Henry III to Henry VI (the years covered by the *CPR*). This does not mean 160 separate individuals, since around a third of the cases are multiples of the same name, where the legal proceedings have simply rumbled on, sometimes for decades. But that still leaves around one hundred individuals over a two-hundred-year period who were, in effect, 'certified idiots'. The style of the patent rolls is, unsurprisingly for a legal document, fairly repetitive, with the vast majority of entries following the same format: the name of the person examined for idiocy, the name(s) of the guardian appointed, the specifics of the property in question and the duration of any wardship (generally until the next heir was of age). One of the earliest cases in the rolls, from 1253, already set the tone for the kind of entries to follow:

> Delivery to John de Lessinton of Richard de Newhus, an idiot, with his wife, to keep so long as the said Richard live; and for their sustenance the king has committed to him his land of Neuhus of the inheritance of the idiot, which land by judgment of the court the king has retained in his hands for the security of the heirs; on condition that the said John do not waste, diminish or in any way alienate anything thereof to the loss or disherison of the heirs, but that, after the death of the said Richard, it revert to his heirs free and quit of the said John and his heirs.[98]

The problem with the shorthand wording 'idiot' is that it does not clarify as to whether the person so described is mentally disabled due to a developmental disorder (what modern psychiatry classes as ID), or mentally disabled due to a degenerative disorder or the effects of trauma (common today as Alzheimer's or head injuries). In the above case, Richard de Newhus could have been a person with congenital IDs, but more likely he was someone affected later in life, a supposition in part informed by the fact that he appears to have been older, since he was married, and most of the cases relating to 'idiocy from birth', and therefore ID in modern parlance, concern younger individuals who were not yet married, i.e. their mental condition had been noticed and acted upon before they were old enough to marry and could therefore potentially alienate the property. Where the patent rolls speak of 'idiot since birth' or such similar phrasing, we appear to be on firmer ground. Another problem with the wording used is the inference made by the modern editors of the patent rolls: sample checks conducted on three cases indicate that the preferred medieval terminology for what the modern editors translated as 'idiot' was in fact *fatuus*, or *fatuus a nativitate*. *Fatuus* is a perfectly recognisable and unambiguous medieval word, and in fact preferable to the more problematic *idiota*, so that the modern translation is not too far off the mark. However, for reasons outlined above, someone could still be a *fatuus* for reasons unconnected to ID. Strictly speaking, therefore, only those cases which relate to idiocy from birth should be counted as indicators of ID.

Of the roughly one hundred individuals associated with idiocy in the CPR, around twenty cases specifically mention idiocy from birth, ranging in date from 1290 to 1446, so that these twenty people are the only definite instances where the equation with ID can be made. In addition, around the same number of cases mention idiocy in people who (should) have just inherited, are not married yet or have similar indicators of a still young age – in these instances the equation with ID is uncertain but very plausible. That means, in much abbreviated terms, that some 60 per cent of idiocy cases in the patent rolls relate to unspecified idiocy (most likely acquired cognitive disability), as opposed to only 20 per cent of possible (let alone definite) ID.

Establishing whether someone was an idiot or not was done by a commission appointed by the king, and often in the presence of the reigning monarch himself, an activity which would have been of interest to the king, since he personally would have been given the wardship (and hence the income from lands and other properties) of the person certified as a lifelong idiot. Such is demonstrated by the following case, which sought to ascertain the type of idiocy, i.e. whether it was a permanent condition or not – although, frustratingly for the historian, this record, as so many medieval sources, has nothing to say on *how* the commission decided for or against idiocy. 'Commission to … hold inquisition as to whether John Thymelby has been an idiot from birth, whereby the ward of his lands and tenements would belong to the king, or whether he afterwards fell into such infirmity, so that such ward would not belong to the king.'[99] There are hints that the system might be abused by parties with a vested interest. In this case from 1379 it is not entirely clear whether Walter Graunger, who is described as too 'impotent', that is, (mentally or physically) weak, to travel and appear before the council in person, is, in fact, mildly intellectually disabled but competent enough to manage his estate, or whether a greedy sovereign is simply trying to exploit the financial returns from a dubious situation.

> Commission to … examine whether Walter Graunger of Wynterburn Clencheston, co. Dorset, who is too impotent to appear before Council, is an idiot, he having petitioned the king, complaining that although he has sense enough to take care of himself and his lands, yet under colour of an inquisition before Walter Cyfrewast, late escheator in that county, procured by his

oppressors, he has been found an idiot from birth, and his lands, ... have been seized by the said escheator.[100]

As with the majority of patent roll entries, the definite idiocy cases, too, follow a standard pattern. An early and succinct example from 1290 is the following: 'Appointment of Juliana, mother of Henry son of John de Holewell, to the custody of his body and lands in the county of Hertford, as it appears by the inquisition before Ralph de Hengham and his fellows, justices of the King's Bench, that he has been an idiot from his birth.'[101] Later entries become more detailed, especially with regard to the property in question. The legal procedure involved examination of someone suspected of being an idiot by a panel of officials, either judicial or governmental, depending on the location, which they had to attend in person, as this entry shows: 'Appointment of William de Shareshull and Thomas Moigne to take John Warre of Rolleston, who is said to have been an idiot from his birth, and bring him before the council at London for examination as to his state.'[102]

Being deemed an idiot from birth was not considered an impediment to marriage, as a case from Cornwall in 1324 demonstrates: Christina had been married to Edmund de Wilyngton and was now widowed; she was supposed to have been presented to an official 'as an idiot from birth, whereby the custody of her lands ought to belong to the king', but she was rescued and abducted by ten men; all eleven (the men and Christina) were now being sought for by a sergeant at arms to be taken before the king.[103] A similar case is cited by Turner. In 1399 'Ralph Dollebeare ravished and carried off by force of arms an idiot named Joan [Tremollou]'.[104] Whether she was a true 'idiot' in the modern sense of ID, or in the vaguer medieval sense, this case certainly indicates the easy victimisation and abuse of people who were mentally impaired.

The question of heredity is one that fascinated nineteenth-century scientists but not medieval legalists; however, by chance some hints of what may possibly be hereditary ID are glimpsed in the patent roll records. One case involves grants to Adam de Skyrewyth, king's watchman, of custody of the lands and person of John de Danthorp 'an idiot from birth' and of 'William Berchet, nephew and one of the heirs of the said idiot, but who, as appears by an inquisition ... is also an idiot'.[105] More family connections with idiocy in siblings appear in the case of the Walraunds, John, Robert and Isabella, the two brothers being described as idiots.

> Grant to Joan, late the wife of Alan Plugenet, of the custody of the manor of Wynefrode, so long as the same is in the king's hands, for the sustenance of John Walraund, an idiot, brother and heir of Robert Walraund, deceased, also an idiot, brother and heir of Isabella Walraund, deceased, upon whose death the late king

[Edward I] granted the custody of the manor of Wynefrode to Alan Plugenet and subsequently to his widow, the same Joan, in whose hands as executrix of her husband the custody then was, to hold at pleasure for the like purpose.[106]

There certainly does not seem to have been a notion of the passing on of ID from one generation to the next as one will find in the nineteenth and twentieth centuries, and hence neither does one find medieval concerns over the degeneration of society as a whole if 'idiots' are allowed to breed.

In contrast, questions of heredity provoked a rather over-excited response in the historiography. One late example, from 1968, may suffice, if anything, to remind us of the sea-change in attitudes in a comparatively recent time.

> By far the commonest form is mere low intelligence resulting not from specific damage or malformation of the brain but from the considerable variation in inherited intelligence which seems to be inevitable in a freely breeding population. It is usually assumed that disorders in whose causation heredity plays an important part become more prevalent in a population as its care for its sick and handicapped members becomes more general and effective. Theoretically, this makes it more likely that its more eccentric or stupider members will survive and breed.[107]

Ironically, for someone like Walker, who no doubt held a positivist view of history, it is that very antithesis of modernity, the Middle Ages, that was rather effective at caring for 'disabled' members of society. One need think only of hospitals and alms-houses, the ubiquitous donation of alms to the needy as an act of charity, to see that people with ID stood a good chance to 'survive and breed', so that, following this line of argument, medieval instances of 'low intelligence' among the population as a whole should have been higher than today. Walker further bemoaned the loss of asylums, arguing that 'the modern tendency to regard the return of the patient to the community as the proper aim of hospital psychiatry is busily reducing whatever eugenic effect the institution used to have'.[108] I cite this to remind the reader how far, thankfully, we have moved on since then.

Possible heredity in a direct line is evidenced in a Cornish family in the *CPR*. William Chambernon had two daughters, Elizabeth and Katharine, who inherited the estate. 'Elizabeth has been from birth and still is an idiot', which did not prevent her, however, from marrying William Polglas within three days of her father's death – or had that better be called being married off? William Polglas 'accordingly received for 11 years and more the profits of a moiety of the said manors and lands, amounting to 200 marks yearly, which should by reason of her idiocy have been the king's'. William and Elizabeth had a son, Richard, 'an idiot from his birth', and a daughter, Margaret (presumably not disabled), who was married off to John Herle. On the death of William Polglas, Elizabeth was, 'within two days, married to one John Sergeaux, who, for 16 years and more, received the profits of a moiety of the said manors and lands'. When Katharine, the non-disabled daughter of William Chambernon, died without heirs, her share fell to her sister, Elizabeth, so that Elizabeth's husband, John Sergeaux, became beneficiary of all the Chambernon estates. The whole convoluted family saga then turns to Elizabeth's son-in-law, John Herle, who

> knowing that the said Richard was an idiot from birth, agreed with John Sergeaux for a sum of money to keep Richard in his custody, and married his sister the said Margaret, and because he knew that, if Richard survived his mother Elizabeth, and should be found, on examination, to be an idiot, all the manors and lands aforesaid would be seized into the king's hands, and neither he nor the said Margaret, his wife, would enjoy the same whilst Richard lived, he abducted and removed him to some place unknown, so that the jurors know not whether he is alive or dead.

When John Sergeaux died, leaving the idiot Elizabeth a widow for the second time, John Herle 'took the said Elizabeth into his custody with the manors, lands &c. and has held them' to the date of the patent roll entry.[109] Two generations of idiocy in the same family meant a nice little earner for opportunists like John Herle. The case also provides some rare evidence of the longevity of people with mental impairments, a topic which modern studies seem to have frequently assumed was non-existent, since the stereotype has it that most people with ID would not survive for long, due to lack of medical care for concomitant physical diseases. Elizabeth seems to point to a different story. The escheat records (which incidentally refer to *a tempre nativitatis sue Elizabeth ... fuit fatua et pura ideota*) relate that Elizabeth was married for some thirty-five years to two husbands, and since the death of her second husband had been in wardship for eight years, making a total of forty-three years.[110] If we assume that she was married off in her teens, for argument's sake around the age of sixteen, that would make her age approximately sixty years old, and to all intents and purposes the records indicate that at the time of writing she was still very much alive and well – not exactly the short-lived 'congenital idiot' of the modern imagination.

In 1302 the escheator found William Berchaude to be 'manifestly an idiot (*idiota & non compos mentis sue*), and has been so from his birth (*tempore nativitatis*)'; furthermore, William did not enjoy lucid intervals; and William, who died in 1336, was described as *fatuus et idiota*. In William's family something identifiable as ID may have been hereditary, since William's maternal uncle,

John Danethorp, was also considered to be an idiot from birth. With regard to this, Turner believes: 'It is not impossible to find multiple members of one medieval family who all had some type of mental disorder. It is, however, impossible from the scant evidence given in each record to make any kind of judgment as to what precisely this phenomenon indicates genetically, socially, or culturally, especially when each person was labeled differently.'[111] But in this case, although I agree with Turner that precise diagnosis is impossible, it does seem to indicate some form of ID.

Non-standard circumstances in legal cases seem to have stumped the judicial experts. At York in 1212 one finds the case of a *stultus* who for reasons unknown had falsely confessed to theft, which was referred to the king and recorded in the plea roll: 'The King must be consulted about an idiot who is in the prison because in his witlessness he confessed that he is a thief, although in fact he is not to blame.'[112] In a record of a discussion in 1353, Skipwith, one of Edward III's itinerant judges, told his colleagues of the indictment for homicide of a man who could neither speak nor hear, and rather helplessly inquired what one should do in such a situation (*Skipwith dit a les Justices que ... un fuit endict de mort de un home qui ne puit ne parler ne oier, &c. que serra fait*).[113] The problem was that, unless proven to be an 'idiot', this man would have been presumed to be rational, and hence culpable of his crime, but without an effective communication method, neither one nor the other could be ascertained. And then there was always the suspicion that the accused was feigning mental or sensory disability in an attempt to obtain more lenient treatment. Stupidity or madness was allegedly faked to excuse crime, in the following case, that of heresy. Nicholas Eymerich, who was inquisitor for Aragon in the late fourteenth century, wrote a manual in which he listed faked mental disorder as one of 'ten ways in which heretics seek to hide their errors'. Of the various methods, the ninth way of evading a question was by feigning stupidity or madness, so that, as with the insanity clause for homicide, culpability could not be assigned.[114] And then there is the most curious case of what appears to be a practical joke gone wrong. The *CPR* recorded the following incident from 1265:

> Pardon, at the instance of Thomas de Ferrariis, to William Pilche of Sonky, an idiot, for the death of Augustine le Fevere of Maunnecestre, as it appears by testimony of Robert de Stokeport, coroner in the county of Lancaster, and other trustworthy persons that the said William was passing along the high road by night when he was met by the said Augustine, in the disguise of a terrible monster uttering groans and refusing to speak though adjured in God's name, on account of which the said William rushed upon him as a monster and killed him.[115]

The text tantalisingly alludes to the possibility that William's mental condition was known and Augustine deliberately tried to frighten William for amusement – a case of 'baiting the village idiot'? Regardless of the exact psychiatric diagnosis of his cognitive disability, William Pilche was deemed not responsible for his actions and therefore not culpable of murder. Incidentally, this is the only case of an 'idiot' murdering someone whom Hurnard cited in her seminal study of pardon for homicide, explaining that fewer cases of feeble-minded persons requiring pardon were found 'probably because they seldom attacked others.'[116]

Problems and pitfalls of legal terminologies

For the English medieval legal tracts (such as Bracton, and the various surviving individual cases in the records from the thirteenth to fifteenth centuries) Clarke observed that there were a striking number of variations in phraseology, which on the one hand demonstrated a strong awareness of the existence of mental incapacity or disability, but on the other hand indicated lack of a systematic approach to mental disorder, so that individual phrases in specific cases will certainly have meant something to the people (witnesses, officials, scribes) recording the case but not necessarily to others. 'The lack of [terminological] firmness was doubtless partly due to the infrequency of such cases, and there seems no instance where a medical appraisal was available and taken into account.'[117] But one should note that the medical texts of the period are even less precise or terminologically 'firm' than the legal ones, in part connected with the intractability of many mental afflictions, so that Clarke's expectation of medical input betrays a very modern attitude retrospectively projected onto the medieval evidence, since we nowadays expect medical experts to provide evidence on in/sanity in legal proceedings, whereas medieval courts held far more autonomy in this regard. As Pickett put it so succinctly on the different approaches to and interpretations of insanity by legal and medical writers: 'Varieties of legal insanity are varieties in degree; varieties of medical insanity are varieties in kind.'[118]

In his historical semantics introduction, Walker had pointed to the fluidity of legal terminology, citing the profusion of words like 'lunacy', 'insanity' or 'idiocy', which are interspersed with medieval terms which may be translated as 'frenzy', 'madness', or the phrases *non compos mentis*, *de non saine memoire* and *fatuitas a nativitate*: 'Apart from the very ancient distinction between 'folly from birth' and the other forms of disorder, these terms were usually interchangeable, and it would be a mistake to relate any of them to some more precise subdivision of mental illness.'[119] But Turner's thorough statistical analysis of English legal records between the thirteenth and fifteenth centuries is important because it proves that 'medieval scribes and administrative officials did not use their terminology randomly. The various terms for mental illnesses and incompetence had specific meanings for those authors and their audiences, and they chose the right term for each condition as they assessed it.'[120] Another way of looking at it is to regard the purpose of the legal language as employing a catch-all phraseology to cover all eventualities of mental incompetence, and to use differentiation only to make sure that *all* these conditions are covered, since the main interest of the law is property, not pathology.

Legal agency: idiocy and infancy

As we have seen with regard to the philosophical notion of agency, lack of reason entailed lack of will, and without will there could be no agency. From looking at the language of legal texts, it seems that such philosophical concepts had been ported across in an unadulterated fashion. 'What the madman shared with the infant was not a recognized disease or malady or measured deficiency. It was, rather, the unfitness of both for citizenship, and the fact that punishment would do nothing to improve them.'[121] The free citizen had the capacity, under the discipline of law, for freedom of action. While a child had such capacity, which just needed to develop, the profoundly retarded *ideotus* lacked the very capacity itself. In his examination of canon law, Pickett had argued that persons are responsible only for human acts, namely such actions that are caused by voluntary acts which are moved by the will and assented to by reason – but people with ID allegedly lack reason. Or, expressed from the causality of sin, something is sinful only when both will and reason deliberately engage in pursuit of an act that should not be performed.[122] For canon law, we find the phrase 'mens vero alienata furore, cum sui compos non sit, eorum, que admittit, reatum non contrahit, quia facultatem deliberandi non habuit'.[123] This was in connection with the invalidity of agreements made by people who were *non compos mentis*. The Irish *Law of Aicill*, mentioned above, had argued for a kind of series of developmental milestones in the cognitive development of children, citing the ages of seven and fourteen as markers. This was found in other jurisprudence, too. In English twelfth-century laws and in the borough customs children are categorised legally as minors not just by age, but by their capacity for understanding, moral knowledge and level of intellect, determinations which have implications for the criminal responsibility of those deemed under-age. 'The age of "discretion" was ascertained by the familiar counting and yard measuring tests, which might be regarded as the forerunners of modern psychological theories of intelligence testing.'[124]

Similar concepts existed in a Castilian law code of the thirteenth century, the *Siete Partidas*, which stated that seven was the age when children 'begin to possess intelligence'; however, this is part of a process and not a completed state, since between the ages of seven and fourteen the child has 'no perfect mental capacity, and, on the other hand, is not entirely lacking in it'.[125] In his 'reading' or lecture at the Inns of Court in 1495, Thomas Frowyk argued that children, that is, people under the age of fourteen, could not be found to be idiots.[126] This is presumably so since the natural state of childhood is to be 'without discretion', hence all children are naturally 'idiotic', but of course they grow out of it once they mature.

The notion of the innocence, therefore of the inability to be sinful, and in legal parlance the criminal inculpability of the mentally disabled, was succinctly expressed in the *Ethics (Scito teipsum)* of Peter Abelard. Writing before 1140, Abelard stated that 'sin is said to be that contempt of God or consent to evil from which little children and the naturally foolish are immune; since they have no merits and, as it were, lack reason, nothing is imputed to them as sin' (*peccatum dicitur ipse Dei contemptus uel consensus in malum, ut supra meminimus, a quo paruuli sunt immunes et naturaliter stulti, qui cum merita non habeant tamquam ratione carentes nichil eis ad peccatum inputatur*).[127] The insane and children cannot sin, they are innocent, but that is precisely because they lack reason, which in other respects is one of the defining characteristics of a human being – while they are morally protected, the overall humanity of children and the insane is, arguably, somewhat dubious.

McDonagh had elaborated as follows on English legal notions of idiocy:

> In the fourteenth century, the legal term 'idiot' meant exactly what it said in Greek: a private man. When the term was affixed to an individual by the Court of Chancery after an investigation into the defendant's ability to perform such tasks as handle money and identify lineage, it meant that person was no longer considered a 'public individual' capable of holding any degree of authority at the indulgence of the Crown; instead, he was demoted to the lowly status of an *idiota*, who does not hold a public office and is thus level with peasants and (most) women.[128]

While there is a vestige of the tiniest grain of truth in this, in that, no doubt, *idiota* did find its way into English legal usage via its original Greek meaning of a private person, the interpretation as given here is just an expression of wishful thinking, dreaming of a kind of golden age prior to the IQ test, where individual worth was not measured against perceived levels of rationality or intellect. But, as the numerous cases from the legal records cited above actually demonstrate, if one bothers to read them in their full context, there was far more to the notion of *idiota* than just being 'demoted to the lowly status': one need only recall the oft-cited case of Emma de Beston, who is described as having the countenance of an idiot, or those people who were referred to as idiots from birth (*idiota a nativitate*), for it to become obvious that designating someone as *idiota* was about more than just public responsibility for holding property. If that were the only criterion, then any other disinherited people or those stripped of their holdings for, say, rebellion, would also have been labelled *idiota*, which of course they were not. It may not fit in the ideology of a prerational, pre-modern past, but, as the medieval evidence from a variety of normative texts (legal, theological, philosophical, medical) demonstrates, concepts of individual intelligence not only existed but were strongly tied in to expected levels of rationality to be achieved at specific developmental 'milestones', as the various legal codes cited above demonstrate.

Medieval legal tracts, as well as medical theories, made only limited differentiation and categorisation of mental pathologies, and argumentation in both areas relied on a few simple, well-trodden cases. Most likely this was so because the customary family provision of care and custody exerted social pressures which made care and custody a community matter – something the medieval authorities needed to become involved in only when either family provision was unavailable or the afflicted person's behaviour exceeded the capabilities of a family, as with the violently insane. In cases where people held property, those with mental disability or mental illness ran the risk of exploitation for financial gain, but otherwise encounters with the legal systems of the day were minimal. For medieval jurisprudence, the main concern was about establishing two criteria: whether a person was 'reasonable' enough to conduct their affairs and manage their property, and whether a person could be held responsible for their actions. Medieval laws, like the Roman before them, were concerned with defining mental afflictions for the purposes of establishing whether someone was criminally culpable or not, and if they could marry, inherit or hold property – all on an individual case basis. 'All the major European legal systems which provided for the mad defined insanity in functional rather than in diagnostic terms. The law cared less whether a man was manic or melancholic than whether he was capable of responsibility for his behavior or, to be more precise, capable of acting within the law.'[129]

And, finally, what are we to make of the case of John Cousin, described in the *CPR* as *fatuus*? 'John Cousin, an idiot (*fatuus*), as above, with a hackney, under the price of 40s., and 40s. for his expenses.'[130] This was one of a number of licences granted in December 1367 for foreign travel, embarking from the port of Dover, to be commenced within one month, and limiting the amount of cash that could be taken out of the country – all precautions due to the war with France. For comparison, the value of the horse, and the personal expenses (40s.) equate to what had been granted on 26 November that same year to a yeoman, William Frere. What kind of 'idiot' was John Cousin? If he was mentally challenged, what was he doing travelling abroad in times of conflict, by himself, in charge of his own affairs? Could it be that, rather than reflecting his frame of mind, the title *fatuus* referred to a job description? Was Mr Cousin in fact a professional entertainer, a performing fool? In his case we do not have enough evidence for an answer, but the following chapter will take a closer look at the construction and concept – or not – of the intellectually disabled as courtly fools.

Notes

1 Jonathan Andrews, Asa Briggs, Roy Porter, Penny Tucker and Keir Waddington, *The History of Bethlem* (London and New York: Routledge, 1997), 95–6.

2 *Wills and Inventories from the Registers of the Commissary of Bury St Edmund's and the Archdeacon of Sudbury*, ed. Samuel Tymms, Camden Society (London: 1850), 25.

3 Judith Z. Abrams, *Judaism and Disability: Portrayals in Ancient Texts from the Tanach through the Bavli* (Washington, DC: Gallaudet University Press, 1998), 124.

4 Abrams, *Judaism and Disability*, 139.

5 George Rosen, *Madness in Society: Chapters in the Historical Sociology of Mental Illness* (Chicago: University of Chicago Press, 1968), 65.

6 Cited by Abrams, *Judaism and Disability*, 47.

7 Saul M. Olyan, *Disability in the Hebrew Bible: Interpreting Mental and Physical Differences* (Cambridge: Cambridge University Press, 2008), 113.

8 Cited in Abrams, *Judaism and Disability*, 48.

9 Michael W. Dols (ed. Diana E. Immisch), *Majnûn: The Madman in Medieval Islamic Society* (Oxford: Clarendon Press, 1992), 440, citing Yvon Linant de Bellefonds, *Traité de droit musulman comparé*, 3 vols (The Hague/Paris, 1965–73), vol. I, 247–8, vol. III, 262–3.

10 Dols, *Majnûn*, 440.

11 R. C. Pickett, *Mental Affliction and Church Law: An Historical Synopsis of Roman and Ecclesiastical Law and a Canonical Commentary* (Ottawa, Ontario: The University of Ottawa Press, 1952), 21.

12 Rosen, *Madness in Society*, 128, cf Justinian, *Institutiones*, I, 23, 3–4.

13 P. Birks and G. McLeod (trans. and intro), *Justinian's Institutes* (Ithaca, NY: Cornell University Press, 1987), 108 (Latin) and 111 (English).

14 Fergus Kelly, *A Guide to Early Irish Law* (Early Irish Law Series 3) (Dublin: Dublin Institute of Advanced Studies, 1988), 1.

15 Kelly, *A Guide to Early Irish Law*, 65; see *Dictionary of the Irish Language*, compact edition (Dublin: Royal Irish Academy, 1983), s.v. 2 *drúth*.

16 Kelly, *Guide to Early Irish Law*, 85; for these conditions see *Corpus Iuris Hibernici*, ed. D. A. Binchy (Dublin, 1978) [hereafter *CIH*], with illness at 21.24, insane at 20.29, deaf at 1575.13, maimed at 375.9, leprous at 375.8, wasting sickness at 1575.14 (*mac anfobrachta*) and 375.9 (*di andobracht*); useful here Liam Breatnach, *A Companion to the Corpus Iuris Hibernici* (Dublin: Dublin Institute for Advanced Studies, 2005).

17 Kelly, *Guide to Early Irish Law*, 92.

18 Kelly, *Guide to Early Irish Law*, 92, 154; see *CIH* 271.10.

19 Kelly, *Guide to Early Irish Law*, 93; cf. *CIH* 372.21.

20 Kelly, *Guide to Early Irish Law*, 271 appendix I no. 28; *CIH* 2106.34–2107.20 and 2107.21–35.

21 Kelly, *Guide to Early Irish Law*, 93; on contracts see *CIH* 351.26 and 988.8, 21, on incitement *CIH* 7.11–2 and 1264.33, on man and *mer CIH* 20.29, and woman and *drúth CIH* 1276.36–7 and 1575.15.

22 Kelly, *Guide to Early Irish Law*, 93–4; on the text see *CIH* 1276.18, forfeiture *CIH* 1276.21 also 1276.24 and 2107.1. Under the heading 'The Advice to Doíden' it is edited and translated by Roland Smith, *Ériu*, 11 (1932), 66–85.

23 Basil Clarke, *Mental Disorder in Earlier Britain: Exploratory Studies* (Cardiff: University of Wales Press, 1975), 31; cf. the judgements in Bloodlyings, D. A. Binchy, 'Bretha Crólige', *Ériu*, 12 (1938), 1–77, and the judgements of Dian Cecht, D. A. Binchy, 'Bretha Déin Chécht', *Ériu*, 20 (1966), 1–65.

24 Clarke, *Mental Disorder in Earlier Britain*, 32.

25 Kelly, *Guide to Early Irish Law*, 130; cf. *CIH* 2291.36–2292.3.

26 Gershon Berkson, 'Mental Disabilities in Western Civilization from Ancient Rome to the Prerogativa Regis', *Mental Retardation*, 44:1 (2006), 28–40, at 35, citing M. J. Macauliffe, *Gaelic Law: The Berla Laws, or the Ancient Irish Common Law* (Dublin: Hodge Figgis, 1923), 37.

27 Judith S. Neaman, *Suggestion of the Devil: Insanity in the Middle Ages and the Twentieth Century* (New York: Octagon Books, 1978), 109, citing *Senchus Mor*, ed. and trans. J. O'Donovan, T. O'Mahony, W. Neilson Hancock et al. (Dublin: Alexander Thom/ London: Longmans, 1865–1901), III, iiii and II, xxix.

28 Clarke, *Mental Disorder in Earlier Britain*, 54; see D. A. Binchy (ed.), *Studies in Early Irish Law* (Dublin, 1936), 74.

29 Clarke, *Mental Disorder in Earlier Britain*, 34; M. Richards, *The Laws of Hywel Dda* (Liverpool: Liverpool University Press, 1954), 46.

30 Stefan Jurasinski, 'Madness and Responsibility in Anglo-Saxon England', in Tom Lambert and David Rollason (eds), *Peace and Protection in the Medieval West* (Toronto: PIMS, 2009), 99–120, at 100, 111, 115.

31 Stephen Harper, *Insanity, Individuals, and Society in Late-Medieval English Literature: The Subject of Madness* (Lewiston, Queenston, Lampeter: Edwin Mellen Press, 2003), 35–6.

32 Cited by Margaret McGlynn, 'Idiots, Lunatics, and the Royal Prerogative in Early Tudor England', *The Journal of Legal History*, 26:1 (2005), 1–20, at 4.

33 A. Luders, T. E. Tomlins, J. France et al. (eds), *Statutes of the Realm*, 11
    volumes in 12 (London: George Eyre and Andrew Strahan, 1810–28), at vol. I,
    226.

34 Summarised by Andrews et al., *History of Bethlem*, 96; A. Luders et al (eds),
    Statutes of the Realm, 11 volumes in 12 (London: George Eyre and Andrew
    Strahan, 1810–28), at vol. I, 226.

35 Richard Neugebauer, 'Medieval and Early Modern Theories of Mental Illness',
    Archives of General Psychology, 36 (1979), 477–83, his seminal article, was an
    expanded version of his earlier piece 'Treatment of the Mentally Ill in Medieval
    and Early Modern England', *Journal of the History of the Behavioural Sciences*, 14
    (1978), 158–69.

36 J. Cowell, Ideot, in *The Interpreter of Words and Termes* (London, 1701).

37 *An Exposition of Certaine Difficult and Obscure Words and Termes* (London, 1615),
    fol. 117v.

38 Neugebauer, 'Medieval and Early Modern Theories of Mental Illness', 479.
    In a reworking of his article, Neugebauer admits that it is likely 'that some
    proportion of idiots in fact suffered from deficits of postnatal origin.' (Richard
    Neugebauer, 'Mental Handicap in Medieval and Early Modern England: Criteria,
    Measurement and Care', in David Wright and Anne Digby (eds), *From Idiocy
    to Mental Deficiency: Historical Perspectives on People with Learning Disabilities*
    (London: Routledge, 1996), 22–43, at 32).

39 Christopher Goodey, *A History of Intelligence and 'Intellectual Disability': The
    Shaping of Psychology in Early Modern Europe* (Farnham: Ashgate, 2011), 142.

40 Goodey, *A History of Intelligence*, 142.

41 *Borough Customs*, ed. Mary Bateson, 2 vols, Selden Society 18 and 21 (London:
    Bernard Quaritch, 1904 and 1906), vol. 2, 155–7.

42 For evaluation of *Prerogativa Regis* see Wendy J. Turner, *Care and Custody of the
    Mentally Ill, Incompetent, and Disabled in Medieval England* (Turnhout: Brepols,
    2013).

43 Richard C. Scheerenberger, *A History of Mental Retardation* (Baltimore and
    London: Brookes, 1983), 36, who based his surmises on W. Ireland, *On Idiocy and
    Imbecility* (London: Churchill, 1877).

44 Andrews et al., *History of Bethlem*, 97. The source is TNA, C 140/11/33, an inqui-
    sition post mortem from the third year of the reign of Edward IV. Joan, Countess
    of Kent (1406–90) was remarkably long lived, which *might* speak against her
    having had a form of developmental ID (for example, as pointed out in Chapter
    1, people with Down syndrome often have physical diseases which shorten their
    lifespan). Too many modern commentators have taken the medieval labelling
    of idiocy in the source at face value (e.g. Gwen Seabourne, *Imprisoning Medieval
    Women: The Non-Judicial Confinement and Abduction of Women in England,
    c.1170–1509* (Farnham: Ashgate, 2013), 58, who erroneously stated Joan died in
    1463), instead of questioning the motives for calling someone an idiot.

45 Andrews et al., *History of Bethlem*, cf. *Calendar of Plea and Memoranda Rolls* ...

of the City of London, 1458–1482, ed. P. E. Jones (Cambridge: Cambridge University Press, 1961), 5.

46 Henry de Bracton, *De Legibus et Consuetudinibus Angliae*, edited by George E. Woodbine and translated by Samuel E. Thorne, 4 vols (Cambridge, MA: Harvard University Press, Belknap Press/ London: Selden Society, 1968–77), vol. 4, 177–8.

47 Bracton, *De Legibus*, vol. 4, 143.

48 Bracton, *De Legibus*, vol. 2, 286.

49 Bracton, *De Legibus*, vol. 4, 356.

50 Bracton, *De Legibus*, vol. 4, 351; similar additional phrase at vol. 2, 24.

51 Bracton, *De Legibus*, vol. 4, 308–9.

52 Bracton, *De Legibus*, vol. 2, 424.

53 Simon Kemp, *Medieval Psychology* (New York: Greenwood Press, 1990), 126; cf. Anthony M. Platt and Bernard L. Diamond, 'The Origins and Development of the "Wild Beast" Concept of Mental Illness and Its Relation to Theories of Criminal Responsibility', *Journal of the History of the Behavioral Sciences*, 1 (1965), 355–67.

54 *Fleta*, ed. and trans. Henry G. Richardson and George O. Sayles, 3 vols, Selden Society Publications 72, 89, 99 (London, 1955, 1972, 1984), at vol. 72, 21 in parallel Latin/English.

55 *Fleta*, Richardson and Sayles, vol. 99, 181–2.

56 *The Mirror of Justices*, ed. William Joseph Whittaker, intro. F. W. Maitland, Selden Society 7 (London: B. Quaritch, 1895), xlix.

57 Book II Of Actions, chapter II Of Judges, *Mirror of Justices*, 44.

58 Book II Of Actions, chapter XXX Of Essoins, *Mirror of Justices*, 83.

59 Book II Of Actions, chapter III Of Plaintiffs, *Mirror of Justices*, 45.

60 Thomas Green, 'Societal Concepts of Criminal Liability for Homicide in Mediaeval England', *Speculum*, 47:4 (1972), 669–94, at 669.

61 Daniel N. Robinson, *Wild Beasts and Idle Humours: The Insanity Defense from Antiquity to the Present* (Cambridge, MA and London: Harvard University Press, 1996), 99, citing F. Pollock and F. Maitland, *The History of English Law Before the Time of Edward I* (Cambridge: Cambridge University Press, 1968), vol. II, 480.

62 Book IV Of Judgment, chapter XVI Of the Judgement of Homicide, *Mirror of Justices*, 136.

63 Book IV Of Judgment, chapter XVI Of the Judgement of Homicide, *Mirror of Justices*, 137.

64 According to editorial note, the introduction of this ruling was ascribed to Robert, 'a favourite and a justice of Henry III'. Robert may have been the instigator of the *Prerogativa Regis*.

65 *Mirror of Justices*, 138–9.

66 Book II Of Actions, chapter XXVII Of Contract, *Mirror of Justices*, 73.

67 Book I chapter xi, *Britton*, ed. and tran. Francis Morgan Nichols, 2 vols (Oxford: Clarendon Press, 1865), vol. I, 42.

68 Book I chapter xiv, *Britton*, Nichols, vol. I, 52.

69   Book I chapter xxiii, *Britton*, Nichols, vol. I, 98.

70   Book II chapter iii, *Britton*, Nichols, vol. I, 223, 227.

71   Book III chapter ii, *Britton*, Nichols, vol. II, 20.

72   Book III chapter xxii, *Britton*, Nichols, vol. II, 155.

73   Book III chapter xxii, *Britton*, Nichols, vol. II, 155.

74   Book VI chapter v, *Britton*, Nichols, vol. II, 339.

75   Book VI, chapter x [CXXVI], 1, *Britton*, Nichols, vol. II, 356.

76   'Dumme, denen ihre Verwandten, die ihre Pfleger sind, ihr Gut mit dem Gericht abgenommen haben und sie es mit ihrer Dummheit dazu haben kommen lassen.' Walter Fandrey, *Krüppel, Idioten, Irre. Zur Sozialgeschichte behinderter Menschen in Deutschland* (Stuttgart: Silberburg-Verlag, 1990), 15, citing Freisinger Rechtsbuch, ed. Hans Kurt Claußen (Weimar, 1941), 183.

77   Book I.3, *The Saxon Mirror*, trans. Maria Debozy (Philadelphia: University of Pennsylvania Press, 1999), 69–70; Lehnrecht 1.IV, *Sachsenspiegel. Landrecht und Lehnrecht*, ed. Friedrich Ebel (Stuttgart: Reclam, 1999), 32.

78   Book III.3, *Saxon Mirror*, 117; Landrecht 3.III, *Sachsenspiegel*, 118.

79   Cited by Aleksandra Nicole Pfau, 'Madness in the Realm: Narratives of Mental Illness in Late Medieval France' (PhD diss., University of Michigan, 2008), 20; see Adolf Tobler and Erhard Lommatzsch, *Altfranzösisches Wörterbuch. Adolf Toblers nachgelassene Materialien bearbeitet und mit Unterstützung der Preussischen Akademie der Wisenschaften*, 11 vols (Berlin: Weidmann, 1925–,) vol. 5, 1353.

80   Pfau, 'Madness in the Realm', 119–20; *Coutumes de Beauvaisis*, ed. Amédée Salmon, 3 vols (Paris: Picard et Fils, 1970–74), vol. 2, chapter 34, §1061; *The Coutumes de Beauvaisis of Philippe de Beaumanoir*, ed. and trans. F. R. P. Akehurst (Philadelphia: University of Pennsylvania Press, 1992).

81   Cited in Pfau, 'Madness in the Realm', 125; *Coutumes de Beauvaisis*, ed. Salmon, vol. 2, chapter 56, §1624.

82   Pfau, 'Madness in the Realm', 127.

83   H. H. Beek, *Waanzin in de Middeleeuwen: Beeld van de Gestoorde en Bemoeienis met de Zieke* (Haarlem: De Toorts/ Nijkerk: G.F. Callenbach, 1969), 114 and 298.

84   Beek, *Waanzin in de Middeleeuwen*, 114, case in Archives nationales de France, série JJ, dated 1394, register 146, letter 169.

85   Beek, *Waanzin in de Middeleeuwen*, 141 and 309, appendix IV no. 2, case in Archives nationales de France, série JJ, dated 1414, register 167, letter 187.

86   Beek, *Waanzin in de Middeleeuwen*, 114 and 298, appendix IV no. 2, case in Archives nationales de France, série JJ, dated 1350, register 80, letter 214.

87   *Calendar of Inquisitions Miscellaneous (Chancery), Henry III–Henry V*, 7 vols (London: HMSO, 1916–68) [hereafter *CIM*], vol. 4, 127–8, no. 227.

88   Neugebauer, 'Medieval and Early Modern Theories', 481, citing *CIM*, vol. 4, 1275.

89   *Calendar of the Patent Rolls Preserved in the Public Record Office, 1216–1509*, Public Record Office, 52 vols (London: HMSO, 1891–1901) [hearafter *CPR*], Edward III, vol. 10, 44–5, 17 May 1354, Westminster.

90   Harper, *Insanity, Individuals, and Society*, 57.

91 *Calendar of Inquisitions Post Mortem and Other Analogous Documents Preserved in the Public Record Office*, 20 vols (London: HMSO, 1904–70) [hereafter *CIPM*], vol. 6, 436–9, no. 703; vol. 14, 305–14, no. 325; and vol. 10, 189–93, no. 211.

92 Wendy J. Turner, 'Defining Mental Afflictions in Medieval English Administrative Records', in Cory James Rushton (ed.), *Disability and Medieval Law: History, Literature, Society* (Newcastle-upon-Tyne: Cambridge Scholars Publishing, 2013), 134–56, at 139–40.

93 Turner, 'Defining Mental Afflictions', 140–1.

94 Turner, 'Defining Mental Afflictions', 140; The National Archives [hereafter TNA]: PRO C 60/234, m. 7 and *Calendar of Fine Rolls*, vol. 15, Henry VI, 1422–1430 (London: HMSO, 1935), 180, also TNA: PRO C 60/235, m. 21 and *Calendar of Fine Rolls* vol. 15, 192.

95 Turner, 'Defining Mental Afflictions', 141; TNA: PRO C 134/13, m. 1 and C 66/109, m. 25.

96 Turner, 'Defining Mental Afflictions', 142; TNA: PRO C 137/51, m. 57 and C 60/211, m. 12.

97 Turner, 'Defining Mental Afflictions', 142; TNA: PRO C 135/141, m. 32.

98 *Calendar of the Patent Rolls Preserved in the Public Record Office, 1216–1509*, Public Record Office, 52 vols (London: HMSO, 1891–1901) [hereafter *CPR*], Henry III, vol. 4, 206, membrane 6, 3. July 1253, Southwick.

99 *CPR*, Henry VI, vol. 1, 299, membrane 18d, 26 May 1425, Westminster.

100 *CPR*, Richard II, vol. 1, 358, membrane 33d, 18 February 1379, Westminster.

101 *CPR*, Edward I, vol. 2, 339, membrane 41, 28 January 1290, Westminster.

102 *CPR*, Edward III, vol. 8, 525, membrane 26d, 26 March 1350, Westminster.

103 *CPR*, Edward II, vol. 4, 396, membrane 25, 28 February 1324, Westminster.

104 Wendy Turner, 'Silent Testimony: Emotional Displays and Lapses in Memory as Indicators of Mental Instability in Medieval Emglish Investigations', in W. Turner (ed.), *Madness in Medieval Law and Custom* (Leiden and Boston: Brill, 2010), 81–95, at 92; *CIM*, vol. 7, 8, no. 11.

105 *CPR*, Edward I, vol. 4, 123, membrane 32, 11 March 1303, Westminster; also discussed in Constance Bullock-Davies, *Menestrellorum Multitudo: Minstrels at a Royal Feast* (Cardiff: University of Wales Press, 1978), 52–3, pointing out that the grant was distinctly to Adam's advantage, tantamount to making him the owner, and an example of the esteem a royal watchman was held in.

106 *CPR*, Edward II, vol. 1, 53, membrane 22, 16 March 1308, Westminster.

107 Nigel Walker, *Crime and Insanity in England: Vol. 1. The Historical Perspective* (Edinburgh: Edinburgh University Press, 1968), 9.

108 Walker, *Crime and Insanity in England: Vol. 1*, 9.

109 *CPR*, Richard II, vol. 6, 15–16, membrane 25, 5 July 1396, Westminster.

110 Wendy Turner, 'Town and Country', in W. Turner (ed.), *Madness in Medieval Law and Custom* (Leiden and Boston: Brill, 2010), 17–38, at 34, citing *CIM*, vol. 6, 59–60, no. 127.

111 Turner, 'Defining Mental Afflictions', 142–3; TNA: PRO C 133/106, m. 17;

TNA: C 135/44, m. 2; *CIPM*, Edward I, vol. 4, 78, also at *CIPM* Edward III, vol. 7, 171.

112 Walker, *Crime and Insanity in England*, 19; *Select Pleas of the Crown*, vol. I, Selden Society Publications (London, 1887), 66: 'Loquendum cum rege de quodam stulto qui est in prisona eo quod per demenciam cognovit se esse latronem sed non est culpabilis.'

113 From the *Liber Assisarum* for 26 Edward III, plea 27; cited Walker, *Crime and Insanity in England*, 219 and 239n2.

114 Nicholas Eymerich, *Directorium inquisitorum F. Nicholai Eymerici Ordinis Praedicatorum, cum commentariis Francisci Pegnae sacrae theologiae ac iuris utri- usque doctoris* (Venice, 1595). See Sabina Flanagan, 'Heresy, Madness, and Possession in the High Middle Ages', in Ian Hunter, John C. Laursen and Cary J. Nederman (eds), *Heresy in Transition: Transforming Ideas of Heresy in Medieval and Early Modern Europe* (Aldershot: Ashgate, 2005), 29–41, at 41.

115 *CPR*, Henry III, vol. 5, 407, membrane 22, 18 February 1265, Westminster; Eliza Buhrer, '"But what is to be said of a fool?" Intellectual Disability in Medieval Thought and Culture', in Albrecht Classen (ed.), *Mental Health, Spirituality, and Religion in the Middle Ages and Early Modern Age* (Berlin: De Gruyter, 2014), 314–43 also treats William Pilche of Sonky as a mentally disabled person.

116 Naomi D. Hurnard, *The King's Pardon for Homicide Before A.D. 1307* (Oxford: Clarendon Press, 1969), 169.

117 Clarke, *Mental Disorder in Earlier Britain*, 61.

118 Pickett, *Mental Affliction and Church Law*, 2.

119 Walker, *Crime and Insanity in England*, 3.

120 Turner, 'Defining Mental Afflictions', 145.

121 Robinson, *Wild Beasts and Idle Humours*, 34–5.

122 Pickett, *Mental Affliction and Church Law*, 3–7.

123 *Decretum Gratiani*, ed. E. Friedberg, *Corpus iuris canonici*, I (Leipzig, 1879), C. 15 q. 1 p. c. 2 Par 3.

124 Anthony Michael Platt, 'The Criminal Responsibility of the Mentally Ill in England, 1100–1843' (M.Crim. thesis, University of California, Berkeley, 1965), 18–19; cf. Mary Bateson (ed.), *Borough Customs*, Selden Society 21 (London: Quaritch, 1906), vol. 2, 159 for the test performed at Shrewsbury of knowing a good from a bad penny.

125 Robert I. Burns and Samuel Parsons Scott, *Las Siete Partidas*, vol. 4, *Family, Commerce and the Sea* (Philadelphia: University of Philadelphia Press, 2000), 881 and 957.

126 Margaret McGlynn, 'Idiots, Lunatics, and the Royal Prerogative in Early Tudor England', *The Journal of Legal History*, 26:1 (2005), 8.

127 *Scito teipsum*, ed. D. E. Luscombe, *Peter Abelard's Ethics* (Oxford: Clarendon Press, 1971), 56 Latin; 57 English. See also Jean Porter, 'Responsibility, Passion, and Sin: A Reassessment of Abelard's Ethics', *The Journal of Religious Ethics*, 28:3 (2000), 367–94.

128 Patrick McDonagh, *Idiocy: A Cultural History* (Liverpool: Liverpool University Press, 2008), 6.

129 Neaman, *Suggestion of the Devil*, 68. This is echoed nearly four decades later by McGlynn, 'Idiots, Lunatics, and the Royal Prerogative', 1: 'Lawyers had little interest in the specifics of the illness, but were concerned with its implications for the property and person of the insane man or woman.'

130 *CPR*, Edward III, vol. 14, 72, membrane 4d, 3 December 1367, Westminster.

6

FOOLS, PETS AND ENTERTAINERS: SOCIO-CULTURAL CONSIDERATIONS OF INTELLECTUAL DISABILITY

'Take that idiotic expression off your face.'
'I can't help it,' replied Švejk solemnly. 'I was discharged from the army for idiocy and officially certified by a special commission as an idiot. I'm an official idiot.'
The gentleman of the criminal type ground his teeth:
'What you're accused of and you've committed proves you've got all your wits about you.'[1]

Thus, during the First World War the fictitious good soldier Švejk of the eponymous novel is ejected from the army and classified as an idiot. His idiocy, as the above passage implies, is feigned, since he only acts the part of the fool because it suits him. In medieval terms, Švejk is an artificial fool. The natural fool has the same kind of idiotic freedom that Švejk the good soldier has come to possess by his deliberate act of imitation (or deception?), which therefore renders him an early twentieth-century reincarnation of the medieval artificial fool. In his case the proverbial ignorance is bliss. The distinction between natural and artificial fools is one 'that in Europe was understood and applied from as early as the twelfth century, but, in a wider context, goes back to the earliest recorded beginnings of the fool's history'.[2] Natural fools might further be subdivided into 'innocents', possibly people who in politically incorrect but plain language were 'slow-witted' or 'mentally retarded', and the madman-fools who may have been congenitally or spasmodically insane. Therefore, in searching for the person with ID amongst fools and jesters we need to be aware that court fools can be, firstly, an artificial fool, who is mentally 'normal' but acting out a role, and secondly, a natural fool, who in turn may either be mentally ill or have intellectual or learning disabilities. For the purposes of the present volume, my interest obviously lay in finding people only of the latter category, but that entailed carefully and discerningly sifting through the evidence on court fools overall.

A differentiation between the natural (*nâtürleichen tôren*) and artificial (*willetôre*) fools had been made by Konrad von Megenberg (as discussed in Chapter 3). The split between the natural and the simulating fool refers to the social type of the court fool, a figure whose origins are shrouded in the mists of historiography, but who can be evidenced for the twelfth, if not the tenth or eleventh centuries.[3] In German literary texts one also finds the distinction between natural fools and *Schalksnarren* (artificial court fools) from about the twelfth century, where the fool feigning madness acts as imitator of the mentally ill or debilitated person.

In the later fourteenth century, Langland had already castigated the work-shy, shirking, artificial fools, who 'Fyndeth out foule fantasyes and foles hem maketh/ And [han] wytt at wille to worche yf thei wolde' (Devise false tales and make themselves fools/ But have wit and strength to work if they wished).[4] Such fake fools abuse people's charity:

> But thoo that feynen hem foolis, and with faityng libbeth
> Ayein the lawe of oure lord, and lyen on hemselue,
> Spitten and spuen and speke foule wordes,
> Drynken and dreuelen and do men for to gape,
> Likne men and lye on hem that leneth him no [g]iftes.
> (But those that pose as fools and perform frauds
> Against the laws of our lord, and lie about themselves
> Spitting and spewing and speaking foul words
> Drinking and drooling and making men gape
> Mocking and slandering those who give them no gifts)[5]

For Langland, the *sottis* who sit in the ale-house and drink themselves into a stupor, becoming like beasts, are differentiated from infants and genuine fools, and those whose inward wit fails (*yonge fauntes [and] folis, with hem failith Inwyt, over whom the devil has no power*). 'But with children and fools the fiend has no power/ Over any acts they perform, which might otherwise be wicked' (*Ac in fauntis ne in folis the [fend] hath no might/ For no werk that thei werche, wykkide other ellis*).[6] Natural fools, the witless and innocent, are distinguished from the artificial fools, the professional 'wise fools' (*fooles sages*), flatterers and liars, who are the fiend's disciples since by their tales they entice men to sin and harlotry (*That fedeth [maintain] fooles sages, flatereris and lieries ... Right so flatereris and fooles arn the fendes disciples/ To entice men thorugh hir tales to synne and harlotrie*).[7] Thus, by the end of the fourteenth century 'diametrically opposed views of the Fool were apparent by that time; for whereas the church continued its protection of the witless man, an awareness developed of the need to distinguish such men from their mimics who were beginning to profit from the idiot's immunity from work in the houses of the great'.[8]

Ahistoricity of fools and idiots

An ahistorical stereotype still abounds concerning the linkage between persons with ID and so-called freak shows. 'During the Middle Ages, and thereafter, people with deformities and mental disabilities were frequently displayed for money at village fairs on marketing days, and peasant parents are known to have toured the countryside displaying for money recently born infants with birth defects.'[9] Not a shred of evidence is cited in support of this tale, but the idea may derive from an article on monstrous births[10] – an example of the perpetuation of myths and how they take on a life of their own. Another myth views the past through rose-tinted spectacles. In the fifteenth century the 'mentally defective were not then isolated in institutions but supported as harmless dependents in villages, courts and country houses. The toleration and freedom which their defects assured them inspired some of the sane to assume their outer guise and to seek the support of available patrons by amusing them with comical stupidities and impudent witticisms.'[11] This is a story of the more tolerant, easy-going Middle Ages. It also places the keeping of natural fools first, before the rise of the practice of keeping artificial fools, a view no longer sustainable, based on the evidence amassed by, for example, Southworth.[12] In fact, it seems the other way around, that artificial fools were the earlier entertainers and the naturals came later, and always in far lesser numbers. German historians also of course mentioned the differentiation between artificial and natural fools; according to one historiographical trope the latter were laughed at for their disabilities, whilst nevertheless the sick had their place amidst society, in contrast to the modern isolation in asylums and clinics.[13] Here the past evokes a golden age before institutions, where integration into the community somehow outweighed the ridicule and suffering of 'fools'.

Notions about the lack of reason supposedly reinforced and legitimated an inferior position in this world, leaving those considered to have an ID on the margins of social life and subject to a charity ultimately undertaken for the salvation of the giver, rather than for the welfare of the recipient. Social aspects are thus never far from a discussion of ID. Modern society expects specialist educational and/or care provision for people with ID, to the point of segregation from the mainstream. Although numerically not quantifiable (we simply do not possess the statistical data for the medieval period that nineteenth- and twentieth-century disability historians have), it does seem that the first dedicated 'institutions' in the modern sense for intellectually disabled people originated in the Middle Ages, such as the earliest hospital settings in England and Spain. One should recognise, however, that institutionalisation was the exception rather than the norm. This goes for many things, not just ID, in that the assumed prime unit of contact, support or, if necessary, care was firstly the (extended) family, and secondly one's local community. Though for the medieval period we certainly cannot speak of the 'integration' of intellectually disabled people in the modern sense, there will nevertheless have been a greater visibility of such people in all areas of society, in all walks of life.

A prime example here is the (late) medieval practice in royal, noble or simply wealthy households, of keeping entertainers, commonly known as 'fools'. People with all sorts of mental and physical impairments, not just the 'natural' fools, could sometimes – but neither always nor exclusively – find employment as entertainers in courtly circles. For example, during the years 1304–28 the accounts of countess Mahaut of Artois and Burgundy recorded the presence of a dwarf and a 'fool' of diminutive stature.[14] And according to the *Marienburger Tresslerbuch*, between 1399 and 1409 the court of the Grand Master of the Teutonic Knights played host to a stuttering herald, a blind poet or minstrel, some dwarfs, various cripples and a lame man who demonstrated how he moved himself about on two wheels (perhaps a wheeled trestle reminiscent of the hand trestles so often depicted as used by mobility-impaired people).[15] Therefore, for the later medieval period one may look to economic sources, i.e. the account books of royalty and larger households, which mention fools, and some of these fools are described in such a way as can infer ID. The account books are a classic example of a source which previous historians have already edited, used or analysed, but for completely different research questions, since they were rarely interested in ID, but in noble household expenditure in general.

Court fools, idiots and social theories of dominance

As we have seen in previous chapters, one social consequence for people with ID was that they permanently retained a child-like status in the eyes of their social superiors, on the one hand judged according to mitigating circumstances, i.e. they could not be held responsible for their criminal or 'sinful' actions, but on the other hand subject to the authority, rule and discipline of their superiors, i.e. parents or guardians. The patronisation of certain human members of a pre-modern household, such as children, women, servants and entertainers – and thus dwarfs and fools – has been compared to the abuse of power that is also exercised over non-human creatures, commonly referred to as pets; all of these could simultaneously be highly valued and severely controlled, trained to be obedient, entertaining playthings while also held in some affection. This is a topic first discussed by Tuan's essayistic exploration on dominance, affection and pets that deserves much greater recognition in scholarly circles.[16] Dominance may of course be cruel, exploitative and create the victim, but affection is dominance's anodyne, creating the pet. 'Affection mitigates domination, making it softer and more acceptable, but affection itself is possible only in relationships of inequality. It is the warm and superior feeling one has toward things that one can care for and patronize.'[17] Affectionate dominance over nature can be exemplified by the way in which various cultures have treated gardens, fountains, plants, animals, children, women, slaves, dwarfs and fools. All of these have been modified, trained, tamed and acted upon – they are passive, while agency is enacted by the dominator.

In the early modern period, beggars, rural labourers and black slaves, as well as the 'mad', were all deemed closer to animals than to humans, and with that demoted to pet-like status.[18] Zijderveld wrote of his encounter with Peppi, a man acting as factotum in a Viennese apartment block in the late 1960s, that he was 'a relic of a bygone age', who still shared many of the characteristics of the traditional household fool. On Peppi's death he commented: 'He is missed as one misses a dog which has died after having loyally shared one's life for many years.'[19] Zijderveld further noted that artificial fools may, in historically correct if politically incorrect fashion, be compared to 'expensive pets', 'mentioned in one breath with dogs, falcons and monkeys … court jesters were pets – very much loved, but usually not loved as real human beings so much as dog, cats or horses'.[20] On pets in general Tuan observed: 'Pets are a part of one's personal entourage. They are physically and emotionally close to their owner. They can be taken for granted and yet are never out of their owner's mind for long.'[21] Pets and fools thus share a common ground, both being affectionately dominated by their masters.

Explanatory myths are necessary to justify this power imbalance. The domination of the 'normally' intelligent over intellectually disabled people is an example of such myth-making, since, following Goodey's argument, the creation of intelligence as a concept allows the creation of the myth of intellectual differences. Similarly, Tuan already pointed out that people who exploit nature seldom realise that they are harming the plants and animals that they are dominating and, in contrast to people who exploit other humans for profit or pleasure, this does not cause uneasy consciences. Therefore, to overcome the unease of human dominion, the dominators need some kind of justification, some kind of rationale. One form of justification is the enforcement of dichotomies, e.g. between culture and nature, mind and body; once hierarchical structures have been imposed, those with power can use the positive binaries (culture and mind) to dominate those perceived negatively (nature and body). 'Men of power, arrogating to themselves the attributes of mind and culture, find it pleasing to have around them humans of a lesser breed – closer to nature – on whose head they may lay an indulgent hand.'[22]

Differences in physical appearance and in the intellectual capacities believed to be associated with them were used as justification for domination and subservience, a topic more often associated with racism.[23] But physical differences, so-called characteristics, can also be used to point out mental differences. One may just think of the so-called typical facial features of people with Down syndrome. Pseudo-scientific categories, e.g. physiognomy, have been used to ascribe mental differences to people on the basis of the shape of their head, facial features and expressions.[24] At a popular level today, such pseudo-science is alive and well.

As Tuan wrote, human pets 'are people whom their self-designated superiors regard as powerless, not fully human, and in some way entertainingly peculiar'.[25] Since people with ID are regarded as permanent children, they are in effect powerless, as compared to the fully human adults around them, just as children are comparatively powerless in relation to adults. And the various philosophical and scientific arguments generated over the centuries practically all reinforced the status of people deemed to be intellectually disabled as not fully human. According to concepts which treat children as not yet fully human, the permanent childishness of people with ID renders them stuck in a kind of pre-human condition. Peculiarity as entertainment seems to be the one element out of the three – powerlessness, sub-humanness, entertainment – that Tuan mentioned which is more subject to cultural change and different mentalities. The entertainment value of dwarfs and fools fluctuated with the fashions, if the sparse sources allow such a generalising statement at all, so that in imperial Roman times as well as the Renaissance the keeping of dwarfs and fools was popular among the higher echelons of society, whereas for the early Middle Ages there seems to be no evidence, and in the high Middle Ages dwarfs and fools – as different from minstrels and/or jesters – seem to be conspicuous by their rarity.

As to the question why there were fewer fools in the earlier Middle Ages and more in the later, a simple economic speculation may provide the answer. In brief, it is to do with the availability of resources, how many 'unproductive' people can be carried by an economic unit, or how many such people the unit/household wants to carry. Evidence for this is in the multifunctional jobs of the early fools (minstrel, gamekeeper, groom etc.) that they held in addition to 'playing the fool'. The specialisation of the later fools, as only and exclusively fools, is a sign of the shifting of economic resources within aristocratic households. If we follow the analogy between fools and pets, as was put forward in Tuan's dominance and affection theory, the same may be said about the specialisation in the keeping of pet animals. Take dogs as an example: from what we know, early medieval households tended to keep 'working dogs' (guard dogs, hunting dogs, sheep dogs etc.) but very few 'lap dogs', the latter becoming more popular and more frequently mentioned in the sources as the Middle Ages progressed. The lap dog, in contrast to the working dog, has no utilitarian function whatsoever, in fact consumes resources rather than contributing to production, so that the keeping of such animals is a sign of its status as pet. And following Tuan's analogy, the later medieval fool, who has no function other than 'playing the fool' (regardless of whether as an artificial or a natural), becomes pet-like in the lack of economic or productive function. Keeping fools, pets, or what were sometimes called 'parasites' is a sign of courtly sophistication, not just in the cultural but also in the economic sense, since without the material foundations to support them, fools, pets or parasites would not have existed.

That the same attitude could be shown toward pets and people, specifically courtly fools, emerges from an edict passed at the Reichstag held at Augsburg in 1500, which ordered that all those persons who kept fools should ensure that they kept them in such a fashion that they did not bother or molest other people[26] – an order that might just as easily have been passed concerning the keeping of domestic animals such as dogs. What little we know about real-life fools who are documented only at the very end of the period under consideration does corroborate the theory of fools as quasi-pets. Claus von Rannstedt, also known as Claus Narr, who prompted a copious literary output in German including a farce by Hans Sachs, was fool to the electors of Saxony, literally becoming a living heirloom for some fifty years. He started his career after having been discovered as a child while his lord was travelling through his domains. He served first the Elector Ernst of Saxony (d. 1486), then Albrecht of Saxony (d. 1500), was then 'loaned' to the archbishop of Magdeburg, on whose death in 1513 he was returned to Saxony, where he performed for Frederick III the Wise (d. 1525) and John the Steadfast, then, after 1530, becoming lost to the documentary record. Most of the anecdotes transmitted about Claus Narr describe him as someone who was mentally deficient, eccentric and appeared to vegetate in a world of delusions and phantasms.[27] But his career appeared to span almost five decades, so whatever condition he may have had was one that did not affect longevity.

The presence of a natural fool is attested at the court of Wernher von Zimmern (1420–83), one of the earliest counts of Zimmern, described in the *Zimmerische Chronik*, who kept a foolish childish poor person, a senseless fool (*dorechten, kindischen armen Menschen, einen unbesinnten dor*).[28] For comparison with Tuan's theory of fools as pets, one may note this advice from the

Zimmerische Chronik: 'Fools need to be driven and drilled, else they spoil or become idle' (*Die narren muessen getriben und geiebt sein, oder sie verderben oder verliegen sonst*). Beek cited this to mean that fools need to be trained,[29] with the Dutch word *dressuur*, derived from the French *dressage* meaning training, and still used as the technical term for a certain type of equestrian sport, making the link even more obvious. Fools and animals thus stand in close relationship to each other in yet another aspect: they are trained, not educated.

Tuan pondered some intriguing questions concerning the difference between past and present attitudes towards 'deformity and dementia'; premodern potentates appear to have been amused and reassured, while we commiserate with or even feel threatened by disability. One plausible suggestion is that the 'social distance' between the two actors was just right: 'a little closer and the potentate would have found the deformity painful, a little farther apart and the potentate might lose that measure of sympathy which made both the charitable impulse and amusement possible'.[30] Given the socio-cultural conditions of the time, it is therefore understandable (the emic approach), even if by modern standards no longer acceptable (the etic approach),[31] that fools, dwarfs and entertainers were 'kept' as objects of compassion and charity rolled into one. Court followers, that is, having – or keeping – people at one's court, might be a phenomenon more readily associated with the early modern period, but the high Middle Ages already had the 'needy', the poor who were given alms, or, like the English kings in the thirteenth and fourteenth centuries, – a permanent staff of so-called *oratores*.[32] All of these were people with the reciprocal duty, for having been given alms, i.e. charity, of praying for the soul of the donor. With a change in the way rulers, or the potentates in Tuan's phrase, saw themselves toward the later Middle Ages, and with changing perceptions and definitions of the poor and the needy, that reciprocal arrangement also changed.[33] When prayers by the recipients of alms were no longer valued so highly, other factors could attain higher value, such as the entertainment factor. Courtly entertainers, dwarfs and fools replaced needy, poor and disabled people in the attention of potentates. Medieval court fools are therefore seen by many commentators, not just Tuan, to resemble affectionately treasured but dominated pet animals in the property of a lord.

Classical antiquity and the origin of 'fools'

Greek and Roman antiquity had depicted 'fools' in imagery, focusing on physiognomy, pathology and pandering to the grotesque, before depicting them in texts.[34] Polemon, a compiler of physiognomical traditions, wrote on facial features and corporal gestures as indicators of character and described 'stupid' persons in his *Physiognomika*.[35] From the first century AD we have the example of Harpaste, a feeble-minded female slave, one of the *moriones* that were so popular in aristocratic Roman society, who was part of the inheritance that his first wife left to Seneca, and to whom Seneca expressed revulsion.[36] In one *Epistle to Lucilius* Seneca wrote that Harpaste suddenly became blind, adding 'strange but true', she does not know she is blind, and keeps asking the overseer to let her go, she says, because the house is so dark.[37] Contemporary with Seneca's detached observations are the biting satires in the *Epigrams* of Martial (c. 41–c. 104). Already here is the definition of the true *morio* as the one who behaves 'realistically' stupid and not overdrawn or exaggerated. 'His stupidity does not lie, is not feigned by wily art./ He that is witless to excess has his wits.'[38] The physiognomy of *moriones* is remarked upon, with a pointy head allegedly identifying the real fool. 'Ah, but this one with the pointed head and/ long ears that move like donkeys' are wont to do,/ who denies that he is the son of Cyrta the natural?'[39] In this context it is interesting to note that in an article on the first detailed records of exhibiting the mentally retarded at freak shows, which were published in America in the 1850s, Bogdan pointed out that it seems that the 'exhibits' were mainly microcephalic people. 'One reason for this is that the appearance of such people, when accented with shaved heads and the other trappings show men gave them, lended [*sic*] most readily to the exotic presentation that was part and parcel of the flamboyant humbug of the world of amusement.'[40] This is an important aspect of the visibility of disability, since a 'normal-looking' mentally retarded person would not have given spectators much to look at. One may compare both Martial and the phenomenon of the spectacular freak show with what Konrad of Megenberg (see Chapter 3 above) had to say on the physiognomy and the head shape of natural fools. Thus, for Martial the market value of the natural fool exceeds that of the fake *morio*. 'He was described as a natural. I bought him for twenty thousand./ Give me back my money, Gargilianus. He's no fool [lit.: he knows].'[41] And in his *Annals* Tacitus described the procurator of Cappadocia, Julius Pelignus, as a man despised alike for his feeble mind as for his deformed body (*ignavia animi et deridiculo corporis iuxta despiciendus*); but he was an intimate of the emperor Claudius, in turn a man who 'used to beguile the dullness of his leisure with the society of jesters' (*conversatione scurrarum iners otium oblectaret*).[42] In contrast, the emperor Alexander Severus (r. 222–35) got rid of the many *moriones* in his household whom he had inherited from his predecessors, by gifting them to the Roman people, thereby offloading the economic 'problem' of caring for and maintaining such 'unproductive' persons from the imperial coffers onto the public purse.

All the dwarfs, both male and female, fools, catamites who had good voices, all kinds of entertainers at table, and actors of pantomimes he made public property; those, however, who were not of any use were assigned, each to a different town, for support, in order that no one town might be burdened by a new kind of beggars.[43]

Chrysostomos (347–407), one of the Church fathers, remarked on the custom of keeping 'fools': 'we live in luxury, and waste our substance on harlots and parasites and flatterers, and even on monsters, idiots, and dwarfs; for men convert the natural defects of such into matter for amusement' (*Homily* 3 on 1 Timothy 1:14). The practice is commented on again at *Homily 17* on 1 Timothy 6:12.

And is it not a foolish desire, when men like to keep idiots and dwarfs, not from benevolent motives, but for their pleasure, when they have receptacles for fishes in their halls, when they bring up wild beasts, when they give their time to dogs, and dress up horses, and are as fond of them as of their children? All these things are foolish and superfluous, nowise necessary, nowise useful.[44]

Chrysostomos might have been talking about pets. As Tuan had observed, a pet 'is a diminished thing, whether in the figurative or in the literal sense', with the pet inessential for the material daily needs, more an object of vanity and pure pleasure.[45] The idea of the dwarf-fool as pet was already remarked upon by Welsford with regard to the Roman *morio*: 'his chief appeal was not intellectual but sensational, and that among the female population at any rate he corresponded to our modern lap-dogs and teddy-bears.'[46]

Medieval court fools

According to Welsford, the distinction between natural and artificial fools 'goes back to at least the twelfth century'.[47] In fact, if the evidence in Martial's epigrams is anything to go by, it goes back at least to the early Roman empire. With regard to the custom of keeping court fools, Welsford's statement that 'the earliest indubitable references to medieval court-fools date from the twelfth century' has often been cited.[48] Based on that pioneering work, later social historians such as Southworth provided more clarity on the matter. When the origin and supposed derivation of this custom is critically analysed, most scholars conclude that so far no seamless chain of tradition can be ascertained from antique, Celtic or other pre-medieval fools, until the emergence of the first documented proto-fools in the eleventh or twelfth centuries.[49]

Concerning the Old Irish, Norman and Plantagenet courts, one encounters only examples of artificial fools, as it appears there is little evidence in the earlier medieval period for the presence of people with ID at either the Irish or English courts, although 'it should not be supposed that they were altogether absent from the courts of the Anglo-Saxon, Norman or early Plantagenet kings.'[50] This argument is based on the fact that in the sources, which are mainly of a financial nature (account rolls), persons who were paid for their entertainment skills were very often also employed in other roles. For example, these early minstrel-fool-jesters (note how difficult it is to untangle what become later categories of entertainer) could also be employed as huntsmen, messengers or waferers. Since to be a messenger one had to be able to accurately and securely relay a given message, it is most unlikely that an entertainer-cum-messenger was mentally incompetent. A further distinction can be gleaned from such financial sources, and that is the presence or absence of 'keepers'. The earlier minstrel-fools were most likely artificial fools, since they were in control of their property (often granted to them on retirement), receiving wages, and had servants of their own, in contrast to natural fools, who (as was shown in Chapter 5 above) were legally incompetent and therefore did not manage property but were themselves 'managed' by keepers.[51] An example of a minstrel-fool might be Rahere (d. 1144), the founder of St Bartholomew's, London, who had a vision while in Rome which prompted him to commence his hospital project. He was an entertainer in courtly circles, and 'owtward pretendid the cheyr [look] of an ydiotte'[52] to gain publicity and raise awareness, as we might say, but also, according to Clarke, 'to disguise his purpose a little to get useful cooperation from people'.[53] Rahere is therefore a prime example of the artificial fool, and a very pro-active and manipulative one at that.

When the fools have a 'keeper' who handles all the finances for them, organises clothes for them etc., this is probably a sign of 'fools' who are genuinely intellectually disabled, and incompetent to look after their own affairs. In the nineteenth century Canel had already tried to distinguish between the two types, based on the presence of 'keepers', but Welsford thought that this was impossible, following a careful study of the accounts. 'The fools in France and England seem always to have had attendants, but the terminology does not necessarily enable us to distinguish the body-servant from the warder, though sometimes it is clear that it is the latter who is under consideration.'[54] For the early period Southworth cited one possible isolated example of an innocent, Jacomin who is termed *stultus et histrio regis* ("king's fool and player"), who had a special outfit made for him in 1260'.[55] Elsewhere it is mentioned that a royal 'order was given to Richard de Ewell and Hugh de Treni, buyers of the King's Wardrobe, that they shall have an outfit suitable made for Jacomin, the King's Fool and Minstrel (*istrio*)'[56] – the wording is ambiguous, since the buyers of the king's wardrobe could be officials overseeing all clothing expenses at court, not just especially for a mentally incompetent person. Southworth presumed that because Jacomin replaced two earlier fools whose names indicate knightly background, and the accounts name him by only his single, proper name, without locative or patronymic, Jacomin may have been of humbler status than the previous two, and on this alone suggested that Jacomin may have been mentally impaired.

The problem is, as so often, the reticence of the sources to provide any more detail that might allow us to determine whether persons like Jacomin may or may not have had ID. Southworth suggested that if the artificial fools 'are assumed to have modelled their behaviour on genuine madmen or "simpletons", the precedence of the latter may be taken for granted'.[57] This is a spurious argument. Just because artificial fools model their behaviour on natural fools, it does not automatically follow that natural fools were kept as courtly entertainers – one can readily think of an alternative explanation, whereby the artificials copy natural fools whom they have observed in society as a whole. Southworth admitted that it was difficult if not impossible to distinguish the naturals from the artificial minstrel-fools; supposedly the naturals behaved more 'simple-mindedly' and the artificials more 'frantically'. 'It is only on the basis of the type of payments they received, and other contextual details, that we are able to separate them.'[58]

With Henricus Stultus, the fool of the Count of Savoy, who in 1299 received 12d. as a gift of the Lord Edward (the future king Edward II), plus another 10d. via William de Hertfeld on the order of Edward, for gaming (*ad ludendum ad talos*),[59] one may assume that *stultus* in this case does not imply ID, but a job description, since it begs the question what kind of gaming activity would warrant a payment of 22d. if it were rather basic and not very entertaining. Robertus Fatuus, court fool to Queen Eleanor, appeared in accounts and received payments between 1289 and 1317/18, thus he was a long-serving retainer. Of interest, and ambiguity, is the payment in 1289 of 3s. made 'to the groom/page of Alianor de Saukeuyle, for cash on account [i.e. money borrowed] for Robert the Fool [lit. 'for cash given to him on account] for a game of dice'.[60] Does this imply that Robert was too incompetent to handle cash by himself? Possibly a similar case occurred in 1311/12, when 20s. were paid 'to John de Mendlesham, groom (*garcio*) of Robert le Fol'. However, in the same accounting period, 20s. were given directly 'to Robert le Fol, to buy himself a targe for performing [the sword and buckler dance] in the presence of the King'.[61] Hence in this case Robert was deemed mentally competent enough not only to buy his own equipment but also to perform a rather difficult and potentially dangerous sword dance. Robert is also named as Robin le Fol in accounts of 1290/91, where he appears under a new master, the Count of

Brittany, following the death of Queen Eleanor, and travelling overseas to Brittany with him.[62] The famous payroll of 1306 (when a great feast was held at Whitsun for the knighting of Edward of Caernarvon, the future Edward II), which included payments of wages and expenses to scores of royal, baronial and foreign 'guest star' minstrels and entertainers, appears not to have included payment for the fool, Robert, formerly of Queen Eleanor.[63] Can one assume from this omission that on an important, spectacular and magnificent occasion such as this feast, the fool was regarded as an ambiguous entertainer, unreliable, too impulsive perhaps, too unruly to conform, and hence was not present?

One of many fools during the reigns of Edward II and Edward III all confusingly called Robert, this being the third Robert, had a *garcio* (boy or valet) to look after him in 1313.[64] A 'keeper' for the fool is often cited as evidence that this fool was a 'natural', who needed someone to look after him due to mental incompetence, but in this case, as in many others, the presence of a servant is inconclusive. Many people of otherwise quite lowly status had servants, and many of the 'artificial' fools had servants paid for them out of the royal accounts. Robert III may or may not have been a person with ID – the evidence is just too ambiguous. An item formerly believed to be a wardrobe account of Eleanor of Castile, but more recently suggested by Bullock-Davies to stem from the reign of Edward III and relating to Queen Philippa's accounts, concerned a payment for making a robe for Roger Sutor, 'master, guardian or keeper' of Robert the Fool.[65] Judging by the date of the entry, this Robert the Fool may be a different individual from the older Robert who had been fool to Queen Eleanor; this later Robert could perhaps have been a person with ID, if the role that Roger Sutor had really was that of master, guardian or keeper, and not of servant to Robert.

As with the questions of keepers versus servants, the fact that a royal fool was pensioned off to a monastery, as were Robert Bussard in 1307 to Meaux and 'William Chewepayn, otherwise called Robert le Fol' (Robert VI) to St Albans in 1361,[66] simply indicates that royal retainers were in the enviable position of being beneficiaries of an early form of pension plan[67] and did not have to worry about provisions for their retirement – again, such evidence can point either way.

Perhaps we are on firmer ground with the case of Jakeman, described as an 'idiot', who was retained by alms from the household of Edward III's queen, Philippa of Hainault, and who had a 'keeper' at Westminster who still received an allowance in 1374, five years after Philippa's death, for Jakeman's maintenance: '9th September. – To Reginald Baker, of the town of Westminster, in money paid to his own hands of the King's alms, for the support of Jakeman, an idiot, in the retinue of the late Queen of England, by direction of the Treasurer and Chamberlains of the Exchequer, – 1*l.* 6*s.* 8*d.*'[68] This suggests that Jakeman was mentally incompetent enough to warrant having someone appointed to look after his financial affairs, and, as Southworth convincingly argued, the fact that the maintenance came out of the royal alms fund makes it unlikely that Jakeman was one of the royal wards under the terms of the *Prerogativa Regis*.

Triboulet, court fool to René of Anjou, was commemorated in a medal struck for the occasion (Figure 1) and in a marble relief. Triboulet died in 1466, so that art historian Tietze-Conrat suggested that the marble relief, which is life size, might have been made for his tomb. What is notable about his portrait is that Triboulet had a tiny head of distinctive shape, sometimes referred to as a 'tower head', emphasised by the profile view. The 'tower'-shaped skull formation on its own does not imply any form of ID (the composer Gustav Mahler's skull was the same shape). 'But in the case of the jester

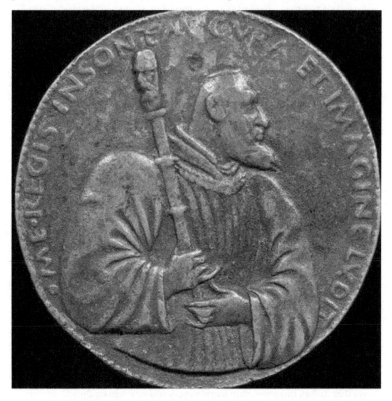

1 Medal possibly portraying Triboulet, fool to René of Anjou, made 1461–66

this tower head is microcephalic, and it is the combination of exceptional shape and exceptional smallness which makes the profile of this man so unforgettable.'[69] According to the account books of René of Anjou, Triboulet had a 'keeper', since on 4 August 1447 'Jacquet, gouverneur de Triboulet' was paid 'X gros pour une barrete roge, au dit Triboulet par commandement du Seigneur'.[70] This ties in with the observation that if fools were deemed too incompetent to handle money, payments show up in the accounts as being made to their 'keeper' and not to the fool in person.

During the reign of Henry VII, more fools leave traces of their presence in the records, but whether this reflects a predilection of Henry's or simply better preservation of records is an open question. One such fool, simply named as Dik, is a likely candidate for a genuine natural fool. He 'was clothed by John Flee of the Wardrobe in 1493, and again in the following year, at a total cost of £2 16s 7d, received neither wages nor rewards, and the only other references to him (in 1495/96) relate to the payment of wages to his "master" – plainly a keeper'.[71] A new era for royal fools seems to begin at this point, since in 1502/3 we find the first mention of the official title 'Keeper of the King's fools' (*Kepar of oure foole*), given to William Worthy, known as Phypp.[72] With the establishment of this office, and the end of the medieval period, verifiable 'natural' fools start appearing in greater numbers at the English (and other European) royal courts. Between 1498 and 1500 there are payments throughout to 'the foles master', which implies their keeper, and at Henry VII's funeral in 1509 the then holder of the title 'kinges fole', called Mr Martin, was accompanied by 'Phypp hys master', on which Southworth commented sardonically: 'Plainly, the need was felt for the restraining presence of his keeper on such a solemn occasion.'[73]

There was a striking gender imbalance in 'employment' of fools. Notable by their almost complete absence throughout the period under discussion were female fools, whether of the artificial or the natural variety. 'Even taking into account the occasional dwarf, female fools were rarely to be met with in European courts during the Middle Ages and seldom appear in the psalters.'[74] (Figure 2) Southworth found one female medieval fool, Artaude du Puy, fool in 1374 and 1376 to Jeanne, queen of Charles V of France.[75] Since it is not clear from the sources, which mention only the usual payments, what kind of fool Artaude was, one cannot make any inferences as to her mental condition. Welsford noted two female entertainers from the French court of the 1380s: a Dame Alice who was dwarf to Charles VI's queen Isabeau, as well as 'Johanne the Queen's female fool'.[76] Together with the psalter illumination reproduced here, that makes three possible female fools and one female dwarf.

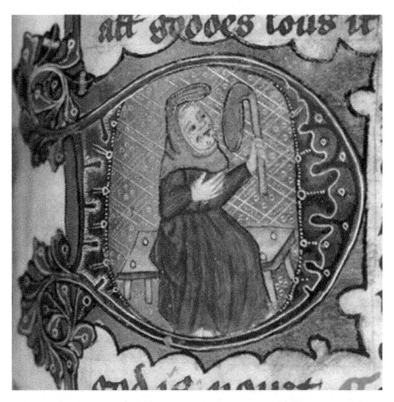

2 Rare depiction of a female fool, with lolling tongue, wearing a feather, as initial for Psalm 52, from Richard Rolle, *Commentary on the Psalter*, made in England, late 14th century

Foolish behaviour

Natural and artificial fools may be differentiated, but both have in common the idea that their folly should be harmless. 'If he was really an idiot, his stupidity amused and diverted his master. If he was an artificial fool, his assumed "innocence" lowered him beyond the reach of vengeance and left him free to speak his mind.'[77] In German, *Narr* could be used as a term that lumped together the character traits of stupidity, senselessness, intellectual limitations but also mental illness, so that foolishness does not just entail comic ridicule; instead, the fool could be dangerous and downright nasty. This perception is borne out by the Swabian dialectal *narret* or *nerrsch werden*, still in use today, which mean someone beside themselves with anger.[78] Contrary to the stereotypical image of the natural fool as someone generally harmless, placid and, especially, non-violent (often seen in contrast to the *furiosi* or *phrenetici* of the medieval discourse of mental illness), fools as real-life intellectually disabled persons can react just as violently as any other 'normal' person. 'Individuals with intellectual disability, particularly those with more severe intellectual disability, may also exhibit aggression and disruptive behaviors, including harm of others or property destruction.'[79]

Since the pre-modern reaction to (perceived) violence often tends to be with violence, it may not surprise to note that medieval treatment of fools was not always sensitive. Fools, like children and animals, had to be chastised, and since their verbal skills were deficient, the chosen means was corporal punishment. In fourteenth-century French royal payroll accounts one finds evidence not just for the existence of fools as courtly entertainers but also, more disturbingly, in the laconic language of administration, for their – by modern standards – brutal treatment. One payroll cites money to be given to a 'king of the ribauds [ribalds]' for 'beating Agnes the fool'.[80] Figure 3 depicts what may be a microcephalic fool being beaten by his keeper; older art history interpreted this image to represent a Jew (symbolic of the old law) being corrected by a Christian (the new law), but more recently it has been suggested that it might portray the court fool of John the Good (1319–64).[81] Unsubstantiated, but in keeping with the times (1930s) when Swain was writing, is this sentiment with regard to the harsh treatment of kept fools: 'One is glad that the stories of domestic fools seems to indicate that they were most often mentally defective'[82] – as Southworth has demonstrated, actually they were more often artificials. The ridicule a medieval court fool was subjected to is evident in the following anecdote, where Borra, jester to Ferdinand of Aragon, was made the butt of a particularly vicious 'joke'. In 1414 at the coronation banquet, Borra was seized by a theatrical figure of Death, caught by a rope thrown around him, and hoisted up as if to meet Death. 'The fool was so terrified that he urinated, and the urine ran onto the heads of those who were sitting below. According to the report, the King watched all this and was greatly amused, as were all the others.'[83] This crude and inhumane 'joke' could have been enforced on any kind of jester – it need not take a natural fool to be so scared by the situation as to react in such a way – considering that, as court fool, one's position was constantly at the whim and mercy of one's master, so that this is not necessarily evidence for Borra's being a person with ID.

Speculum Laicorum, an English collection of exempla made at the end of the thirteenth century, includes an episode concerning foolish behaviour which just might be reflecting real life, both the practice of keeping a domestic fool as well as possibly a report of the kind of 'irrational' behaviour a person with ID might exhibit.

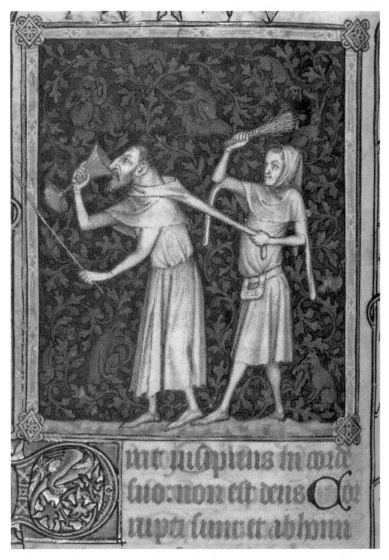

3 A microcephalic fool being beaten by his keeper? Initial to Psalm 52, from the
Psalter of Bonne of Luxembourg, c. 1348/49

They tell the story that once there was in the house of a certain rich man a fool named Philip, to whom his master one day gave a new shirt. When he put it on, Philip ran through the hall and other rooms of the house asking who he was, for Philip the fool did not know himself in his new shirt.

(Fertur quod in domo cujusdam divitis fuit quidam stultus nomine Philippus, Cui una die dominus suus dedit novam tunicam. Qua induta, discurrit per aulam et ceters domus officinas requirens quis esset, Philippus stultus non cognoscens seipsum propter novam tunicam)[84]

The story ultimately has a didactic and moral purpose, since the senseless running around of the fool is likened to the lovers of material things who are blinded by these deceptions and do not heed the salvation of their soul. But one can also detect the grain of a true description in this episode of the bewilderment that a person with ID might face when confronted with a new, unfamiliar thing. The fool's inane babblings that might sometimes hide a deeper meaning or express unexpected truths, as well as practical jokes and physical acrobatics, were the chief forms of entertainment he was expected to provide. As Swain pointed out, 'records of the spontaneous chatter of household fools of course do not exist'.[85] Which is why we need to look obliquely at surviving sources such as the *Speculum Laicorum*, since they occasionally shed some light on what sayings or behaviour real fools may have manifested.

In their behaviour, fools often affected a kind of childishness. As we saw in the discussion of philosophical notions, perennial childhood was the hallmark of the fool. Deprecating comments were made by Wulfstan, in his *Sermon on False Gods*, on the pagans who are so stupid that

they took it for wisdom to worship the sun and the moon as gods on account of their shining brightness … But they might have readily discerned, *if they had the power of reason,* that he is the true God

(Hi namon eac him ða þaet to wisdome … þaet hy wurðedon him for godas þa sunnan 7 ðone monan for heora scinendan beorhtnesse … Ac hy mihton georne tocnawan, gif hi cuðon þaet gescead, þaet se is soð God).[86]

Wulfstan presents a caricature of the pagans' simplicity and childish attraction to bright, shiny things – like the later European explorers taking glass beads to their encounters with the natives. The Old English *tocnawan* means as much as 'knowing, recognising', and *gescead* 'significance, importance, understanding', in extended sense, *gesceadwisness* 'wisdom'; relics of this meaning survive in the modern German *gescheit* 'clever, intelligent, brainy, bright, wise, prudent, sensible', with the phrase *Sei doch gescheit* meaning 'do be sensible', hence 'do not be a fool'. The child, unlike the fool, has the positive potential of gaining not just age but also wisdom, hence inclusion in the secular and divine hierarchy, which is denied the fool, who remains stupid throughout his life.[87] Permanent childishness is the identifier of the 'genuine' fool. Triboulet (of the known portrait) was described as at the age of thirty being just like at his birth, aping everyone.[88] King Henry III of England was reputed to be a simple man, according to the Franciscan chronicler Salimbene, who relates the anecdote that one day a jester cried aloud in Henry's presence

> 'Hear ye, hear ye, my masters! Our king is like unto the Lord Jesus Christ.' 'How so?' asked the King, hugely flattered. 'Because our Lord was as wise at the moment of His conception as when he was 30 years old: so likewise our King is as wise now as when he was a little child.'[89]

Henry III was, despite his alleged simplicity, just as prone to fury and outbursts of temper as other rulers, so that he ordered the hapless jester to be strung up. But the royal servants solidarised with one of their own and only went through the motions of the punishment, miming an execution, and told the (un)lucky fool to keep out of the way until the king had forgotten the affair. What of a reversion to childishness? Thomas Aquinas has famously been called the 'dumb ox'. It is then a coincidence or not to observe that according to his *Life* by the 'faithful testimony' of his friend Reginald, who was with him in his last days, the last confession Aquinas made was like that of a 'five year old boy'.[90]

Court fools amused not just because of their acted performances but because of 'mental deficiencies or physical deformities'.[91] The performative aspects of the natural fools are important. It is their very physicality – no contradiction to ID not being a physical impairment – that is emphasised, the observance of their 'wrong' bodies (physiognomy, shape, clothing) and the 'wrong' things they do with their bodies (inappropriate behaviour, gestures) that marks out the natural from the artificial fools.[92] Physicality was also a theme for Velten's article on court fools and laughter, which mainly concerned humorous stories associated with the comic actions of 'Gonella', who may have been one or several people of that name, starting with a jester of the early fourteenth century (see cover image for a representation of 'Gonella'). Velten stated that, at the latest from the twelfth century onwards, mentally afflicted persons, the so-called natural fools (called in the sources *stulti, fatui* or more rarely *moriones*), were brought to the courts often as children, where they provided entertainments together with the physically deformed such as cripples and dwarfs. Velten took the evidence for this statement from the secondary literature, in this instance Swain's *Fools and Folly*; but there is no primary material to back it up. Velten is more convincing, pointing out that artificial fools, who deliberately act their dramatics or histrionics, influence the contemporary image and discourse of the court fool to a far greater degree

than the natural fools, which they achieve by their appearance, their demeanour and the staging of comic performances. The only other notable comment
which has direct relevance to the theme of fools as people with ID is that both
the natural and the artificial fools entertain courtly society not just by verbal,
voiced and musical modes of expression, but to a great degree with the aid of
their bodies.[93]

Konrad Bitschin (c. 1400–c. 1470), author of an instruction manual for
marriage, *De vita coniugali*, in chapter 28 advised young men against immod-
erate use of bodily movement; limbs are to be gestured with sparingly, and
attention is to be drawn only to those body parts that are performing the
appropriate work at the right time. 'Making such gestures, which are not
serving the intended purpose, therefore only proceeds from a foolish sense
or from an elation of the mind or from some other internal vice, such as from
melancholia or inertia [listlessness, apathy or sloth] (*Ideo agere gestus operi non
deservientes intento vel procedit ex mentis insipientia vel elatione animi aut aliquo
alio vitio, scilicet melancholiae vel inertiae*).'[94]

In the context of misuse of gesture, one may point out that children naturally are more active than adults (not just humans; as any pet keeper will know,
younger animals are more active than older ones), so that the stereotype of the
'fidgety' child seems to be a transcultural and diachronic commonplace. The
norms of polite, refined society, whether medieval courtly or Enlightenment
salon, demanded control of one's movements and gestures, so that part of the
education of children involved instilling in them proper decorum. The difference between then and now, however, appears to be that while in the past
the movement drive of children was accepted as part of being a child, modern
society has increasingly pathologised this behavioural trait. Thus argues Smith,
author of a recent book on hyperactivity, who presents hyperactivity as a
uniquely late twentieth-century disorder, suggesting that the fidgety children
of the past (e.g. *Zappelphilipp* in *Struwwelpeter* [by Herbert Hoffmann, 1845])
cannot be equated with the typical hyperactive child of the second half of the
twentieth century, the decades that created attention-deficit disorder as an
educational problem to be solved by medication.[95]

Incorrect gestures were already criticised in Proverbs 6:12–13: 'A naughty
person, a wicked man,/ Walketh with a froward mouth./ He winketh with his
eyes, he speaketh with his feet,/ He teacheth with his fingers' (*homo apostata
vir inutilis graditur ore perverso/ annuit oculis terit pede digito loquitur*). Here it
is the apostate, the unbeliever, like the atheist fool of Psalm 52, who uses perverted forms of miscommunication. On teaching children proper rhetorical
skills, Quintilian, the Roman educationalist, emphasised that children learn
not to imitate the shrill voice of a woman, the wavering voice of an old man,

the stagger of a drunk or the cringing of slaves (*servili vernilitate inbuatur*).[96] Grimacing was regarded as something low and slavish – people with ID also 'make faces'. And in the twelfth century, Peter the Chanter, in *Verbum abbreviatum*, advised that the correct form of rhetoric involves learning to speak without making unnecessary gestures.[97]

The stutter of fools was believed to be a characteristic of their lack of linguistic abilities.[98] Imitation of the stammering language, or of the childish speech, of the natural fool can be found in a literary character feigning madness and acting the fool. Tristan in the Middle High German continuation of the *Tristan*-romance by Heinrich von Freiberg, composed c. 1285–90, first greets the queen with an imitated stutter: 'go go go go go go got/ grüeze iuch, vrouwe, sunder spot'; then at a later encounter addresses the queen in a kind of reduced childish grammar: '"vriuntel machen, vriuntel machen!"/ sprach er und begonde lachen:/ "Nimmer tuon, nimmer tuon!"'.[99] These lines seemingly reflect a realistic picture of the speech pattern of a retarded, infantile 'idiot'. *Vriuntel* means to be friendly, and in an extended sense to have a sexual relationship.[100] An *Etymology* of about 1300 defined *cachinor* as 'one who from ancient times is said to laugh immoderately and without intelligence. The definition could cover the idiot or the idiot's mimic and no strong condemnation is implied apart from the degrading aspects of such behaviour.'[101] The passage is accompanied by an illustration of a prancing figure, naked except for a two-eared hood, bauble and symbolic sword (could this provide evidence for the fool as entertainer modelling his behaviour on the fool as 'innocent'?), meaning that the inane laughter and lack of intelligence of the natural become the behavioural characteristics that the artificials, the entertainers, deliberately imitate. In the fifteenth century, the poet John Lydgate (c. 1370–c. 1451) described the natural fool as the person with 'face unstable, gazing East and South/ with loud bursts of laughter he interrupts his speech/ He gapes like a rook, with jaw wide open/ Like a captured Jay enclosed in his cage' (*fface vnstable, gasyng Est and South,/ With loude lauhtres entrith his language/ gapeth as a rook, abrood goth iowe and mouth/ lyk as a iay enfomyned in hys cage*).[102] Schmitt discussed the gestures made by the taunters and mockers of Christ at the Flagellation and Crucifixion in paintings of the later fifteenth century.[103] Can these gestures of poking out tongues, finger in mouth, general grimacing, be seen not just as revival of the antique notion of slaves as being particularly prone to such 'bad' gesturing, but also as linking the facial movements of people with ID with such negative associations?

Stereotypes of social class, especially alleged rusticity, also abounded in connection with ID. The medieval peasant often was an object of contempt and derision to his contemporaries, described as rough, dirty, boorish and foolish. One may note here the image of the 'stupid' peasant, referring to the entire class of peasants, not just individuals, as being mentally less able than their social superiors. 'Peasants were supposed to be stupid, an enduring image of the countryman common across boundaries and time.'[104] *Boorish*, of course, is the adjective pertaining to the awkward and coarse behaviour of the peasant farmer (Old English *bûr*, *gebûr*), which in its pejorative usage dates from the sixteenth century, thereby demonstrating the post-medieval continued stereotyping of the rural population.[105]

In the context of the oblation of peasant children into monasteries, or generally the reception of former peasants by monastic houses, the early twelfth-century Cluniac abbot Peter the Venerable compared these rustics to mental defectives and to people 'not useful for anything'.[106] Peter forbade the continued reception of oblates at Cluny without the express permission of the abbot, because of the great number of peasants, infants, old men and mental defectives the monastery had been receiving, which Peter deemed a majority. Ulrich of Cluny (also known as Ulrich of Zell, d. 1093) famously described the practice of oblation in the second half of the eleventh century as one whereby parents can offload supernumerary – or superfluous – children onto a monastery. As examples he simply gave too great a number of offspring ('they have a houseful, so to speak, of sons and daughters'); but also the 'defec- tives', those 'who have any defect which would make them less desirable in the secular world', so that the well-intended origins of institutional oblation have been perverted 'by the greed of parents, who, for the benefit of the [rest of the] family, commit to monasteries any hump-backed, deformed, dull or unprom- ising children they have'.[107] Intellectually less able children are regarded to be among the 'undesirables'. However, the reference to 'dull or unpromising' children needs to be treated with caution. Note here that in a modern edition of this text the Latin (*non carent sanitate corporali et membrorum integritate, ab his ipsis qui sunt ita semihomines uel ita semiuiui*) speaks of the exact opposite, namely of 'those who are not lacking in bodily health or integrity of limbs, but who are half-men or half-alive', rather than of the hump-backed or deformed. If it is still to be interpreted as a reference to people with ID, then the allusion to 'half-men or half-alive' (*semihomines uel ita semiuiui*) is strong language indeed.[108] Although one must consider that Ulrich was writing polemic, and had an axe to grind against the practice of oblation, which he criticised per se, nevertheless one cannot dismiss out of hand the presence of some disabled children in earlier monasteries.

One consequence of such attitudes was that monasteries became more exclusively upper class towards the thirteenth and fourteenth centuries, and certainly the monastic reform orders (Cistercians, Praemonstratensians etc.)

did not help. The Dominican and Franciscan mendicant orders, as preachers and proselytisers, obviously had a vested interest in education, learning and, hence, intelligence. But by raising standards for entry requirements they were becoming more exclusive, too.[109] The occasional 'simple-minded' member of a convent could nevertheless be found, for instance the lay sister in a thirteenth-century nunnery, noted in the register of Archbishop Eudes of Rouen for the visitation records of his archbishopric (6 November 1259): 'We visited the nuns at Bondeville [a Cistercian priory for nuns]. In residence were thirty-two nuns, of whom two were novices; three lay brothers; and seven lay sisters, two of whom were simple-minded [*fatue*].'[110] Eudes' record is purely matter of fact, without further comment. Therefore it appears that he may have regarded it as not terribly noteworthy to have 'simple-minded' people present in the convent, or at least as a situation that required no further action on the part of the episcopal visitation (whereas other situations do, mainly financial).

The unlearned, rustic person as quasi mentally disabled, in fact almost as a person with learning difficulties in the modern sense, is presented in the story of a novice in the *Formicarius* of Johannes Nider (d. 1438). Henricus Kaltysen, doctor of theology and Dominican inquisitor, related the story to Nider. In the Dominican convent of Buscoducensus (Low Countries?) was a youth of about thirteen years who had been placed there by his parents. The novice became demonically possessed, the symptoms of which state included raptures, but also a miraculous knowledge of Latin (*locutus est bene latine quod prius nescivit*). The local people, especially the women, thought this was a miracle, but the friars knew better that the boy was previously a rude rustic (*Fratres igitur, qui iuvenem prius rudem nimis esse noverant*) and interpreted this as an evil doing. After being exorcised

the boy was again a rustic as before but with a difference: his face took on an unwonted and horrible aspect and such a doltish expression that it was unclear that he could attain the degree of literacy required for the priesthood
(Juvenis autem, ingenio rudis, prout ante, relictus est, et ex praesentia horrendi Daemonis etaimnum aspectum quendam praefert insolitum, verius ingratum et horribilem. Quinimo tam hebes est ingenio, ut, etiam dispensatione praevia, valde dubium sit, an litteraturam attingere valeat).[111]

Perhaps the meaning of this parable is that transgression of status (from rude rustic to Latinate intellectual) is damnable, so the moral of the story rams home the dangers of such upward mobility, making the boy appear even more 'stupid' than before and questioning his career prospects. With this story we may now turn to the problem of literary evidence.

Foolish literature

Literary historians have looked at the figure of the fool in a short metrical romance entitled *Kyng Robert of Cicyle*, composed at the end of the fourteenth century in Midlands dialect and surviving in ten manuscripts.[112] This has been termed a 'vital document for the study of the medieval court fool' because, 'allowing for the fact that it is a work of fiction, the poem appears accurately to reflect aspects of the historical practice of fool-keeping'.[113] The problem is that most of the more detailed evidence for the 'practice of fool-keeping' tends to come from literary texts, i.e. works of fiction, while the strictly historical evidence, in the shape of courtly accounts, informs on purely the bare bones (i.e. the fact that a fool was kept at a given court, expenses for food, clothing and so forth) but say next to nothing about how this person was treated, what kind of entertainment they were meant to provide, let alone whether they were a natural or an artificial fool. Rare glimpses of how a court actually employed a fool, such as the report on Borra, are few and far between. Interestingly, Walsh emphasised the pet-like status of a fool in the poem of *Robert of Cicyle*, but without referencing Tuan's seminal work: 'The "entertainment" Robert provides to the court is similarly one-dimensional like that of a pet animal: no song, music, dance, witty banter, or even innocent babble, but simply the delusional rantings of a psychotic.'[114] Walsh took this very depiction, which could also be regarded as an exaggerated picture, to argue for its veracity on the grounds that it does not mince words, does not sentimentalise. But yet again, the suspicion is aroused that this is a circular argument, using a literary text to argue for historicity, when most of the historic evidence in turn appears to be derived from the same works of fiction.

Additionally we have the problem of the late-medieval fool-literature which skews the picture. At the end of Middle Ages a literature of stories and morality tales featuring folly became popular, including a long list of vices or faults which were now blamed not on neglect of any of the Christian virtues (e.g. pride, lack of charity) but on a general, unspecific unreason, a kind of *Zeitgeist* of unreason. In literature, folly took centre stage, for example in Jacob Van Oestvoren's *Die Blauwe Schute* (1413),[115] Lydgate's 'The Ordre of Folys' (1460) or Sebastian Brant's *Narrenschiff* (1494), where madness takes all of humanity aboard the foolish ship on a communal odyssey. The immense popularity of the *Narrenschiff*, which unleashed an economic boom in the conceptual fool, resulted in an almost inflationary usage, which had repercussions for the social semantics of the term.[116] The evil reign of madness is railed against by Thomas Murner in *Die Narrenbeschwörung* (1512), makes entry into academic texts in Jakob Wimpfeling's *Monopolium Philosophorum* (Heidelberg, 1480) and Jodocus Gallus' *Monopolium et societas, vulgo des Lichtschiffs* (Strasbourg, 1489). Beek, too, observed that this kind of literature does not actually help us much in gaining an understanding of the mentally ill or disabled, since the fool here has become only a cliché for moralistic discourse.[117] Therefore folly in all its manifestations came by the end of the fifteenth century to connote social outsiders, and the categorisation of different groups as fools corresponded to their marginal status. 'From the fifteenth century onwards, the face of madness never ceased to haunt the imagination of the West.'[118]

The case of the Psalm-fool

The fool of the Psalms is another such chimera. Kolve, the eminent Chaucerian scholar, had argued that some of the fools depicted in relation to Psalms 14 and 52[3] could be portraying persons with ID. With regard to the iconography, the art historian Groß pointed out that, in contrast to the portraits of natural fools at court, which attempt to focus on physical and, especially, facial characteristics (think of the above-mentioned 'Gonella' or 'Triboulet'), the many illustrations to Psalm 52 showing the *insipiens* depict a figure identifiable only by clothing and other material attributes (the stick or marotte), but not by physical or personal characteristics.[119] The tension between text (Psalm 52 refers to the deliberate folly of the atheist) and image (the manuscript illuminations tend to portray people loosely categorised as mentally afflicted) stems from the observations that the 'wrong' characters are used to illustrate the text. By rights, the illustrations should depict people capable of reason who act imprudently or unwisely, since according to theological notions one must have reason in the first place for reason to succumb to sin, but the choice of using a fool, madman or congenital idiot as illustration contradicts this. The choice of depiction may have derived from the association – and conflation – of several words all meaning 'fool' in the widest sense, the *insipiens*, *stultus* or *fatuus* of psalter Latin, but the innocent fool does not illustrate the meaning of the text. 'Where the text speaks of human folly, these images present a radical dysfunction or deficiency of mind.'[120] The development of psalter iconography led to a standardised cycle of eight psalter illustrations becoming adopted, following the Paris University Bible of around 1205–30, which then spread across northern Europe.[121] One may go even further with regard to this argument and draw attention to the contemporary concerns with rationality, the intellect, philosophy, discussions on the nature of humanity, the soul etc., all of which coincide at the end of the twelfth and the in early thirteenth centuries, crystallising first in Paris, then later in Oxford, with the (re)discovery of the Aristotelian philosophic corpus. Is it any coincidence that the word *idiota* first becomes used in the modern sense of mentally disabled around the 1220s (see Blund's tractate on the soul), while even a generation or so earlier, in the 1170s, *idiota* was still used as a job description for an entertainer in the story of Petrus idiota?

There is an intriguing mention of a miracle with a person labelled as an *idiota* as main protagonist, which at first sight might provide the one piece of evidence for the healing of a person with ID. But on closer inspection this emerges to be something of a red herring, since the term *idiota* is a job description and not a medical diagnosis. In the miracles of Thomas Becket written 1172x75 by William of Canterbury, the story is told of a jester, called Petrus idiota, who was stunned by a fall in the hospice of Crondall near Winchester. Petrus had missed dinner because he was too busy getting other guests to laugh at his words and actions (*quia verbis vel operibus alienis risus excitabat*), so that he ran to the kitchen, slipping on the wet ground and bashing his head; this caused a massive tumour of his jaw, which, this being after all a miracle story, was successfully cured by a phial of Thomas Becket. Petrus regained his powers of speech and ate and drank as if nothing had happened. The narrator concluded as a moral to the story: 'Et venit stupor super stuporem', which literally translates as 'and stupor fell on the stupid one', but might also be read as 'astonishment fell on the insensible one'.[122] That would mean astonishment at the miracle befalling the rather 'silly' Petrus. Note that the miracle refers only to the healing of the effects of the accident, not of whatever prior mental state Petrus was in, hence the assumption that Petrus idiota was another artificial fool.

In the mid-fourteenth century court fools and jesters began to replace the feeble-minded and insane persons depicted in the psalters (Figure 4). Kolve pointed out the absurdity of asking a moron, an idiot or a madman if God exists or not, since the credulity of such people means that they will say anything, wherefore the depictions of these kinds of people as the atheistic philosophical fool actually miss the point.[123] For the use of such imagery, Kolve argued that Psalm 52 is 'not a portrait of a non-believer ... but rather an apotropaic image of one'[124] which is similar in function to the gargoyles and other monsters on cathedrals. However, Kolve treated the depictions of idiots/ fools and madmen as interchangeable, missing the point that the madman is textually far more appropriate, since to be mad one must have started out at some point in one's life with the capacity for reason. The psalter fool is a fool precisely because he misuses his reason to say that there is no God, whereas the born fool never had such capacity in the first place. The fool as madman, rather than fool as intellectually disabled, may be depicted in the psalter initial of a somewhat disturbingly portrayed monk with mouth agape (Figure 5).

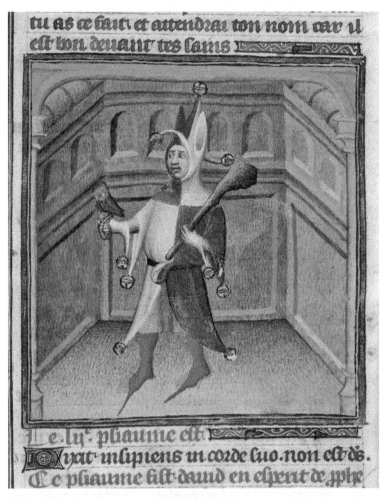

4 A court fool in typical jester costume, as illustration to the initial 'Dixit insipiens' of Psalm 52, Guyart des Moulins, *Bible historiale*, made in central France, 1411

Historians have also proposed a much closer connection between the theological fool of the Psalms and the mirror image of such a fool as foil, even antitype, to the prototype of the just and sagacious ruler.[125] However, this theory also misses a crucial point, namely that at around the same time that the fool of the Psalms is coming to literary and iconographic prominence (the thirteenth century), the philosophical texts emerging from the new institution of the university are coming to distinguish those who refuse to know (the Psalm-fool)

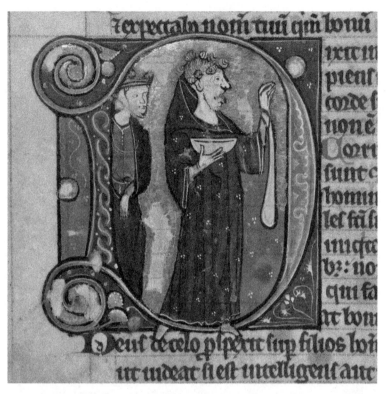

5 Psalter image of a mad fool, here depicted in a monk's habit with shaven head and curled forms instead of hair, mouth agape, in the background the figure of a queen looking on, detail of historiated initial 'D'(ixit) to Psalm 52, made in northern England between 1270–80

from those who cannot know (the natural born fool). Therefore the fool of the psalms is the atheist, not a mentally disabled person![126] In the Middle Ages we 'have not yet arrived at a situation comparable with that which confronted eighteenth-century apologists, for whom the individual who denies that there is a God is not a literary fiction, the "Fool" of the Psalms, but a person who really needs to be convinced'.[127] In other words, turning this observation around, the medieval interpretation of the Fool of the Psalms is one of only fictional, symbolic character and is, as has been argued above, a metaphorical fool and not a reflection of any 'real' people deemed foolish, or deemed by extension to be intellectually disabled.

So where does this leave us with regard to the question of fools and ID? The only thing we can be certain about is the ambivalence of the fool. On 19 June 1313 King Edward II watched a performance in Pontoise, France, recorded in the royal accounts, which included payments 'to Bernard le Fol [the Fool] and 54 of his fellow actors, coming naked (*nudis*) into the presence of the king, and dancing (*cum tripudio*)'.[128] It is highly probable that Bernard bore the name 'fool' as a title, not that he was intellectually disabled. Neither was a court jester invariably mentally ill. 'Many were undoubtedly skilled comedians whose witty banter and astute grasp of social and political trends allowed them to provide both entertainment and commentary. It is equally clear, however, that medieval courts often kept people whose comic function was far from voluntary, and who might today be categorized as mentally ill or mentally disabled.'[129] The last word on the topic of fools is best left to Welsford, the pioneer of their academic study, not least because it reminds us that older historiography can still teach us valuable insights: 'The Fool, in fact, is an amphibian equally at home in the world of reality and the world of imagination.'[130]

Notes

1 Jaroslav Hašek, *The Good Soldier Švejk*, trans. Cecil Parrott (London: Penguin, 1974), 20.

2 John Southworth, *Fools and Jesters at the English Court* (Stroud: Sutton, 1998), 5.

3 Dirk Matejovski, *Das Motiv des Wahnsinns in der mittelalterlichen Dichtung* (Frankfurt-a-M.: Suhrkamp, 1996), 28; Matejovski notes at 72 and 314n49 that in modern research the dating of the appearance of courtly fools is disputed.

4 Langland, *Piers Plowman*, C-text version, Prologue, lines 37–8. For this and subsequent references to the poem, see *Piers Plowman: A Parallel-Text Edition of the A, B, C and Z Versions: Text*, ed. A. V. C. Schmidt (London: Longman, 1995).

5 *Piers Plowman*, B-text version, Passus X, lines 39–45.

6 *Piers Plowman*, A-text version, Passus X, lines 58, 64–5.

7 *Piers Plowman*, B-text version, Passus XIII, lines 422, 429–30.

8 Sandra Billington, *A Social History of the Fool* (Brighton: Harvester Press/New York: St. Martin's, 1984), 20.

9 David A. Gerber, 'Volition and Valorization in the Analysis of the "Careers" of people Exhibited in Freak Shows', *Disability, Handicap and Society*, 7:1 1(992), 53–69, at 57–8.

10 Ottavia Niccoli, '"Menstruum quasi monstrum": monstrous births and menstrual taboo in the sixteenth century', in E. Muir and G. Ruggiero (eds), *Sex and Gender in Historical Perspective* (Baltimore, MD: Johns Hopkins University Press, 1990), 5.

11 Barbara Swain, *Fools and Folly during the Middle Ages and the Renaissance* (New York: Columbia University Press, 1932), 2, 53.

12 Southworth, *Fools and Jesters*.

13 Lutz S. Malke (ed.), *Narren. Porträts, Feste, Sinnbilder, Schwankbücher und Spielkarten aus dem 15. bis 17. Jahrhundert* (Leipzig: Faber & Faber, 2001), 12.

14 Archives du departement de Pas-de-Calais, Series A, 316, fol. 14; Series A, 293, fol. 20; cited in Sharon Farmer, 'A Deaf-Mute's Story', in Miri Rubin (ed.), *Medieval Christianity in Practice* (Princeton, NJ: Princeton University Press, 2009), 203–9, at 207.

15 J. Brandhorst, 'Spielleute – Vaganten und Künstler', in Bernd-Ulrich Hergemöller (ed.), *Randgruppen in der spätmittelalterlichen Gesellschaft* (Warendorf: Fahlbusch, 2nd edn, 1994), 169n41.

16 Yi-Fu Tuan, *Dominance and Affection: The Making of Pets* (New Haven, CT: Yale University Press, 1984, new edition, 2004).

17 Tuan, *Dominance and Affection*, 2, 5.

18 Keith Thomas, *Man and the Natural World: Changing Attitudes in England, 1500–1800* (Harmondsworth: Allen Lane, 1983), 44.

19 Anton C. Zijderveld, *Reality in a Looking Glass: Rationality through an Analysis of Traditional Folly* (London: Routledge and Kegan Paul, 1982), vii.

20 Zijderveld, *Reality in a Looking Glass*, 93, 182n12, 112.

21 Tuan, *Dominance and Affection*, 162.

22 Tuan, *Dominance and Affection*, 167.

23 Philip Mason, *Patterns of Dominance* (London: Oxford University Press, 1971); Barrington Moore, Jr, *Injustice: The Social Basis of Obedience and Revolt* (New York: M. E. Sharpe, 1978).

24 C. F. Goodey, 'Blockheads, Roundheads, Pointy Heads: Intellectual Disability and the Brain Before Modern Medicine', *Journal of the History of the Behavioral Sciences* 41:2 (2005), 165–83.

25 Tuan, *Dominance and Affection*, 153.

26 Claudia Gottwald, *Lachen über das Andere: Eine historische Analyse komischer Representationen von Behinderung* (Bielefeld: transcript Verlag, 2009), 82.

27 Werner Mezger, *Hofnarren im Mittelalter: Vom tieferen Sinn eines seltsamen Amts* (Konstanz: Universitätsverlag Konstanz, 1981), 74.

28 Angelika Groß, *'La Folie'. Wahnsinn und Narrheit im spätmittelalterlichen Text und Bild* (Heidelberg: Carl Winter Universitätsverlag, 1990), 101, after *Zimmerische Chronik*, ed. Hansmartin Decker-Hauff, 3 vols (Stuttgart, 1964), vol. I, 259.

29 H. H. Beek, *Waanzin in de Middeleeuwen: Beeld van de Gestoorde en Bemoeienis met de Zieke* (Haarlem: De Toorts/Nijkerk: G.F. Callenbach, 1969), 25; *Die Zimmerische Chronik* III, ed. K. A. Barack (Tübingen, 1869), 576.

30 Tuan, *Dominance and Affection*, 159–60.

31 For a discussion of the conceptual differences between emic, looking from the inside out, and etic, looking from the outside in, see Irina Metzler, *Disability in Medieval Europe: Thinking about Physical Impairment during the High Middle Ages, c.1100–1400* (New York and London: Routledge, 2006), 9–10, 33.

32 Irina Metzler, *A Social History of Disability in the Middle Ages: Cultural*

Considerations of Physical Impairment (New York and London: Routledge, 2013), 160, 200.

33 Metzler, *A Social History of Disability*, 196–8.

34 Danielle and Michel Gourevitch, 'Terres cuites Hellénistiques d'inspiration médicale au Musée du Louvre', *Presse Médicale*, 71 (1963), 2751–2, catalogued 267 terracotta figurines in the Louvre with pathological features, of which 34 were described as having the features of diverse idiots ('faciès d'idiots divers'); William E. Stevenson, *The Pathological Grotesque Representation in Greek and Roman Art* (Ann Arbor, MI: University Microfilms International, 1978), 184–5, 192–5 on the depiction of 'stupid' people with microcephaly, hydrocephalus and cretinism.

35 *Physiognomika*, A5.6.10, B29.58.60, text and trans. in Simon Swain (ed.), *Seeing the Face, Seeing the Soul: Polemon's* Physiognomy *from Classical Antiquity to Medieval Islam* (Oxford: Oxford University Press, 2007).

36 Herbert Graßl, 'Zur sozialen Position geistig Behinderter im Altertum', in Ingomar Weiler and Herbert Graßl (eds), *Soziale Randgruppen und Außenseiter im Altertum. Referate vom Symposion 'Soziale Randgruppen und Antike Sozialpolitik' in Graz (21. bis 23. September 1987)* (Graz: Leykam, 1988), 107–16, at 110.

37 *Epistle to Lucilius* Book 5, letter 50,2: 'Harpasten, uxoris meae fatuam, scis hereditarium onus in domo mea remanisse. Ipse enim auersissimus ab istis prodigiis sum: si quando fatuo delectari uolo, non est mihi longe quaerendus: me video. Haec fatua subito desiit uidere. Incredibilem rem tibi narro, sed ueram: nescit esse se caecam; subinde paedagogum suum rogat ut migret, ait domum tenebricosam esse.' *Sénèque, Lettres a Lucilius*, tome II, ed. F. Préchac (Paris: Les Belles Letres, 1963), 34.

38 Martial, *Epigrams*, XIV, 210: 'Non mendax stupor est nec fingitur arte dolosa./ Quisquis plus iusto non sapit, ille sapit.' See M. Garmaise, 'The *Morio* in Martial's Epigrams, with emphasis on 12.93', *Scholia*, 11 (2002), 55–64.

39 Martial, *Epigrams*, VI, 39: 'Hunc vero acuto capite et auribus longis,/ quae sic moventur ut solent asellorum,/ quis morionis filium negat Cyrtae?'

40 R. Bogdan, 'Exhibiting Mentally Retarded People for Amusement and Profit, 1850–1940', *American Journal of Mental Deficiency*, 91 (1986), 120–6, at 125.

41 Martial, *Epigrams*, VIII, 13: 'Morio dictus erat: viginti milibus emi./ Redde mihi nummos, Gargiliane: sapit!'

42 Tacitus, *Annales* 12.49, available at http://www.perseus.tufts.edu/hopper/.

43 *Historia Augusta*, The Life of Severus Alexander 34,2: 'Nanos et nanas et moriones et vocales exsoletos et omnia acroamata et pantomimos populo donavit; qui autem usui non erant singulis civitatibus putavit alendos singulos, ne gravarentur specie mendicorum', trans. David Magie (Loeb Classical Library, 1924), vol. II, 243.

44 Available at www.newadvent.org/fathers (accessed 5 December 2012).

45 Tuan, *Dominance and Affection*, 139.

46 Enid Welsford, *The Fool: His Social and Literary History* (London: Faber & Faber, 1935, repr. 1968), 59.

47 Welsford, *The Fool*, 119.

48 Welsford, *The Fool*, 114.

49 Edgar Barwig and Ralf Schmitz, 'Narren. Geisteskranke und Hofleute', in Bernd-Ulrich Hergemöller (ed.), *Randgruppen in der spätmittelalterlichen Gesellschaft* (Warendorf: Fahlbusch, 2nd edn, 1994), 220–52, at 235.

50 Southworth, *Fools and Jesters*, 48.

51 Southworth, *Fools and Jesters*, 46.

52 N. Moore, *The Book of the Foundation of St Bartholomew's Church in London* (London, 2nd edn, 1923), 12–13; an English translation was made c.1400 from the twelfth-century Latin original, both copied into the same MS B.L. Cotton Vespasian B ix.

53 Basil Clarke, *Mental Disorder in Earlier Britain: Exploratory Studies* (Cardiff: University of Wales Press, 1975), 144.

54 A. Canel, *Recherches Historiques sur les Fous des Rois de France* (Paris, 1873); Welsford, *The Fool*, 119.

55 Southworth, *Fools and Jesters*, 42; *Calendar of Close Rolls Henry III, 1259–61*, 321, for 25 December.

56 Constance Bullock-Davies, *A Register of Royal and Baronial Domestic Minstrels, 1272–1327* (Woodbridge: Boydell, 1986), 74.

57 Southworth, *Fools and Jesters*, 48.

58 Southworth, *Fools and Jesters*, 53.

59 Bullock-Davies, *Register of Minstrels*, 71, citing TNA PRO E101/355/17.

60 Bullock-Davies, *Register of Minstrels*, 167, citing British Library MS Cotton Nero C.viii, fol. 83v.

61 Bullock-Davies, *Register of Minstrels*, 168, citing British Library MS Cotton Nero C.viii, fol. 85r.

62 Bullock-Davies, *Register of Minstrels*, 171.

63 Constance Bullock-Davies, *Menestrellorum Multitudo: Minstrels at a Royal Feast* (Cardiff: University of Wales Press, 1978), 12.

64 Bullock-Davies, *Register of Minstrels*, 167, citing British Library Cotton Nero C.viii, fols 83v.

65 Bullock-Davies, *Register of Minstrels*, 201, citing British Library MS Cotton Galba E.iii, fol. 188v.

66 Southworth, *Fools and Jesters*, 54, 56.

67 See Metzler, *Social History of Disability*, 132–9.

68 Southworth, *Fools and Jesters*, 57, cf. *Issues of the Exchequer: Being a Collection of Payments Made out of His Majesty's Revenue, from King Henry III to King Henry VI inclusive ...*, ed. Frederick Devon (London, 1837), 197.

69 Erica Tietze-Conrat, 'A Relief Portrait by Francesco Laurana', *Allen Memorial Art Museum Bulletin*, 12:3 (1955), 87–90, at 89.

70 Cited Tietze-Conrat, 'A Relief Portrait by Francesco Laurana', 90.

71 Southworth, *Fools and Jesters*, 61; cf. Sydney Anglo, 'The Court Festivals of Henry VII: A Study Based upon the Account Books of John Heron, Treasurer of the

Chamber', *Bulletin of the John Rylands Library*, 43:1 (1960), 12–45, at 28 for clothing expenses, 29 for monthly wages of 10s paid to 'Dik the foles master', and 30 for 'Dik the foles master in rewarde' 6s 8d.

72 Southworth, *Fools and Jesters*, 61; Welsford, *The Fool*, 119, 158.

73 Southworth, *Fools and Jesters*, 63.

74 Southworth, *Fools and Jesters*, 100.

75 Bernard Guenée, 'Fou du roi et roi fou. Quelle place eurent les fous à la cour de Charles VI?', *Comptes-rendus des séances de l'Académie des Insriptions et Belles-Lettres*, 146 (2002), 649–66, at 652.

76 Welsford, *The Fool*, 118.

77 Swain, *Fools and Folly*, 54.

78 Mezger, *Hofnarren im Mittelalter*, 54.

79 *DSM-5*, 40.

80 Alfred Canel, *Recherches historiques sur les fous des Rois de France* (Paris: Alphonse Lemerre, 1873), 21ff, cited by Judith S. Neaman, *Suggestion of the Devil: Insanity in the Middle Ages and the Twentieth Century* (New York: Octagon Books, 1978), 133.

81 Charles Sterling, *La peinture médiévale à Paris: 1300–1500* (Paris: Bibliothèque des arts, 1987), 110.

82 Swain, *Fools and Folly*, 58.

83 Clifford Davidson, 'Introduction', in Clifford Davidson (ed.), *Fools and Folly* (Kalamazoo, MI: Medieval Institute Publications, 1996), 1–8, at 8n16, citing Peter Meredith and John E. Tailby (eds), *The Staging of Religious Drama in Europe in the Later Middle Ages* (Kalamazoo, MI: Medieval Institute Publications, 1983), 95.

84 Jean-Théobald Welter, *Le Speculum Laicorum: Edition d'une collection d'exempla, composée en Angleterre à la fin du XIIIe siècle* (Paris, 1914), 11, cited by Swain, *Fools and Folly*, 59 Latin, 205 English paraphrase.

85 Swain, *Fools and Folly*, 60.

86 Modern English: *Anglo-Saxon Prose*, ed. and trans. Michael Swanton (London: Dent, 1975), 123; Old English: Dorothy Bethurum (ed.), *The Homilies of Wulfstan* (Oxford: Clarendon Press, 1957), 221–2.

87 Mezger, *Hofnarren im Mittelalter*, 54.

88 Beek, *Waanzin in de Middeleeuwen*, 25, citing A. Canel, *Recherches historiques sur les fous des rois de France* (Paris, 1873), 162.

89 G. G. Coulton, *From St Fancis to Dante: Translations from the Chronicle of the Franciscan Salimbene (1221–1288)*, reprt with intro. E. Peters of 2nd edn 1907 (Philadelphia: University of Pennsylvania Press, 1972), 247; Latin in *Cronica fratris Salimbene de Adam ordinis Minorum*, ed. O. Holder-Egger, Monumenta Gemaniae Historica Scriptores vol. 32 (Hanover: Hahn, 1905-13), 305.

90 John Saward, *Perfect Fools: Folly for Christ's Sake in Catholic and Orthodox Spirituality* (Oxford: Oxford University Press, 1980), 84, citing Bernard Guido, *Vita* xli, in *Fontes Vitae S. Thomae Aquinatis*, ed. D. Prümmer (Toulouse, 1912), 206.

91 Welsford, *The Fool*, 55.
92 Lutz S. Malke (ed.), *Narren. Porträts, Feste, Sinnbilder, Schwankbücher und Spielkarten aus dem 15. bis 17. Jahrhundert* (Leipzig: Faber & Faber, 2001), 14.
93 Hans-Rudolf Velten, 'Komische Körper: Zur Funktion von Hofnarren und zur Dramaturgie des Lachens im Spätmittelalter', *Zeitschrift für Germanistik*. Neue Folge, 11:2 (2001), 292–317, at 295, 296–7, 301.
94 *Konrad Bitschins Pädagogik. Das vierte Buch des enzyklopädischen Werkes 'De vita coniugali'*, ed. Richard Galle (Gotha, 1905), cited by August Nitschke, *Bewegungen in Mittelalter und Renaissance. Kämpfe, Spiele, Tänze, Zeremoniell und Umgangsformen* (Historisches Seminar Band 2) (Düsseldorf: Schwann, 1987), 125.
95 Matthew Smith, *Hyperactive: The Controversial History of ADHD* (London: Reaktion, 2012).
96 *De institutione oratoria*, I, 11 and XI, 3, 90.
97 Peter the Chanter, *Verbum abbreviatum*, in PL, vol, 205, col. 35; see Jean-Claude Schmitt, *Die Logik der Gesten im europäischen Mittelalter*, trans. Rolf Schubert and Bodo Schulze (Stuttgart: Klett-Cotta, 1992), 59.
98 Swain, *Fools and Folly*, 39ff.
99 Heinrich von Freiberg, *Tristan*, ed. Danielle Buschinger (Göppinger Arbeiten zur Germanistik 270) (Göppingen, 1982), lines 5175–6 and 5239–41, cited in Matejovski, *Motiv des Wahnsinns*, 231, 232.
100 Matthias Lexer, Mittelhochdeutsch Taschenwörterbuch (Stuttgart: Hirzel, 38th edn, 1992), s.v. *vriunt*.
101 Billington, *A Social History of the Fool*, 4; Exeter College, Oxford, MS 42, fol. 12r.
102 Billington, *A Social History of the Fool*, 10 for modern English, 126n17 for Middle English transcription of Bodleian Library MS Laud. 683, lines 41–4; cf. 'The Order of Fools', in *Early English Poetry, Ballads, and Popular Literature of the Middle Ages*, ed. J. O. Halliwell et al. (London: Percy Society, 1840), vol. II, 165.
103 Schmitt, *Logik der Gesten*, 246–7.
104 Paul Freedman, *Images of the Medieval Peasant* (Stanford, CA: Stanford University Press, 1999), 150. I have discussed this in Metzler, 'Afterword', in Wendy J. Turner (ed.), *Madness in Medieval Law and Custom* (Leiden and Boston: Brill, 2010), 197–217, at 207.
105 T. F. Hoad, *The Concise Oxford Dictionary of English Etymology* (Oxford: Clarendon Press, 1986), s.v. *boor*.
106 Statuta 35, *Statuta Petri Venerabilis Abbatis Cluniacensis IX*, in *Consuetudines benedictinae variae (saec. XI–saec. XIV)* (*Corpus consuetudinum monasticarum* 6) (Siegburg, 1975), 86, cited by John Boswell, *The Kindness of Strangers: The Abandonment of Children in Western Europe from Late Antiquity to the Renaissance* (New York: Pantheon Books, 1988), 299 and 320.
107 Ulrich of Cluny, *Epistola nuncupatoria*, PL, vol. 149, cols 635–6, cited in trans. by Boswell, *Kindness of Strangers*, 300.

108 Susan Boynton and Isabelle Cochelin, *From Dead of Night to End of Day: The Medieval Customs of Cluny/Du coeur de la nuit à la fin du jour: Les coutumes clunisiennes au moyen âge* (Leiden: Brill, 2005), 329–47, at 330–1. Mirko Breitenstein, *Das Noviziat im hohen Mittelalter* (Münster: Lit Verlag, 2008), 89–90 discusses the question of disabled children as oblates in the light of recent historiography, and concludes that oblation occurred despite of, not because of, disability.

109 See Angela Montford, *Health, Sickness, Medicine and the Friars in the Thirteenth and Fourteenth Centuries* (Aldershot: Ashgate, 2004).

110 *The Register of Eudes of Rouen*, trans. S. M. Brown and ed. J. F. O'Sullivan (New York and London, 1964), 395.

111 [*Formicarius*], Liber III, cap. I, Johannes Nideri, *Visionibus as Revelationibus...* (Helmestadii: Pauli Zeisingii, 1692), 291–2.

112 Edition in *Middle English Metrical Romances*, Walter Hoyt French and Charles Brockway Hale (eds) (1930, reprt New York: Russell and Russell, 1964), vol. II, 933–46.

113 Martin W. Walsh, 'The King His Own Fool: *Robert of Cicyle*', in Clifford Davidson (ed.), *Fools and Folly* (Kalamazoo, MI: Medieval Institute Publications, 1996), 34–46, at 34.

114 Walsh, 'The King His Own Fool', 37.

115 Zijderveld, *Reality in a Looking Glass*, 75 for more on this poem, written in emulation of a rhymed charter for a non-existant guild.

116 Matejovski, *Motiv des Wahnsinns*, 30.

117 Beek, *Waanzin in de Middeleeuwen*, 28.

118 Michel Foucault, *History of Madness*, ed. Jean Khalfa, trans. Jonathan Murphy and Jean Khalfa (London and New York: Routledge, 2006), 14.

119 Groß, *'La Folie'*, 107.

120 V. A. Kolve, 'God-Denying Fools and the Medieval "Religion of Love"', in Lisa J. Kiser (ed.), *Studies in the Age of Chaucer* 19 (Columbus, OH: The New Chaucer Society, The Ohio State University, 1997), 3–59, at 13–14.

121 See Günther Haseloff, *Die Psalterillustration im 13. Jahrhundert. Studien zur Geschichte der Buchmalerei in England, Frankreich und den Niederlanden* (Kiel: n.p., 1938), which remains the main study.

122 Miracles of Thomas Becket, ed. J. C. Robertson, *Materials for the History of Thomas Becket*, Rolls Series 67 (London: Longman, 1875), vol. I, 207–8, Book II miracle 47 *De cadente idiota*.

123 Kolve, 'God-Denying Fools', 16, also 16n18 on *sely* in Middle English as 'innocent, blessed or happy'.

124 Kolve, 'God-Denying Fools', 19.

125 Barwig and Schmitz, 'Narren. Geisteskranke und Hofleute', 235.

126 Prime example of a modern study on the fool as atheist – not a word about disability here – is Dorothea Weltecke, *'Der Narr spricht: Es ist kein Gott'. Atheismus, Unglauben und Glaubenszweifel vom 12. Jahrhundert bis zur Neuzeit* (Frankfurt-a-M: Campus, 2010).

127 G. R. Evans, *Philosophy and Theology in the Middle Ages* (London and New York: Routledge, 1993), 52.

128 Bullock-Davies, *Register of Minstrels*, xiii and 9; cf. idem, *Menestrellorum Multitudo*, 26, 55–60; also discussed in Valerie Allen, *On Farting: Language and Laughter in the Middle Ages* (New York and Basingstoke: Palgrave, 2007), 164.

129 Sylvia Huot, *Madness in Medieval French Literature: Identities Found and Lost* (Oxford: Oxford University Press, 2003), 44.

130 Welsford, *The Fool*, xii.

7

RECONSIDERATIONS: RATIONALITY, INTELLIGENCE AND HUMAN STATUS

The medieval worship of reason is still in force. Our highest praise for an argument or a course of action is that it is rational. Our most serious diagnosis of the physical condition of a patient is that he is 'irrational,' a term which evokes sad and sage nods from the listener.[1]

The construction of a link between psychological and social inferiority may be traced back to ancient Greece. Considering medieval writers' frequent reference to 'authorities' such as Plato and Aristotle, antique aspects of ID certainly underpinned and influenced medieval notions. But no medieval philosopher or theologian was exclusively or solely Aristotelian; they all, even Aquinas, mixed in Platonism to a greater or lesser degree, Nemesius being a very good example of this. Goodey regarded the twelfth century as forming the beginnings of European social administration which, together with late-medieval scholasticism, initiated the formal human science disciplines in the modern era, and claimed that a major conceptual change occurred in the high Middle Ages. 'It is only from 1200 onwards that the objective framework becomes fused, and confused, with the subjective ability, in a single procedure.'[2] With the rise of clerical and intellectual culture, reason became ever more important. The dominance of the clerks in all walks of life advanced from the middle of the twelfth century onwards, affecting tighter definitions of orthodoxy and heresy, the development of administrative techniques giving rise to the power of the bureaucrats, in turn multiplying the demand for trained clerks and the influence such men could wield. In the 1140s the intelligentsia emerged from the burgeoning schools of Paris and Bologna (later to become universities), to which students came from all across Europe and which created 'in effect members of an international managerial elite'. The 'dialectical reasoning that was the hallmark of the schools' furthermore left its mark on the legal and governmental developments of the time, so that analytical thinking and logical polarities became part and parcel in the methods of solving everyday problems of jurisprudence and rule.[3] As the author of the English legal collection known as *Glanvill* made categorically clear, a case is either criminal or civil, and more generally a thing is either this or not this, but no longer a fuzzy intermediate. Such wider developments in society affected the perception of people with mental deficiencies, who could now be classed as rational or not rational, having reason or deprived of reason, and were no longer placed in a nebulous, ill-defined but accommodating zone on a spectrum. Logical, abstract definitions demanded that people, as well as theological, juridical or philosophical problems, were categorised as either/or, rational or irrational, clever or stupid.

The differentiation of levels of intelligence was even ascribed to demons. In the later twelfth century William of Newburgh, in *Historia Rerum Anglicarum*, mentioned a holy man named Ketell who classified demons on a scale ranging from the relatively harmless, considered 'small, contemptible, impotent in strength and dull in understanding' (*parvos ac despicabiles, impotentes viribus et sensu hebetes*), to the 'large, robust and crafty' (*daemones magnos, robustos, et callidos*).[4] Note the opposing terms dull of understanding and crafty, and the use of the less-common term *hebes* to denote lack of mental competence.

Thirteenth-century turning point?

The thirteenth century was the turning point; not, *pace* Goodey, because suddenly the neo-Aristotelian scholastics rediscovered and misrepresented Aristotle's phrase about man being a rational animal, but because they started using the tools of rationality to describe, order, categorise, label, interpret, calculate and so forth. The thirteenth century saw the invention of the alphabetically organised encyclopaedia (Bartholomaeus Anglicus' book on the properties of things), the systematising of knowledge in general and the application of logic in particular to describe the world. It thus is familiarly modern – we can feel comfortable in liking the thirteenth century, unlike the catastrophic fourteenth that was to follow – because we can see our intellectual ancestry reflected in it. Whereas earlier medieval centuries had produced messy, unordered, even, that worst of insults to modern ears, 'unscientific' texts about the world and humanity's place in it, the thirteenth century saw the outpouring of ordered, standardised, measured and, that highest praise of all, rational scientific texts. That is where the problem lies for the perception of ID. Under the older, more random, more fluid descriptions, each case of 'idiocy' was individually described and, if in a legal context, judged on its own merits against a fairly diverse and mobile set of criteria. That is frustrating for historians, because it does not give us a neat, consistent definition to get our teeth into, but it was probably good for people with IDs. In the absence of definite criteria and diagnostic standards, fewer people were pathologised and more people were just 'getting on with it' in whatever daily life they may have led. Only people with severe mental disabilities, as it is called today, would have been pathologised (the wonders of Gervase of Tilbury or Konrad of Megenberg, perhaps), and those with moderate disabilities may perhaps have been noticed (by lawyers, philosophers or anatomists), while people with mild IDs most likely escaped comment in the written sources completely.

With the thirteenth century and the advent of logic, science and rationality in the modern sense, suddenly the authorities – implying intellectual authorities – started taking a greater interest in trying to define the, until then, rather woolly concepts of fools and idiots, for the simple reason that everything, from the heavenly spheres and the hierarchies of angels down to ants and blades of grass, was being subjected to logical categorisation. Umberto Eco famously wrote that only a medieval scholastic could truly appreciate a card index system – or, to update the metaphor, a database. It was in the fourteenth century, the scholastic learning having become embedded among the cultural baggage, that we can encounter a figure like Konrad of Megenberg, who applied the 'scientific techniques' of his day to the description of the assumed physical traits of congenital idiots (e.g. small and/or pointy heads). Until then, idiots had been noted according to their idiosyncratic characters and behaviour, not their physical appearance. New logic brings new scientific approaches. Physiognomy, despite having been around since at least Aristotle's time, only fully rears its ugly head in the fifteenth century, gaining popularity in the sixteenth, and by the seventeenth century Thomas Willis emerges with his description of mental deficiency according to what would become psychiatric criteria.[5]

The speed of intelligence

Supposedly our society is speeding up. Speed emerged as a cultural issue during industrial modernity, through the rise of capitalist society and the shift to urban settings, defined by the belief in 'progress'; hence the medieval world will have been one of bucolic calm, according to this theory. Cultural acceleration has effects not just on the 'immediacy' of the twenty-first century but on our cultural and moral values. Now, confronted with the phenomenon of social acceleration, we tend to believe that faster is better. Here one may consider the effects of societal celerity on cognition, on thinking and on definitions of intelligence. The stereotype of ID, and its subgroup, learning disability (or learning difficulty, depending on regional preference), dictates a picture of slow, ponderous unintelligence and, in contrast to the dull minds (who in Latin were termed *hebetes*) of the learning disabled, those quick on the uptake are bright, fast learners. William of Conches had already referred to slow thinkers as less intelligent. Speed, sharpness and light are culturally contrasted with being slow, blunt and dull. What about the disparity between the accelerators and those who cannot keep up the speed? Virilio noted that the speed at which something happens may change its essential nature, and that which moves with speed quickly comes to dominate that which is slower.[6] Accordingly, by analogy, those who think faster or have quicker wits are deemed more 'intelligent' than those who think more slowly and take longer to express their thoughts. Society, and with it the expectation of cognitive ability, has accelerated to the detriment of those perceived to be slower. The opposition of slow with fast mental states was an idea based on Empedocles, which Goodey noted in his discussion of the special value placed on the speed of thought processes and how the opposite, slowness of intellectual processes, came to be defined as ID.[7]

Augustine had argued for a comparison between children and so-called *moriones*, a late antique term perhaps best equated with the medieval 'fool', relating the anecdote of a father who on the one hand may be amused by such silliness, while on the other hand he dreads the prospect of his own son turning out to be such a 'fool'. As many of the sources demonstrated, one of the main consequences for people with IDs was that they retained a permanent child-like status, which can have been of benefit (being judged according to mitigating circumstances, or not being held responsible for criminal actions) but also denied them autonomy, leaving them permanently under the authority of others. The legal material, for example, does not make sense unless one accepts, as a modern researcher, that in the Middle Ages there existed a category of people (momentarily disregarding their modern equivalent or nonequivalent) whose mental state was not one of insanity by medieval definition but who were nevertheless deemed not culpable for crimes or not legally competent, on the grounds of cognitive capabilities. Of course, such people cannot be equated exactly with the legal status of people with ID today, but the medieval justification for their lack of legal status implies a deeply rooted concern with cognitive and intellectual faculties. Perhaps of most interest to those commentators who want to make a case for the non-inevitability of ID is the fact that even the *idiotae* could sometimes be reassigned legal capabilities. According to medieval concepts, people can drift in and out of ID, which was not regarded as immutable or fixed as it is today.

Two medieval figures crop up frequently in the historiography of ID: Thomas Aquinas and Konrad of Megenberg. But both are overrated. Aquinas was not as influential in the thirteenth century, or even in the fourteenth, as he became later. During his lifetime his writings were far less accepted, and the neo-Thomism of the nineteenth century onwards really rather skews the picture of what medieval theologians and/or philosophers had to say on ID.[8] The capacity for logical reasoning and abstraction has been singled out as the key elements in a classificatory scheme. Concerning the idea, derived from Aquinas, that the faculty of abstraction is the main criterion that divides the intelligent from the stupid, one must conclude, on the basis of alternative medieval texts, that abstraction, like Aquinas, is overrated. While it is true that with the emergence of scholasticism and the rise of the medieval university greater emphasis than before was placed on literacy, book-learning and the kinds of skills associated with urban living, it would be far too simplistic to date all these events as suddenly springing up out of nowhere around the year 1200. Literacy and book-learning were already praised by commentators during the Carolingian – never mind the twelfth-century – renaissance. If anything, the speed of certain developments increased, but the foundations were in place long before the magic year 1200. As a reading of texts as diverse as Nemesius, Isidore of Seville and even Old Irish legal texts makes apparent, these norma-tive texts contained notions of age-appropriate mental abilities, even if the word they used did not translate as 'rationality'. What the medieval authors describe as *ratio* cannot be equated to rational thinking in the modern sense, but the scholastics used it very specifically as a technical term to describe oper-ations in logic (*ratiocinare*). This is not the same as when a modern psychiatrist asserts that a person lacks rational intelligence. The scholastics of course could perfectly well observe that just because a peasant had not learned how to *ratiocinare*, the peasant was not inherently stupid, but simply had not had the chance to learn it, even if peasants *en masse* might be considered stupid. The tests which medieval administrators asked idiots to perform, such as knowing the day of the week, or naming family members, had nothing to do with the modern idea of abstract thinking. These are practical, everyday matters, not abstractions.

The focus on Konrad of Megenberg is understandable, since, as there is comparatively little on medieval people with ID, modern writers will cherish anything juicy, like his few lines, that they can get their hands on. But Konrad is overrated because too many writers cite him outside of the context of his own times and the influence he had. Since he was writing in the mid-fourteenth century, what he says about ID is valid only from the mid-fourteenth century onwards, not for the earlier medieval period – a mistake which it seems a number of modern scholars make when talking about *the* Middle Ages undifferentiatedly, as if it was a singular and not a plural of eras.

Without denying the validity of sociological models like in-/out-groups, one does need to question the binary oppositions of medieval intellectual (scholastic at one of the emerging universities) versus rustic, stupid peasant. Peasants were admittedly considered lowly, albeit harmless, but, as the third estate (those who work), rather important in a grudging sort of way. Also, they are too irrelevant to be the out-group, or the other, or the 'enemy'. Their apparent stupidity can be used as a literary trope, much like Homer's 'wine-dark sea', to illustrate the point a writer is making, when what the writer really targets is a completely different socio-economic group, namely the nobility, the rulers, the secular movers and shakers. If there are any in the thirteenth century whom a scholastic has to prove himself against, they are the powerful of the world, not the stupid but insignificant peasant. The scholastic as a figure is still too recent to have a firm place, the university still too new to be safe and secure as an institution. Medieval intellectuals were at pains to prove their worth, their importance, to the purse-string holders, clerks were trying to convince secular courts of the value of employing the new university graduates. So it is not the stupid peasant who is the out-group, it is the new clerical intelligentsia who are trying to find a foothold, and in so doing perhaps use the trope of the stupid underclass as a means of emphasising the importance of intellectual abilities, and hence their own worth as intellectuals.

It is sometimes argued that while medieval peasants needed certain skills that one might call intellectual – effective farming requires knowledge of agricultural techniques, even if just empirically – there were still plenty of low-level serfs and servants and, later, landless labourers, who did not need those skills. A landless labourer did not have to maintain a plough (a fairly complex piece of equipment) but simply had to use muscle-power and act on the commands of others. But one should not forget that medieval underclasses were rarely as homogenous or static as sociological textbooks assume. Most medieval workers, whether rural or urban, travelling or settled, landholding or landless, were invariably multi-tasking if not multi-skilled, e.g. work was often tied to specific times of year, people are potters in winter and farmers in spring/summer. Multi-tasking is also valid for servants, with the notion of the specialised low-level servant found only in the super-rich noble households who could afford 'parasites', i.e. the very court fools and jesters described in the previous chapter, or, from the early nineteenth century onwards, with the greater (physical and spatial) separation of master and servant. And we must not forget that all we know of medieval peasants, or even landless labourers, was written by people who were economically and socially superior to them. The stereotyping of one group of people by another is so ubiquitous in history as to be almost meaningless for historical inquiry: as a historian one has to separate the semantic wheat from the chaff. Just because medieval texts, mainly fiction (i.e. courtly romances), mention dirty, snivelling, 'stupid' peasants does not mean that in actuality peasants were viewed as inherently more 'stupid' outside the realm of derogatory remarks. Instead, stories such as those in Piers Plowman paint a picture of the deviousness and duplicity (which implies intelligence!) of the landless, the impoverished and beggars. One may regard the stereotypes of late medieval 'fraudulent' beggars, who seem to be primarily recruited from the group of landless poor, and find that, far from being portrayed as 'stupid', such folk are described as cunningly defrauding, well-meant alms-givers.

A conundrum of miracles and idiocy

The problem of how modern authors have dealt with historic notions of idiocy can be compared with the problems also encountered when looking at historic concepts of Otherness more generally. For instance, a prime difficulty is

> the tendency to treat *alien* or *Other* as if they were stable terms denoting complete and consistent rejection when in fact there were degrees of marginality, so much so, that seemingly contradictory positions could be held simultaneously. Peasants might be regarded as descendants of Ham, as unclean and boorish, and yet as close to God by reason of their oppression and humility.[9]

If close to God, why are there no miracle healings of people with ID? What is special about ID that makes it different from the crippled limbs or blind eyes that saints are always healing? It is not just that Christ did not heal ID, since Christ did not heal toothache either, but saints do. So it must be something concerned with a special status for ID, something that makes it contrary to miracle. Could it be that the very presence of ID in and of itself is already miraculous? Congenital idiocy might be categorised as miracle, because genuine idiocy is so different from normal humanity that it is a miraculous event. This is based on Konrad of Megenberg's discussion of 'prodigies', with his distinction between *wunder menschen* and *wunderleichen laüten*, which, as we saw, followed the wider distinction between *miraculi* and *mirabilia* based on Thomas of Cantimpré. Wondrous things were distinguished according to their causality, so that *mirabilia* are still subject to the divine order and are wondrous only because they are preternatural, while *miracula* are caused through the complete revocation of natural laws by direct divine interference. Therefore it might actually have been regarded as 'wrong' to heal the idiots of their idiocy. Clarke noted that, as of the mid-twentieth century, when he was conducting his research, the Hutterites among modern Christian sects 'take all psychiatric conditions – except the totally intractable such as mental defect and fully established psychotic states and epilepsy – as due to sin, in which all men are held to be born'.[10] This could be an interesting analogy for the medieval period: if mental defect is *not* due to sin, then, unlike mental illness and physical illness/disability, which presumably then *is* regarded as due to sin, mental defect as something sinless is not in need of a cure, hence the complete absence of miracle cures from the gospels and on through medieval times.

There just might be one miracle story that describes the healing of someone we could identify as intellectually disabled, by St John of Beverley, who was bishop of Hexham, then York, and was buried at Hexham in 721. A number of hagiographic works on St John exist, with the following excerpts from the *Miracula Sancti Johannis*, chapter 5 ('About Giles, infirm and disfigured, who was made handsome and healthy through the virtue of the saint') by William Ketell, a clerk of Beverley, of around 1100.[11] Giles came to the shrine for a cure (*recuperandæ salutis gratia*, literally: recovery of health), where 'he suffered the laughter of a great many people, an object of spectacle for everybody (*pluribus risui, uniuersis ostentatui habebatur*)'. This is standard hagiographical language, except that the laughter and ridicule are a rare detail, since most miracle accounts mention pity, not laughter. He was described as a young man of monstrous body and stupid mind (*Iuvenis corpore monstrosus & mente fatuus*). 'Moreover, inside he was just like the outside declared: lacking in all practical understanding; not a boy, yet tending towards childlike games in everything (*Erat autem in interiore homine, ut exterior enuntiabat, totius expers prudentiæ; puerilibus vero, non puer per omnia, intendens lusibus*).' This is the crucial element of the description. The Latin refers to literally lack of prudence, which is similar to the fuller descriptions one can find later in thirteenth-century legal texts on 'idiocy'. Giles was thus 'regarded by everyone as a man who was mad in the head, yet harmful to no one but himself (*ita ut insensati capitis homo ab hominibus æstimaretur, nulli tamen nisi sibi nocuus*)'. Now narrative tropes start getting mixed up in the text. The concept of being harmless except to himself has by the thirteenth and fourteenth centuries become the standard legal definition of the *idiotae*, according to Turner, although it does not necessarily equate to modern ID, which both Turner and I are at pains to point out. One must also remember that Ketell was writing two centuries earlier, i.e. around 1100. But Giles is also described as *insensati capitis*, literally senseless of the head, translated by Wilson as mad in the head, which is wording more commonly used for the insane, who are recognised as such in medieval texts. The fact that William Ketell felt obliged to qualify his phrase *insensati capitis* with a description that despite being 'mad' Giles was harming only himself indicates that Ketell was struggling with his reference points, and trying to accommodate a known, tried and tested medieval description of madness with something that might actually not be madness.

> Indeed the disfigured body bore limbs which were suitable to it: a huge and loathsome head, a skinny neck, thighs, legs and feet just like a boy's, monstrously contorted, and completely useless, namely, the wretched and useless burden of the body, which from childhood had never been of any use but had always been a handicap [literally *oneri*: burden, onerous]
>
> (Informe vero corpus sibi condecentia gestabat membra, caput turpe & magnum, collum gracile, femora, crura, pedes velut pueri prodigiose retorta, officioque suo penitus carentia; infelicem videlicet & infructuosam corporis sarcinam, quæ numquam usui, semper oneri a primævo tempore sibi extiterat).

Here the text falls into the standard miracle narrative wording of the terrible 'before' situation for the protagonist, so that the 'after' is all the more miraculous, concentrating purely on the visible, that is, physical aspects. Giles spent the night in the church, and during the nocturnal celebrations of the clergy his miraculous healing occurred, with all the typical hallmarks of miracle, namely lots of bones creaking, loud noises, contortions, which conform with the standard narrative patterns. Giles, 'unable to bear so much distress, rolled about here and there as though insane (*tantæ vexationis impatiens, hinc & inde velut amens volutaretur*)'. Note the phrase 'as though insane': the author was aware that Giles was not insane but his behaviour in the throes of miracle (ecstatic?) resembled that of one insane. Similar phrases were also used in miracle accounts where the protagonist never had any mental affliction whatsoever. 'And so, in the space of a short time, he acquired good health in both body and mind (*sicque spatio brevi temporis evoluto, corporis animique congrua potitus est valitudine*).' This is such a bland, commonplace description as to be almost meaningless, since similar is used for hundreds of miracles of all sorts of physical and mental afflictions between the eleventh and the fourteenth centuries, therefore one should not make too much of the healing of his mind. The miracle attracted many people who were impressed by the transition of Giles, 'whom they had frequently seen crippled and out of his mind (*quem sæpius viderant debilem & insensatum*)'.[12] Note that *insensatum* literally means senseless, so can veer towards witless rather than mad, but on Turner's spectrum of medieval mental afflictions would sit somewhere in the middle.

In summary, this (emphatically only *possibly*) might constitute the one and only miracle healing of a man who may perhaps have had some form of ID. However, William Ketell is at pains to squeeze this miracle into an established textual tradition of miracle narrative, which means that certain elements are included that add little to the modern understanding of whatever underlying affliction may have been present (such as the creaking limbs or the ecstatic, temporary insanity). As part of the tradition of miracle writing, the language used employs phrases that are commonly used for miracle healings of both the physically afflicted (the ubiquitous crippled, blind, deaf, dumb) and the genuinely insane (as opposed to what we would now call the intellectually disabled). Furthermore, Ketell's narrative has an inner transition within the text: the description commences quite specific and unique, but then descends more and more into hagiographical platitudes – which is something often encountered in miracle stories. By the end of this episode, Ketell has subsumed the individual story into a more general type of miracle, one where the protagonist has a number of both physical problems and mental ones, which in medieval terms are treated as 'insanity'. It is almost as if Ketell struggled to fit something more unusual into the established textual frame of reference.

Fluidity of medieval norms and labels

With regard to fixed identity or labelling of a person, it seems that medieval ways of treating ID were much more fluid than modern ones. In modern society, once someone is diagnosed with a condition, be it Down syndrome, autism, dyslexia, that is a label that sticks, in all life situations. The Middle Ages appear to have been different. The same person may in some life situations have been considered an idiot, in others a normal person. Similar notions are admitted by the psychiatric or pedagogical profession today when it is stated that people with mild to moderate ID can 'function' in a number of situations – so they can pass as normal. Unless someone had extreme and instantly noticeable physical features (such as extreme microcephaly), a medieval person with ID would probably have passed as normal most of the time, they would not have had a label that they carried with them at all times. But the modern system of diagnosing, labelling and then performing remedial actions (special education) means that a person is first and foremost 'Johnny with Down syndrome', no longer 'Johnny next door/the cobbler's son'.

This idea is backed up by Kellenberger, who has an interesting general observation concerning the ancient texts he studied, namely that in marked contrast to our modern society ID is rarely remarked upon, which demonstrates a different kind of conceptual awareness of disability.

> Today intellectual or learning disability is considered a special form of existence which calls for particular ways of treating such people. The dividing line is therefore drawn between those people considered to represent the normative and the disabled who are never adequate for the normative. In contrast, the Bible and many pre-modern cultures draw the dividing line much more 'realistically': between those moments when someone is considered adequate according to

the social norm and those when they are not. Thus it becomes apparent that no individual person can fulfil the normative requirement permanently at all times.[13]

No antique (Roman, Greek, ancient Near Eastern) or medieval European culture existed where some form of labelling for 'idiocy', to use this term as shorthand, was *not* present. There is also ample evidence from ethnology that even so-called 'primitive' traditional cultures have plenty of labels for identifying people whom modern Western culture would call intellectually disabled. The argument that less technologically advanced societies, or cultures where the majority of people did not have formal education in the modern sense, would have been cultures that simply did not notice ID is quite obviously wrong. To put it very colloquially, it seems that across many if not all cultures, everyone knows an 'idiot' when they see one but they cannot pinpoint what it is that makes someone an idiot or why. This might constitute the crucial difference between pre-modern 'idiocy' and the modern concept of ID: the older cultures had a plethora of labels, words, terms that all meant some form of negatively perceived intellectual difference, but (until the seventeenth century) there was no attempt at definition in the precise, biomedical, psychiatric kind of way that modern science does. Trying to be politically correct would be counter-productive, since one would have to brush these historical facts under the carpet and pretend there were no 'idiots' in pre-modern societies. Nor can one pretend that medieval (or other pre-modern cultures) just simply did not recognise intellectual differences. The question of how people regarded as intellectually deficient were treated socially by their respective cultures is of course the big question that interests historians most, but that does not detract from the fact that the labels (in all their, by modern 'scientific' standards, confusing, multifarious and rather woolly terminologies) existed in the first place.

Therefore ID has an ontologically ambiguous status. On the one hand, ID exists as a real state or condition (no one would deny that Down syndrome exists in actuality, regardless of whether one subscribes to the labelling or not), but, on the other hand, ID is defined by a fluctuating set of psychiatric and psychological discourses. As Foucault aptly wrote: 'A term like "imbecility" only operates in a system of approximate equivalences which excludes any precise value.'[14]

In conclusion, I offer some provocative ruminations about the much-discussed custom of keeping fools as entertainment. The exact causes and correlations will need to be worked out by future research, but surely it is no coincidence that at the same time, and in the same geographic regions, that the keeping of court fools started to become popular and commonplace, the 'keeping' of professional intellectuals, that is, humanist men of letters, also became a courtly trend. It was in the Italy of the Trecento that men like Petrarca and Boccaccio were not only able to earn a living through the patronage of noble courts, but also had their intellectual outpourings, their letters, literature and classicising commentary valued in and of itself. But it was also during the Trecento that court fools emerged more frequently in the various sources, not just in Italy, but in France too. Both the very clever and the very foolish were cultivated by the courts. The apparent gulf between the diametrical opposites of idiot and intellectual may be just an illusion, since what unites these disparate points on the cognitive spectrum is their shared dependent status, what Tuan has so aptly described as the status of pets, at the whim of wealthy potentates. Arguably it was – and still is – economic power, not brain power, that *really* mattered.

Notes

1   Judith S. Neaman, *Suggestion of the Devil: Insanity in the Middle Ages and the Twentieth Century* (New York: Octagon Books, 1978), 178.

2   Christopher Goodey, *A History of Intelligence and 'Intellectual Disability': The Shaping of Psychology in Early Modern Europe* (Farnham: Ashgate, 2011), 281.

3   R. I. Moore, *The War on Heresy: Faith and Power in Medieval Europe* (London: Profile Books, 2012), 226, 227.

4   William of Newburgh, *Historia Rerum Anglicarum, Chronicles of the Reigns of Stephen, Henry II and Richard I*, ed. R. Howlett, Rolls Series 82 (London, 1884–85), at vol. 82 part 1, 153; C. S. Watkins, *History and the Supernatural in Medieval England* (Cambridge: Cambridge University Press, 2007), 55.

5   Discussed briefly above in Chapter 3.

6   Paul Virilio, *Speed and Politics: An Essay on Dromology* (New York: Semiotext(e), 1977 [1986]).

7   C. F. Goodey, 'Mental Retardation', in G. Gerrios and R. Porter (eds), *A History of Clinical Psychiatry: The Origins and History of Psychiatric Disorders* (London: Athlone, 1995), 239–50; Goodey, *History of Intelligence*, 39–47.

8   Bernard McGinn, *Thomas Aquinas's 'Summa theologiae': A Biography* (Princeton, NJ: Princeton University Press, 2014), 119–36.

9   Paul Freedman, 'The Medieval Other: The Middle Ages as Other', in Timothy Jones and David Sprunger (eds), *Marvels, Monsters, and Miracles: Studies in the Medieval and Early Modern Imaginations* (Kalamazoo: Western Michigan University, 2002), 1–24, at 10.

10 Basil Clarke, *Mental Disorder in Earlier Britain: Exploratory Studies* (Cardiff: University of Wales Press, 1975), 121. Clarke based this on J. W. Eaton and R. J. Weil, *Culture and Mental Disorders: A Comparative Study of the Hutterites and Other Populations* (Glencoe, IL: Free Press, 1955).

11   I am most grateful to Anne Bailey for drawing my attention to this narrative.
12   *The Life and After-Life of St John of Beverley*, ed. and trans. Susan E. Wilson
     (Aldershot: Ashgate, 2006), 165–6; Latin in William Ketell, *Miracula sancti
     Johannis, Acta Sanctorum* Mai II, dies 7, 174C–180D.
13   'Heute gilt geistige Behinderung als eine besondere Existenzform, die nach einem
     speziellen Umgang mit solchen Menschen ruft. Die Grenze verläuft demnach
     zwischen denjenigen, die selbstverständlich der Norm entsprechen, und den
     Behinderten, welche dieser Norm nie genügen können. Die Bibel hingegen und
     weitere vormoderne Kulturen ziehen die Grenzlinie "realistischer": zwischen den
     Momenten, in denen jemand einer gesellschaftlichen Norm genügt, und jenen, in
     denen ihr jemand nicht genügt. So wird deutlich, dass kein Mensch eine bestim-
     mte Norm stets erfüllen kann.' Edgar Kellenberger, *Der Schutz der Einfältigen.
     Menschen mit einer geistigen Behinderung in der Bibel und in weiteren Quellen*
     (Zurich: Theologischer Verlag Zürich, 2011), 153.
14   Michel Foucault, *History of Madness*, ed. Jean Khalfa, trans. Jonathan Murphy and
     Jean Khalfa (London and New York: Routledge, 2006), 127.

Select bibliography

Abrams, Judith Z., *Judaism and Disability: Portrayals in Ancient Texts from the Tanach through the Bavli* (Washington, DC: Gallaudet University Press, 1998).

Albertus-Magnus-Institut (ed.), *Albertus Magnus und sein System der Wissenschaften. Schlüsseltexte in Übersetzung Lateinisch-Deutsch* (Münster: Aschendorff, 2011).

Andrews, Jonathan, 'Identifying and Providing for the Mentally Disabled in Early Modern London', in David Wright and Anne Digby (eds), *From Idiocy to Mental Deficiency: Historical Perspectives on People with Learning Disabilities* (London: Routledge, 1996).

Andrews, Jonathan, 'Begging the Question of Idiocy: The Definition and Socio-cultural Meaning of Idiocy in Early Modern Britain: Part I', *History of Psychiatry*, 9 (1998), 65–95.

Andrews, Jonathan, Asa Briggs, Roy Porter, Penny Tucker and Keir Waddington, *The History of Bethlem* (London and New York: Routledge, 1997).

[Aristotle] Jonathan Barnes (ed.), *The Complete Works of Aristotle: The Revised Oxford Translation* (Princeton: Princeton University Press, 1984).

Banks, S. E. and J. W. Binns (eds), *Gervase of Tilbury: Otia imperialia. Recreation for an Emperor* (Oxford: Clarendon Press, 2002).

[Bartholomæus Anglicus] *On the Properties of Things: John Trevisa's Translation of Bartholomæus Anglicus De proprietatibus Rerum. A Critical Text*, Vol. I, eds M. C. Seymour and Colleagues (Oxford: Clarendon Press, 1975).

Bartholomaeus Anglicus, *On the Properties of Soul and Body. De proprietatibus rerum libri III et IV*, ed. R. James Long (Toronto: PIMS, 1979) .

Barwig, Edgar and Ralf Schmitz, 'Narren. Geisteskranke und Hofleute', in Bernd-Ulrich Hergemöller (ed.), *Randgruppen in der spätmittelalterlichen Gesellschaft* (Warendorf: Fahlbusch, 2nd edn, 1994), 220–52.

Beek, H. H., *Waanzin in de Middeleeuwen: Beeld van de Gestoorde en Bemoeienis met de Zieke* (Haarlem: De Toorts/ Nijkerk: G. F. Callenbach, 1969).

Berkson, Gershon, 'Intellectual and Physical Disabilities in Prehistory and Early Civilization', *Mental Retardation*, 42 (2004), 195–208.

Berkson, Gershon, 'Mental Disabilities in Western Civilization from Ancient Rome to the Prerogativa Regis', *Mental Retardation*, 44:1 (2006), 28–40.

Bertram, Hans, 'Die Entwicklung der Psychiatrie im Altertum und Mittelalter', *Janus*, 44 (1940), 81–122.

Billington, Sandra, *A Social History of the Fool* (Brighton: Harvester Press/New York: St Martin's, 1984).

Blund, Iohannes, *Tractatus de anima*, ed. D. A. Callus and R. W. Hunt (London: British Academy/Oxford University Press, 1970).

Bonser, Wilfred, *The Medical Background of Anglo-Saxon England* (London: Wellcome Historical Medical Library, 1963).

Borden, Arthur R., *A Comprehensive Old-English Dictionary* (Washington, DC: University Press of America, 1982).

[Bracton] Henry de Bracton, *De Legibus et Consuetudinibus Angliae*, ed. George E. Woodbine, trans. Samuel E. Thorne, 4 vols (Cambridge, MA: Harvard University Press, Belknap Press/London: Selden Society, 1968–77).

Britton, ed. and trans. Francis Morgan Nichols, 2 vols (Oxford: Clarendon Press, 1865).

Brockliss, Laurence and Heather Montgomery (eds), *Childhood and Violence in the Western Tradition* (Oxford and Oakville: Oxbow, 2010).

Brooks, R., 'Official Madness: A Cross-cultural Study of Involuntary and Civil Confinement Based on "Mental Illness"', in Jane Hubert (ed.), *Madness, Disability and Social Exclusion: The Archaeology and Anthropology of 'Difference'* (London and New York: Routledge, 2000), 9–28.

Buck, Carl Darling, *A Dictionary of Selected Synonyms in the Principal Indo-European Languages* (Chicago: University of Chicago Press, 1949).

Bullock-Davies, Constance, *A Register of Royal and Baronial Domestic Minstrels, 1272–1327* (Woodbridge: Boydell, 1986).

Burack, Jacob A., Robert M. Hodapp, Grace Iarocci and Edward Zigler (eds), *The Oxford Handbook of Intellectual Disability and Development* (New York: Oxford University Press, 2012).

Bynum, W. F. and Roy Porter (eds), *Companion Encyclopedia of the History of Medicine*, 2 vols (London and New York: Routledge, 1993).

Clarke, A. D. B. and A. M. Clarke (eds), *Mental Deficiency: The Changing Outlook* (London: Methuen, 1st edn, 1958).

Clarke, Basil, *Mental Disorder in Earlier Britain: Exploratory Studies* (Cardiff: University of Wales Press, 1975).

Cockayne, T. O., *Leechdoms, Wortcunning and Starcraft of Early England,* Rolls Series 35 (London, 1864–66).

Conrad, Lawrence I., Michael Neve, Vivian Nutton, Roy Porter and Andrew Wear, *The Western Medical Tradition 800 BC to AD 1800* (Cambridge: Cambridge University Press, 1995).

Corèdon, C. and A. Williams, *A Dictionary of Medieval Terms and Phrases* (Cambridge: D. S. Brewer, 2004).

Corner, George, *Anatomical Texts of the Earlier Middle Ages: A Study in the Transmission of Culture* (Washington, DC: Carnegie Institution of Washington, 1927).

Daston, Lorraine and Katharine Park, *Wonders and the Order of Nature, 1150–1750* (New York: Zone Books, 1998).

Davidson, Herbert A., *Alfarabi, Avicenna, and Averroes, on Intellect: Their Cosmologies, Theories of the Active Intellect, and Theories of Human Intellect* (New York and Oxford: Oxford University Press, 1992).

Dentan, R. K., 'The Response to Intellectual Impairment among the Semai', *American Journal of Mental Deficiency*, 71 (1967), 764–6.

The Didascalion of Hugh of St Victor, trans. and intro. Jerome Taylor (New York: Columbia University Press, 1991).

Digby, Anne, 'Contexts and Perspectives', in David Wright and Anne Digby (eds), *From Idiocy to Mental Deficiency: Historical Perspectives on People with Learning Disabilities* (London: Routledge, 1996).

Dols, Michael W. (ed. Diana E. Immisch), *Majnûn: The Madman in Medieval Islamic Society* (Oxford: Clarendon Press, 1992).

Dominguez, Emilio J., 'The Hospital of Innocents: Humane Treatment of the Mentally Ill in Spain, 1409–1512', *Bulletin of the Menninger Clinic*, 31, (1967), 285–97 .

Edgerton, R. B., 'Anthropology and Mental Retardation: A Plea for the Comparative Study of Incompetence', in H. Prehm, L. Mamerlynck and J. E. Crosson (eds), *Behavior Research in Mental Retardation* (Eugene: University of Oregon Press, 1968), 75–87.

Evans, G. R., *Philosophy and Theology in the Middle Ages* (London and New York: Routledge, 1993).

Evans, G. R., *Getting It Wrong: The Medieval Epistemology of Error* (Leiden: Brill, 1998).

Fandrey, Walter, *Krüppel, Idioten, Irre. Zur Sozialgeschichte behinderter Menschen in Deutschland* (Stuttgart: Silberburg-Verlag, 1990).

Fidler, Deborah J., 'Child Eliciting Effects in Families of Children with Intellectual Disability: Proximal and Distal Perspectives', in J. A. Burack et al. (eds), *Oxford Handbook of Intellectual Disability*, 366–79.

Fleta, ed. and trans. Henry G. Richardson and George O. Sayles, 3 vols, Selden Society Publications 72, 89, 99 (London, 1955, 1972, 1984).

Foucault, Michel, *History of Madness*, ed. Jean Khalfa, trans. Jonathan Murphy and Jean Khalfa (London and New York: Routledge, 2006).

Ginzberg, E., 'The Mentally Handicapped in a Technological Society', in S. Osler and R. Cooke (eds), *The Biosocial Bases of Mental Retardation* (Baltimore, MD: Johns Hopkins University Press, 1965).

Glare, P. G. W. (ed.), *Oxford Latin Dictionary* (Oxford: Clarendon Press, 1992).

Goodey, C. F., ' Mental Disabilities and Human Values in Plato's Late Dialogues', *Archiv für Geschichte der Philosophie*, 74 (1992), 26–42.

Goodey, C. F., 'Mental Retardation', in G. Gerrios and R. Porter (eds), *A History of Clinical Psychiatry: The Origins and History of Psychiatric Disorders* (London: Athlone, 1995), 239–50.

Goodey, C. F., 'The Psychopolitics of Learning and Disability in Seventeenth-century Thought', in David Wright and Anne Digby (eds), *From Idiocy to Mental Deficiency: Historical Perspectives on People with Learning Disabilities* (London: Routledge, 1996), 93–117.

Goodey, C. F., '"Foolishness" in Early Modern Medicine and the Concept of Intellectual Disability', *Medical History*, 48 (2004), 289–310.

Goodey, C. F., 'Blockheads, Roundheads, Pointy Heads: Intellectual Disability and the Brain Before Modern Medicine', *Journal of the History of the Behavioral Sciences* 41:2 (2005), 165–83.

Goodey, C. F., *A History of Intelligence and 'Intellectual Disability': The Shaping of Psychology in Early Modern Europe* (Farnham: Ashgate, 2011).

Groß, Angelika, *'La Folie'. Wahnsinn und Narrheit im spätmittelalterlichen Text und Bild* (Heidelberg: Carl Winter Universitätsverlag, 1990).

Gross, Charles G., 'From Imhotep to Hubel and Wiesel: The Story of Visual Cortex', in Kathleen S. Rockland, Jon H. Kaas and Alan Peters (eds), *Extrastriate Cortex in Primates* (New York: Springer, 1997), 1–58.

Hacking, Ian, *The Social Construction of What?* (Cambridge, MA and London: Harvard University Press, 1999).

Harper, Stephen, *Insanity, Individuals, and Society in Late-Medieval English Literature: The Subject of Madness* (Lewiston, Queenston, Lampeter: Edwin Mellen Press, 2003).

Harvey, E. Ruth, *The Inward Wits: Psychological Theory in the Middle Ages and the Renaissance* (London: Warburg Institute, University of London, 1975).

Herrtage, Sidney J. H. (ed.), *Catholicon Anglicum*, Early English Text Society, os 75 (London, 1881).

Huot, Sylvia, *Madness in Medieval French Literature: Identities Found and Lost* (Oxford: Oxford University Press, 2003).

Ibn Khaldûn, *The Muqaddimah: An Introduction to History*, trans. Franz Rosenthal, abridged and ed. N. J. Dawood (London: Routledge and Kegan Paul, 1967).

[Isidore] *The Etymologies of Isidore of Seville*, trans. and intro. Stephen A. Barney, W. J. Lewis, J. A. Beach and Oliver Berghof (Cambridge: Cambridge University Press, 2010).

Ivanov, Sergey A., *Holy Fools in Byzantium and Beyond*, trans. Simon Franklin, (Oxford: Oxford University Press, 2006).

Jackson, Mark (ed.), *The Oxford Handbook of the History of Medicine* (Oxford: Oxford University Press, 2011).

Jackson, Stanley W., 'Unusual Mental States in Medieval Europe. I. Medical Syndromes of Mental Disorder: 400–1100 A.D.', *Journal of the History of Medicine*, 27 (1972), 262–97.

Kanner, Leo, *A Miniature Textbook of Feeblemindedness* (New York: Child Care Publications, 1949).

Kanner, Leo, *A History of the Care and Study of the Mentally Retarded* (Springfield, IL: Thomas, 1964).

Kellenberger, Edgar, 'Augustin und die Menschen mit einer geistigen Behinderung. Der Theologe als Beobachter und Herausgeforderter', *Theologische Zeitschrift*, 67 (2011), 56–66.

Kellenberger, Edgar, *Der Schutz der Einfältigen. Menschen mit einer geistigen Behinderung in der Bibel und in weiteren Quellen* (Zurich: Theologischer Verlag Zürich, 2011).

Kelly, Fergus, *A Guide to Early Irish Law* (Early Irish Law Series 3) (Dublin: Dublin Institute of Advanced Studies, 1988).

Kemp, Simon, *Medieval Psychology* (New York: Greenwood Press, 1990).

Kenny, Anthony, *Aquinas on Mind* (London and New York: Routledge, 1993).

Kluge. Etymologisches Wörterbuch der deutschen Sprache, ed. E. Seebold (Berlin and Boston: De Gruyter, 25th edn, 2011).

Knuuttila, Simo, *Emotions in Ancient and Medieval Philosophy* (Oxford: Clarendon Press, 2004).

Kolve, V. A., 'God-Denying Fools and the Medieval "Religion of Love"', in Lisa J. Kiser (ed.), *Studies in the Age of Chaucer* 19 (Columbus, OH: The New Chaucer Society, The Ohio State University, 1997), 3–59.

Konrad von Megenberg, *Das Buch der Natur*, ed. Franz Pfeiffer (Stuttgart, 1861).

Krueger, Derek, *Symeon the Holy Fool: Leontius's 'Life' and the Late Antique City* (Berkeley: University of California Press, 1996).

Liddell, Henry George and Robert Scott, *A Greek–English Lexicon*, revised and augmented Sir Henry Stuart Jones with assistance Roderick McKenzie (Oxford: Clarendon Press, 1940).

McDonagh, Patrick, *Idiocy: A Cultural History* (Liverpool: Liverpool University Press, 2008).

McGlynn, Margaret, 'Idiots, Lunatics, and the Royal Prerogative in Early Tudor England', *The Journal of Legal History*, 26:1 (2005), 1–20.

MacLehose, William F., *'A Tender Age': Cultural Anxieties over the Child in the Twelfth and Thirteenth Centuries*, (New York: Columbia University Press, 2008).

Mann, Stuart E., *An Indo-European Comparative Dictionary* (Hamburg: Helmut Buske, 1984).

Matejovski, Dirk, *Das Motiv des Wahnsinns in der mittelalterlichen Dichtung* (Frankfurt-a-M.: Suhrkamp, 1996).

Metzler, Irina, *Disability in Medieval Europe: Thinking about Physical Impairment during the High Middle Ages, c.1100–1400* (New York and London: Routledge, 2006).

Metzler, Irina, *A Social History of Disability in the Middle Ages: Cultural Considerations of Physical Impairment* (New York and London: Routledge, 2013).

Mezger, Werner, *Hofnarren im Mittelalter: Vom tieferen Sinn eines seltsamen Amts* (Konstanz: Universitätsverlag Konstanz, 1981).

Middle English Dictionary, at http://quod.lib.umich.edu/m/med/med_ent_search.html.

The Mirror of Justices, ed. William Joseph Whittaker, intro. F. W. Maitland, Selden Society 7 (London: B. Quaritch, 1895).

Moore, R. I., *The Formation of a Persecuting Society: Power and Deviance in Western Europe 950–1250* (Oxford: Blackwell, 1987).

Moss, Joanna, Patricia Howlin and Chris Oliver, 'The Assessment and Presentation of Autism Spectrum Disorders and Associated Characteristics in Individuals with Severe Intellectual Disability and Genetic Syndromes', in J. A. Burack et al. (eds), *Oxford Handbook of Intellectual Disability*, 275–99.

Neaman, Judith S., *Suggestion of the Devil: Insanity in the Middle Ages and the Twentieth Century* (New York: Octagon Books, 1978).

Nemesius: On the Nature of Man, trans. with intro. and notes R. W. Sharples and P. J. van der Eijk (Liverpool: Liverpool University Press, 2008).

Neubert, Dieter and Günther Cloerkes, *Behinderung und Behinderte in verschiedenen*

Kulturen. Eine vergleichende Analyse ethnologischer Studien (Heidelberg: Edition Schindele, 2nd edn 1994).

Neugebauer, Richard, 'Medieval and Early Modern Theories of Mental Illness', *Archives of General Psychology*, 36 (1979), 477–83.

Niccols, Alison, Karen Thomas and Louis A. Schmidt, 'Socioemotional and Brain Development in Children with Genetic Syndromes Associated with Developmental Delay', in J. A. Burack et al. (eds), *Oxford Handbook of Intellectual Disability*, 254–74.

Olyan, Saul M., *Disability in the Hebrew Bible: Interpreting Mental and Physical Differences* (Cambridge: Cambridge University Press, 2008).

O'Neill, Ynez V., 'William of Conches and the Cerebral Membranes', *Clio Medica*, 2 (1967), 13–21.

O'Neill, Ynez V., 'William of Conches' Description of the Brain', *Clio Medica*, 3 (1968), 203–23.

O'Neill, Ynez V., *Speech and Speech Disorders in Western Thought before 1600* (Westport, CT and London: Greenwood Press, 1980).

Osborne, Catherine, *Dumb Beasts and Dead Philosophers: Humanity and the Humane in Ancient Philosophy and Literature* (Oxford: Clarendon Press, 2007).

Pfau, Aleksandra Nicole, 'Madness in the Realm: Narratives of Mental Illness in Late Medieval France' (PhD diss., University of Michigan, 2008).

Pickett, R. Colin, *Mental Affliction and Church Law: An Historical Synopsis of Roman and Ecclesiastical Law and a Canonical Commentary* (Ottawa, Ontario: The University of Ottawa Press, 1952).

[Polemon] *Seeing the Face, Seeing the Soul: Polemon's Physiognomy from Classical Antiquity to Medieval Islam*, ed. Simon Swain, with contributions by George Boys-Stones ... [et al.] (Oxford: Oxford University Press, 2007).

Price, B. B., 'The Physical Astronomy and Astrology of Albertus Magnus', in *Albertus Magnus and the Sciences*, ed. James Weisheipl (Toronto: PIMS, 1980).

Price, B. B., *Medieval Thought: An Introduction* (Oxford: Blackwell, 1992).

[Quintilian] *The Institutio oratoria of Quintilian*, trans. H. E. Butler (Loeb Classical Library 124) (Cambridge, MA: Harvard University Press/London: Heinemann, 1980).

Reichert, Folker, *Das Bild der Welt im Mittelalter* (Darmstadt: Primus Verlag, 2013).

Reynolds, Philip L., 'The Infants of Eden: Scholastic Theologians on Early Childhood and Cognitive Development', *Mediaeval Studies*, 68 (2006), 89–132.

Richardson, Kristina L., *Difference and Disability in the Medieval Islamic World: Blighted Bodies* (Edinburgh: Edinburgh University Press, 2012).

Robert Kilwardby O.P.: On Time and Imagination: De Tempore. De Spiritu Fantastico, ed. by P. Osmund Lewry O.P. (Oxford: Oxford University Press, 1987).

Robert Kilwardby O.P.: On Time and Imagination. Part 2: Introduction and Translation by Alexander Broadie (Oxford: Oxford University Press, 1993).

Robinson, N. M., 'Mild Mental Retardation: Does It Exist in the People's Republic of China?', *Mental Retardation*, 16 (1978), 295–8.

Rosen, George, *Madness in Society: Chapters in the Historical Sociology of Mental Illness* (Chicago: The University of Chicago Press, 1968).

Saward, John, *Perfect Fools: Folly for Christ's Sake in Catholic and Orthodox Spirituality* (Oxford: Oxford University Press, 1980).

The Saxon Mirror, trans. Maria Debozy (Philadelphia: University of Pennsylvania Press, 1999).

Scheerenberger, Richard C., *A History of Mental Retardation* (Baltimore and London: Brookes, 1983).

Siegel, Rudolph E., *Galen on Psychology, Psychopathology and Function and Diseases of the Nervous System* (Basel: Karger, 1973).

Siegel, Rudolph E., *Galen on the Affected Parts: Translation from the Greek Text with Explanatory Notes* (Basel et al.: S. Karger, 1976).

Sorabji, Richard, *Emotion and Peace of Mind: From Stoic Agitation to Christian Temptation* (Oxford: Oxford University Press, 2000).

Southworth, John, *Fools and Jesters at the English Court* (Stroud: Sutton, 1998).

Sprunger, David, 'Depicting the Insane: A Thirteenth-Century Case Study', in Timothy Jones and David Sprunger (eds), *Marvels, Monsters, and Miracles: Studies in the Medieval and Early Modern Imaginations* (Kalamazoo: Western Michigan University, 2002), 223–41.

Stainton, Timothy, 'Medieval Charitable Institutions and Intellectual Impairment c.1066–1600', *Journal on Developmental Disabilities/Le journal sur les handicaps du développement*, 8:2 (2001), 19–29.

Stainton, Timothy, 'Reason and Value: The Thought of Plato and Aristotle and the Construction of Intellectual Disability', *Mental Retardation*, 39 (2001), 452–60.

Stainton, Timothy, 'Reason, Grace and Charity: Augustine and the Impact of Church Doctrine on the Construction of Intellectual Disability', *Disability & Society*, 23:5 (2008), 485–96.

Stainton, Timothy and Patrick McDonagh, 'Chasing Shadows: The Historical Construction of Developmental Disability', *Journal on Developmental Disabilities/Le journal sur les handicaps du développement*, 8:2 (2001), ix–xvi.

Swain, Barbara, *Fools and Folly during the Middle Ages and the Renaissance* (New York: Columbia University Press, 1932).

Tuan, Yi-Fu, *Dominance and Affection: The Making of Pets* (New Haven, CT: Yale University Press, 1984, new edition 2004).

Turner, Wendy J., 'Silent Testimony: Emotional Displays and Lapses in Memory as Indicators of Mental Instability in Medieval English Investigations', in W. J. Turner (ed.), *Madness in Medieval Law and Custom* (Leiden and Boston: Brill, 2010), 81–95.

Turner, Wendy J., 'Defining Mental Afflictions in Medieval English Administrative Records', in Cory James Rushton (ed.), *Disability and Medieval Law: History, Literature, Society* (Newcastle-upon-Tyne: Cambridge Scholars Publishing, 2013), 134–56.

Velten, Hans-Rudolf, 'Komische Körper: Zur Funktion von Hofnarren und zur

Dramaturgie des Lachens im Spätmittelalter', *Zeitschrift für Germanistik*. Neue Folge, 11:2 (2001), 292–317.

von Bernuth, Ruth, 'From Marvels of Nature to Inmates of Asylums: Imaginations of Natural Folly', *Disability Studies Quarterly*, 26:2 (2006).

von Bernuth, Ruth, *Wunder, Spott und Prophetie. Natürliche Narrheiten in den 'Historien von Claus Narren'* (Tübingen: Niemeyer, 2009).

Walker, Nigel, *Crime and Insanity in England: Vol. 1. The Historical Perspective*, (Edinburgh: Edinburgh University Press, 1968).

Walsh, Martin W., 'The King His Own Fool: *Robert of Cicyle'*, in Clifford Davidson (ed.), *Fools and Folly* (Kalamazoo, MI: Medieval Institute Publications, 1996), 34–46.

Welsford, Enid, *The Fool: His Social and Literary History* (London: Faber & Faber, 1935, rpt 1968).

William of Conches: A Dialogue on Natural Philosophy (Dragmaticon Philosophiae), trans. Italo Ronca and Matthew Curr (Notre Dame, IN: University of Notre Dame Press, 1997).

Wright, David, *Downs: The History of a Disability* (Oxford: Oxford University Press, 2011).

Wright, David and Anne Digby (eds), *From Idiocy to Mental Deficiency: Historical Perspectives on People with Learning Disabilities* (London: Routledge, 1996).

Zijderveld, Anton C., *Reality in a Looking Glass: Rationality through an Analysis of Traditional Folly* (London: Routledge and Kegan Paul, 1982).

Index